HEALTH AND WELLNESS
ILLNESS AMONG AMERICANS

ISSN 1549-0971

HEALTH AND WELLNESS
ILLNESS AMONG AMERICANS

Barbara Wexler

INFORMATION PLUS® REFERENCE SERIES
Formerly Published by Information Plus, Wylie, Texas

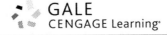

GALE
CENGAGE Learning·

Detroit • New York • San Francisco • New Haven, Conn • Waterville, Maine • London

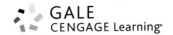

GALE
CENGAGE Learning®

Health and Wellness: Illness among Americans

Barbara Wexler

Kepos Media, Inc.: Paula Kepos and Janice Jorgensen, Series Editors

Project Editors: Kimberley McGrath, Kathleen J. Edgar, Elizabeth Manar

Rights Acquisition and Management: Leitha Etheridge-Sims, Kimberly Potvin

Composition: Evi Abou-El-Seoud, Mary Beth Trimper

Manufacturing: Cynde Lentz

For product information and technology assistance, contact us at
Gale Customer Support, 1-800-877-4253.
For permission to use material from this text or product,
submit all requests online at **www.cengage.com/permissions.**
Further permissions questions can be e-mailed to
permissionrequest@cengage.com

Cover photograph: © Vadim Ponomarenko/Shutterstock.com.

Gale
27500 Drake Rd.
Farmington Hills, MI 48331-3535

ISBN-13: 978-0-7876-5103-9 (set)
ISBN-13: 978-1-4144-8144-9

ISBN-10: 0-7876-5103-6 (set)
ISBN-10: 1-4144-8144-6

ISSN 1549-0971

This title is also available as an e-book.
ISBN-13: 978-1-4144-9726-6 (set)
ISBN-10: 1-4144-9726-1 (set)
Contact your Gale sales representative for ordering information.

Printed in the United States of America
1 2 3 4 5   16 15 14 13 12

FD284

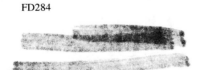

TABLE OF CONTENTS

PREFACE

Health and Wellness: Illness among Americans is part of the *Information Plus Reference Series.* The purpose of each volume of the series is to present the latest facts on a topic of pressing concern in modern American life. These topics include the most controversial and studied social issues of the 21st century: abortion, capital punishment, care for the elderly, crime, the environment, immigration, minorities, social welfare, women, world poverty, youth, and many more. Even though this series is written especially for high school and undergraduate students, it is an excellent resource for anyone in need of factual information on current affairs.

By presenting the facts, it is the intention of Gale, Cengage Learning to provide its readers with everything they need to reach an informed opinion on current issues. To that end, there is a particular emphasis in this series on the presentation of scientific studies, surveys, and statistics. These data are generally presented in the form of tables, charts, and other graphics placed within the text of each book. Every graphic is directly referred to and carefully explained in the text. The source of each graphic is presented within the graphic itself. The data used in these graphics are drawn from the most reputable and reliable sources, such as from the various branches of the U.S. government and from private organizations and associations. Every effort has been made to secure the most recent information available. Readers should bear in mind that many major studies take years to conduct and that additional years often pass before the data from these studies are made available to the public. Therefore, in many cases the most recent information available in 2012 is dated from 2009 or 2010. Older statistics are sometimes presented as well, if they are landmark studies or of particular interest and no more-recent information exists.

Even though statistics are a major focus of the *Information Plus Reference Series*, they are by no means its only content. Each book also presents the widely held positions and important ideas that shape how the book's subject is discussed in the United States. These positions are explained in detail and, where possible, in the words of their proponents. Some of the other material to be found in these books includes historical background, descriptions of major events related to the subject, relevant laws and court cases, and examples of how these issues play out in American life. Some books also feature primary documents or have pro and con debate sections that provide the words and opinions of prominent Americans on both sides of a controversial topic. All material is presented in an evenhanded and unbiased manner; readers will never be encouraged to accept one view of an issue over another.

HOW TO USE THIS BOOK

"Health" describes the condition of being free from disease. "Wellness," however, is an important complement to health that represents a person's overarching efforts to live happily and successfully—emotionally, intellectually, occupationally, physically, socially, and spiritually. This book examines health and wellness among Americans, including the ways in which illness is currently prevented, identified, and treated. Many common types of chronic, degenerative, genetic, and infectious diseases are described, as are the concepts of mental health and illness. Both traditional and selected complementary and alternative medicine are covered.

Health and Wellness: Illness among Americans consists of nine chapters and three appendixes. Each chapter is devoted to a particular aspect of health and wellness in the United States. For a summary of the information that is covered in each chapter, please see the synopses that are provided in the Table of Contents. Chapters generally begin with an overview of the basic facts and background information on the chapter's topic, then proceed to examine subtopics of particular interest. For example, Chapter 8:

Mental Health and Illness defines and distinguishes between mental health disorders and mental health problems. Explored next is the occurrence of mental disorders among adults and children in the United States. The chapter explains that not all mental disorders require treatment and describes the reasons that some people do not seek needed treatment. The remainder of the chapter details the causes and treatment of a variety of mental disorders including autism spectrum disorders, depression, bipolar disorder, schizophrenia, anxiety disorders and phobias, attention deficit/hyperactivity disorder, and disruptive disorders as well as eating disorders. The chapter concludes with a discussion of suicide, which in some instances is a consequence of depression or another serious mental disorder. Readers can find their way through a chapter by looking for the section and subsection headings, which are clearly set off from the text. They can also refer to the book's extensive Index if they already know what they are looking for.

Statistical Information

The tables and figures featured throughout *Health and Wellness: Illness among Americans* will be of particular use to readers in learning about this issue. These tables and figures represent an extensive collection of the most recent and important statistics on health and wellness, as well as related issues—for example, graphics cover the prevalence of overweight and obesity, how Americans assess their own health, leading causes of death in the United States, recommended immunizations, and the symptoms of depression. Gale, Cengage Learning believes that making this information available to readers is the most important way to fulfill the goal of this book: to help readers understand the issues and controversies surrounding health and wellness in the United States and reach their own conclusions.

Each table or figure has a unique identifier appearing above it, for ease of identification and reference. Titles for the tables and figures explain their purpose. At the end of each table or figure, the original source of the data is provided.

To help readers understand these often complicated statistics, all tables and figures are explained in the text. References in the text direct readers to the relevant statistics. Furthermore, the contents of all tables and figures are fully indexed. Please see the opening section of the Index at the back of this volume for a description of how to find tables and figures within it.

Appendixes

Besides the main body text and images, *Health and Wellness: Illness among Americans* has three appendixes.

The first is the Important Names and Addresses directory. Here, readers will find contact information for a number of government and private organizations that can provide further information on aspects of health and wellness. The second appendix is the Resources section, which can also assist readers in conducting their own research. In this section, the author and editors of *Health and Wellness: Illness among Americans* describe some of the sources that were most useful during the compilation of this book. The final appendix is the detailed Index. It has been greatly expanded from previous editions and should make it even easier to find specific topics in this book.

ADVISORY BOARD CONTRIBUTIONS

The staff of Information Plus would like to extend its heartfelt appreciation to the Information Plus Advisory Board. This dedicated group of media professionals provides feedback on the series on an ongoing basis. Their comments allow the editorial staff who work on the project to continually make the series better and more user-friendly. The staff's top priority is to produce the highest-quality and most useful books possible, and the Information Plus Advisory Board's contributions to this process are invaluable.

The members of the Information Plus Advisory Board are:

- Kathleen R. Bonn, Librarian, Newbury Park High School, Newbury Park, California
- Madelyn Garner, Librarian, San Jacinto College, North Campus, Houston, Texas
- Anne Oxenrider, Media Specialist, Dundee High School, Dundee, Michigan
- Charles R. Rodgers, Director of Libraries, Pasco-Hernando Community College, Dade City, Florida
- James N. Zitzelsberger, Library Media Department Chairman, Oshkosh West High School, Oshkosh, Wisconsin

COMMENTS AND SUGGESTIONS

The editors of the *Information Plus Reference Series* welcome your feedback on *Health and Wellness: Illness among Americans*. Please direct all correspondence to:

Editors
Information Plus Reference Series
27500 Drake Rd.
Farmington Hills, MI 48331-3535

CHAPTER 1
DEFINING HEALTH AND WELLNESS

An important first step in preventing illness and disability is learning about health conditions in our families that may put us at increased risk for diseases such as diabetes, heart disease, some cancers, Alzheimer's Disease, mental illness and many others.

—Regina Benjamin, U.S. Surgeon General, in "U.S. Surgeon General Declares Thanksgiving as 'Family Health History Day'" (November 22, 2011)

Many definitions of health exist. Most definitions consider health as an outcome—the result of actions to produce it, such as good nutrition, immunization to prevent disease, or medical treatment to cure disease. The *American Heritage Dictionary* (2011) defines health as fixed and measurable: "The overall condition of an organism at a given time." However, health may also be viewed as the active process used by individuals and communities to adapt to ever-changing environments.

The *Merriam-Webster's Dictionary* (2012) defines health as "the condition of being sound in body, mind, or spirit; *esp*: freedom from physical disease or pain." However, in 1948 the constitution of the World Health Organization (WHO; October 2006, http://www.who.int/ governance/eb/who_constitution_en.pdf) defined health as "a state of complete physical, mental and social well-being and not merely the absence of disease or infirmity." This still widely used definition is broader and more positive than simply defining health as the absence of illness or disability.

Expanding on the WHO definition of health and the commonly understood idea of well-being, the concept of wellness has been defined by the National Wellness Institute (2012, http://www.nationalwellness.org/index.php? id_tier=2&id_c=26) as "a conscious, self-directed and evolving process of achieving full potential [and] is multi-dimensional and holistic, encompassing lifestyle, mental and spiritual well-being, and the environment." Wellness encompasses how people feel about various aspects of their lives. Six interrelated aspects of human life are commonly known to make up wellness:

- Emotional wellness refers to awareness, sensitivity, and acceptance of feelings and the ability to successfully express and manage one's feelings. Emotional wellness enables people to cope with stress, maintain satisfying relationships with family and friends, and assume responsibility for their actions.

- Intellectual wellness emphasizes knowledge, learning, creativity, problem solving, and lifelong interest in learning and new ideas.

- Occupational wellness relates to preparing for and pursuing work that is meaningful, satisfying, and consistent with one's interests, aptitudes, and personal beliefs.

- Physical wellness is more than simply freedom from disease. The physical dimension of wellness concentrates on the prevention of illness and encourages exercise, healthy diet, and knowledgeable, appropriate use of the health care system. Physical wellness requires individuals to take personal responsibility for actions and choices that affect their health. Examples of healthy choices include wearing a seatbelt in automobiles, wearing a helmet when bicycling, and avoiding tobacco and illegal drugs.

- Social wellness is acting in harmony with nature, family, and others in the community. The pursuit of social wellness may involve actions to protect or preserve the environment or contribute to the health and well-being of the community by performing volunteer work.

- Spiritual wellness involves finding meaning in life and acting purposefully in a manner that is consistent with one's deeply held values and beliefs.

The concept of wellness is broader and includes more facets of human life than the traditional definition of health, and the two differ in an important way. When defined as the absence of disease, health may be measured and assessed objectively. For example, a physical examination and the results of laboratory testing enable a physician to determine that a patient is free of disease and thereby healthy.

In comparison, wellness is a more subjective quality and is more difficult to measure. The determination of wellness relies on self-assessment and self-report. Furthermore, it is not necessarily essential that individuals satisfy the traditional definition of good health to rate themselves high in terms of wellness. For instance, many people with chronic (ongoing or long-term) conditions—such as diabetes, heart disease, or asthma—or disabilities report high levels of satisfaction with each of the six dimensions of wellness. Similarly, people in apparently good health may not necessarily give themselves high scores in all six aspects of wellness.

MEASURES OF QUALITY OF LIFE

Quality of life encompasses multiple subjective measures of many interrelated aspects of life. Along with health, quality of life takes into consideration one's work life, housing, schools, neighborhoods, and communities as well as spiritual life, values, and interpersonal relationships. There are many measures of quality of life. For example, the United Nations explains in "The Human Development Index (HDI)" (2011, http://www.undp.org.bz/human-development/the-human-development-index-hdi/) that it has used the Human Development Index (HDI) since 1993 to compare countries in terms of life expectancy, poverty, literacy, education, and other indicators. The WHO (Five) Well-Being Index (http://www.cure4you.dk/354/WHO-5_English.pdf) is a short, self-administered questionnaire that poses five questions about the frequency of positive mood (good spirits and relaxation), vitality (being active and waking fresh and rested), and general interests.

Other measures include the:

- Physical Quality of Life Index, which is used to rank countries and summarizes infant mortality, life expectancy at age one, and basic literacy on a 0 to 100 scale.

- Happy Planet Index, which compares countries based on a combined score of environmental impact and well-being to measure the environmental efficiency with which people live long and happy lives.

- Self-Perceived Quality of Life, which provides a measurement of health-related and nonhealth-related aspects of well-being, such as emotions and physical and mental health indices.

- Popsicle Index, which is the percentage of people in a community who believe that a child can leave his or her home, go to the nearest store to buy a Popsicle,

and return home alone safely; it is a measure of feelings of safety and security.

HEALTH-RELATED QUALITY OF LIFE

In "Health-Related Quality of Life (HRQOL)" (March 17, 2011, http://www.cdc.gov/hrqol/concept.htm), the Centers for Disease Control and Prevention (CDC) defines health-related quality of life (HRQoL) as "those aspects of overall quality of life that can be clearly shown to affect health—either physical or mental." For individuals, an assessment of HRQoL includes measures of health risks and medical conditions; functional status; the presence and extent of social support such as family, friends, and community; and socioeconomic status. HRQoL is a latent trait, which means that it cannot be assessed directly using a single measure; instead, it is measured using a set of indicators. Figure 1.1 shows the predictors and indicators that contribute to the HRQoL measure that the CDC uses in its Behavioral Risk Factor Surveillance System (http://www.cdc.gov/brfss/).

At the population or community level, HRQoL considers resources such as the availability of medical care, conditions such as sanitation and safe food and water supplies, policies such as the provision of nutritious school lunches, and practices such as smoking, physical activity, and use of preventive services that influence a population's health. Tracking and analyzing HRQoL enables the development of public health policy and the allocation of resources to determine the burden of preventable disease, injuries, and disabilities and identifies health needs. It also informs the design of interventions to help individuals and communities with less than optimal perceived health.

HRQoL serves as a key measure of the health of the nation. Healthy People 2020 (http://www.healthypeople.gov/2020/default.aspx), the 10-year agenda for improving the nation's health, names quality of life improvement as a key public health goal. Healthy People 2020 evaluates HRQoL using the following measures:

- The Global Health Measure evaluates physical, mental, and social HRQoL by querying people about self-rated health, physical HRQoL, mental HRQoL, fatigue, pain, emotional distress, and social activities.

- The Well-Being Measures consider how people feel in terms of their health and satisfaction with life, fulfillment of their ambitions and potential, and the quality of their relationships. These measures also assess positive emotions and emotional resilience (how well people endure and manage stress).

- The Participation Measures look at individuals' assessments of the impact of their health on their social participation in education, employment, civic, social, and leisure activities. Participation Measures show that individuals with functional limitations such as vision

FIGURE 1.1

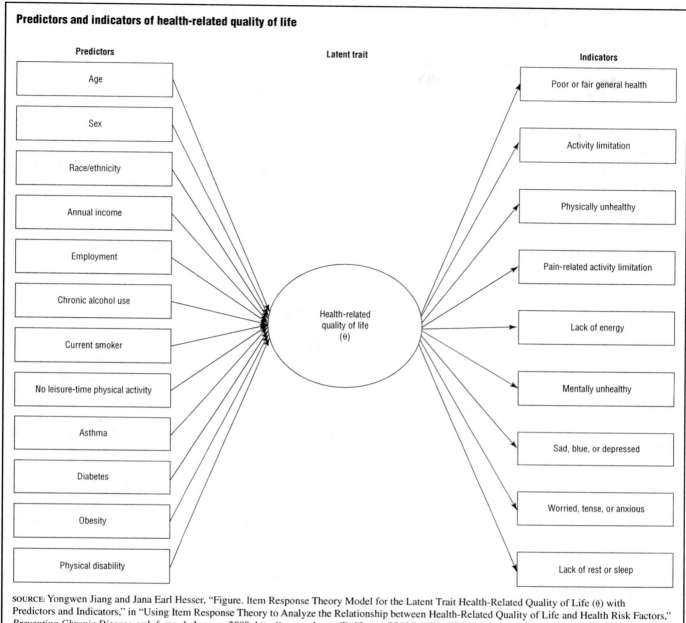

Predictors and indicators of health-related quality of life

| Predictors | Latent trait | Indicators |

SOURCE: Yongwen Jiang and Jana Earl Hesser, "Figure. Item Response Theory Model for the Latent Trait Health-Related Quality of Life (θ) with Predictors and Indicators," in "Using Item Response Theory to Analyze the Relationship between Health-Related Quality of Life and Health Risk Factors," *Preventing Chronic Disease*, vol. 6, no. 1, January 2009, http://www.cdc.gov/Pcd/issues/2009/jan/07_0272.htm (accessed December 14, 2011)

loss, walking problems, or intellectual disability are able to live long, productive lives.

In "Health-Related Quality of Life (HRQOL)," the CDC explains that many measures, such as the Medical Outcomes Study Short Forms, the Sickness Impact Profile, and the Quality of Well-Being Scale, have been used to assess HRQoL and functional status, but because most are time- and labor-intensive to administer, they are not appropriate for population-wide surveillance. The CDC observes that HRQoL is increasingly important in view of Americans' increasing life expectancy. This assessment can be used to help improve older adults' lives as they age.

THE HEALTH OF THE UNITED STATES

A primary indicator of the well-being of a nation is the health of its people. Many factors can affect a person's health: heredity, race or ethnicity, gender, income, education, geography, exposure to violent crime, exposure to environmental agents, exposure to infectious diseases, and access to and availability of health care.

Whereas physicians and other health practitioners observe the influences of these factors as they care for individual patients, epidemiologists (public health researchers who study the occurrence of disease) examine the distribution and rates of diseases and injuries in the population. Practitioners and epidemiologists each apply the scientific method to achieve their objectives, but they use it in varying ways. For instance, in the database step of the scientific method, practitioners use history and physical examination to determine a patient's health, whereas epidemiologists use surveillance and description. Practitioners seek to deliver appropriate treatment to individual patients, whereas epidemiologists recommend actions to prevent the spread of disease or otherwise improve the health of an entire community or population.

Epidemiologists and other public health professionals assess health by determining the incidence and prevalence rates of disease and disability in a given community. Incidence is a measure of the rate at which people without a disease develop the disease during a specific time period, and it describes the continuing occurrence of disease over time. For example, a researcher might report that men in a given community aged 65 years and older have a 2% incidence of heart disease. Prevalence describes a group or population at a specific point in time. For example, the prevalence of high blood pressure found during screening at a health fair on a specific day might be 22%.

Other measures of the health of a population, such as natality (birth) and mortality (death) rates, are known as vital health statistics. This chapter provides an overview of vital health statistics and the health status of Americans.

BIRTHRATES AND FERTILITY RATES

The birthrate is the number of live births per 1,000 women. The fertility rate is the number of live births per 1,000 women between 15 and 44 years of age, which is generally considered a woman's prime childbearing years.

In "Births: Preliminary Data for 2010" (*National Vital Statistics Reports*, vol. 60, no. 7, November 2011), Brady E. Hamilton, Joyce A. Martin, and Stephanie J. Ventura of the CDC report that there were 4 million births in the United States in 2010, down from 4.1 million births in 2009. This number translates to a birthrate of 13.5 births per 1,000 women in 2009, which was down from 14 births per 1,000 women in 2008. (See Table 1.1.) As the number of live births decreased from 1990, the fertility rate also has declined from 70.9 live births per 1,000 women in 1990 to 68.6 live births per 1,000 women in 2008. Hamilton, Martin, and Ventura report that the 2010 fertility rate, 64.1 births per 1,000 women aged 15 to 44 years, was a full 3% below the rate in 2009 (66.2) and the lowest rate reported since the late 1990s.

Birthrates have continued to decline for teenagers aged 15 to 19 years. In 2008 the number of live births per 1,000 teens aged 15 to 17 years was 21.7, down from the last most recent peak of 38.5 in 1991. (See Table 1.1.) Hamilton, Martin, and Ventura report that the rate for teenagers aged 15 to 17 years declined 12%, from 19.6 per 1,000 in 2009 to 17.3 per 1,000 in 2010. For this age group, the rate declined 20% from 2007 through 2010, and 55% since 1991.

In contrast, the birthrate for women aged 25 to 34 years was relatively unchanged between 2005 and 2008. (See Table 1.1.) The birthrate for women aged 35 to 39 years, which increased dramatically between 1980 and 2000, decreased in 2010—from 46.1 births per 1,000 women in 2009 to 45.9 births per 1,000 women. The birthrate for this age group decreased 2% between 2009 and 2010.

Women aged 20 to 29 years continued to have the highest birthrates (90 per 1,000 women in 2010, down 6% from 2009), although the proportion of births to these women has declined in recent years. (See Table 1.1 for the rates for selected years between 1950 and 2008.)

Fertility rates focus on live births to mothers in the primary childbearing age group: 15 to 44 years. In 2008 the fertility rate for American women was 68.6 births per 1,000 women, which was an increase from 2005 (66.7) but a decrease from 1990 (70.9). (See Table 1.1.) Total fertility rates, which offer an index of lifetime fertility among women, not only varied by age but also by race and ethnic origin. In 2008 the fertility rate was higher for Hispanic women (98.8 births per 1,000 Hispanic women aged 15 to 44 years) than for non-Hispanic white women (59.4 births per 1,000). (See Table 1.1.)

Hamilton, Martin, and Ventura report that the fertility rate in 2010 dropped 3% from 2009 to the lowest reported rate since 1987. The fertility rate fell below the replacement level in 2010—replacement is the rate at which a given generation can exactly replace itself, which is estimated to be approximately 2,100 births per 1,000 women. The rate had been above replacement in 2006 and 2007, but has dropped each year since 2007.

Factors other than age, race, and ethnicity can have dramatic effects on fertility and birthrates. For example, even though women who are currently married and living with their husband have much higher fertility rates than those women who have never married or are separated, widowed, or divorced, Hamilton, Martin, and Ventura report that the birthrate for unmarried women had been increasing steadily over the years, from 43.6 births per 1,000 unmarried women aged 15 to 44 years in 2002 to 51.8 births per 1,000 unmarried women in 2007. However, it declined to 49.9 births per 1,000 unmarried women in 2009 and to 47.7 births per 1,000 unmarried women in 2010. Concerning the decline in teen birthrates, the CDC cites successful health prevention programs that include education emphasizing prevention of pregnancy through abstinence (avoiding sexual contact) and contraception (measures to prevent pregnancy) as well as a leveling-off of sexual activity among teens. Hamilton, Martin, and Ventura observe that in 1970 unmarried teenagers accounted for half of all births to unmarried women; in 2010 unmarried teens accounted for just 20% of births to unmarried women.

TABLE 1.1

Crude birth rates, fertility rates, and birth rates, by age of mother, according to race and Hispanic origin, selected years 1950–2008

Race, Hispanic origin, and year	Crude birth rate[a]	Fertility rate[b]	10–14 years	15–19 years Total	15–17 years	18–19 years	20–24 years	25–29 years	30–34 years	35–39 years	40–44 years	45–54 years[c]
All races					Live births per 1,000 women							
1950	24.1	106.2	1.0	81.6	40.7	132.7	196.6	166.1	103.7	52.9	15.1	1.2
1960	23.7	118.0	0.8	89.1	43.9	166.7	258.1	197.4	112.7	56.2	15.5	0.9
1970	18.4	87.9	1.2	68.3	38.8	114.7	167.8	145.1	73.3	31.7	8.1	0.5
1980	15.9	68.4	1.1	53.0	32.5	82.1	115.1	112.9	61.9	19.8	3.9	0.2
1981	15.8	67.3	1.1	52.2	32.0	80.0	112.2	111.5	61.4	20.0	3.8	0.2
1982	15.9	67.3	1.1	52.4	32.3	79.4	111.6	111.0	64.1	21.2	3.9	0.2
1983	15.6	65.7	1.1	51.4	31.8	77.4	107.8	108.5	64.9	22.0	3.9	0.2
1984	15.6	65.5	1.2	50.6	31.0	77.4	106.8	108.7	67.0	22.9	3.9	0.2
1985	15.8	66.3	1.2	51.0	31.0	79.6	108.3	111.0	69.1	24.0	4.0	0.2
1986	15.6	65.4	1.3	50.2	30.5	79.6	107.4	109.8	70.1	24.4	4.1	0.2
1987	15.7	65.8	1.3	50.6	31.7	78.5	107.9	111.6	72.1	26.3	4.4	0.2
1988	16.0	67.3	1.3	53.0	33.6	79.9	110.2	114.4	74.8	28.1	4.8	0.2
1989	16.4	69.2	1.4	57.3	36.4	84.2	113.8	117.6	77.4	29.9	5.2	0.2
1990	16.7	70.9	1.4	59.9	37.5	88.6	116.5	120.2	80.8	31.7	5.5	0.2
1991	16.2	69.3	1.4	61.8	38.5	94.0	115.3	117.2	79.2	31.9	5.5	0.2
1992	15.8	68.4	1.4	60.3	37.5	93.7	113.7	115.7	79.6	32.3	5.9	0.3
1993	15.4	67.0	1.4	59.0	37.4	91.1	111.3	113.2	79.9	32.7	6.1	0.3
1994	15.0	65.9	1.4	58.2	37.2	90.3	109.2	111.0	80.4	33.4	6.4	0.3
1995	14.6	64.6	1.3	56.0	35.5	87.7	107.5	108.8	81.1	34.0	6.6	0.3
1996	14.4	64.1	1.2	53.5	33.3	84.7	107.8	108.6	82.1	34.9	6.8	0.3
1997	14.2	63.6	1.1	51.3	31.4	82.1	107.3	108.3	83.0	35.7	7.1	0.4
1998	14.3	64.3	1.0	50.3	29.9	80.9	108.4	110.2	85.2	36.9	7.4	0.4
1999	14.2	64.4	0.9	48.8	28.2	79.0	107.9	111.2	87.1	37.8	7.4	0.4
2000	14.4	65.9	0.9	47.7	26.9	78.1	109.7	113.5	91.2	39.7	8.0	0.5
2001	14.1	65.3	0.8	45.3	24.7	76.1	106.2	113.4	91.9	40.6	8.1	0.5
2002	13.9	64.8	0.7	43.0	23.2	72.8	103.6	113.6	91.5	41.4	8.3	0.5
2003	14.1	66.1	0.6	41.6	22.4	70.7	102.6	115.6	95.1	43.8	8.7	0.5
2004	14.0	66.3	0.7	41.1	22.1	70.0	101.7	115.5	95.3	45.4	8.9	0.5
2005	14.0	66.7	0.7	40.5	21.4	69.9	102.2	115.5	95.8	46.3	9.1	0.6
2006	14.2	68.5	0.6	41.9	22.0	73.0	105.9	116.7	97.7	47.3	9.4	0.6
2007	14.3	69.5	0.6	42.5	22.1	73.9	106.3	117.5	99.9	47.5	9.5	0.6
2008	14.0	68.6	0.6	41.5	21.7	70.6	103.0	115.1	99.3	46.9	9.8	0.7
Race of child:[d] White												
1950	23.0	102.3	0.4	70.0	31.3	120.5	190.4	165.1	102.6	51.4	14.5	1.0
1960	22.7	113.2	0.4	79.4	35.5	154.6	252.8	194.9	109.6	54.0	14.7	0.8
1970	17.4	84.1	0.5	57.4	29.2	101.5	163.4	145.9	71.9	30.0	7.5	0.4
1980	14.9	64.7	0.6	44.7	25.2	72.1	109.5	112.4	60.4	18.5	3.4	0.2
Race of mother:[e] White												
1980	15.1	65.6	0.6	45.4	25.5	73.2	111.1	113.8	61.2	18.8	3.5	0.2
1981	15.0	64.8	0.5	44.9	25.4	71.5	108.3	112.3	61.0	19.0	3.4	0.2
1982	15.1	64.8	0.6	45.0	25.5	70.8	107.7	111.9	64.0	20.4	3.6	0.2
1983	14.8	63.4	0.6	43.9	25.0	68.8	103.8	109.4	65.3	21.3	3.6	0.2
1984	14.8	63.2	0.6	42.9	24.3	68.4	102.7	109.8	67.7	22.2	3.6	0.2
1985	15.0	64.1	0.6	43.3	24.4	70.4	104.1	112.3	69.9	23.3	3.7	0.2
1986	14.8	63.1	0.6	42.3	23.8	70.1	102.7	110.8	70.9	23.9	3.8	0.2
1987	14.9	63.3	0.6	42.5	24.6	68.9	102.3	112.3	73.0	25.9	4.1	0.2
1988	15.0	64.5	0.6	44.4	26.0	69.6	103.7	114.8	75.4	27.7	4.5	0.2
1989	15.4	66.4	0.7	47.9	28.1	72.9	106.9	117.8	78.1	29.7	4.9	0.2
1990	15.8	68.3	0.7	50.8	29.5	78.0	109.8	120.7	81.7	31.5	5.2	0.2
1991	15.3	66.7	0.8	52.6	30.5	83.3	108.8	118.0	80.2	31.8	5.2	0.2
1992	15.0	66.1	0.8	51.4	29.9	83.2	107.7	116.9	80.8	32.1	5.7	0.2
1993	14.6	64.9	0.8	50.6	30.0	81.5	106.1	114.7	81.3	32.6	5.9	0.3
1994	14.3	64.2	0.8	50.5	30.4	81.2	105.0	113.0	82.2	33.5	6.2	0.3
1995	14.1	63.6	0.8	49.5	29.6	80.2	104.7	111.7	83.3	34.2	6.4	0.3
1996	13.9	63.3	0.7	47.5	28.0	77.6	105.3	111.7	84.6	35.3	6.7	0.3
1997	13.7	62.8	0.7	45.5	26.6	75.0	104.5	111.3	85.7	36.1	6.9	0.3
1998	13.8	63.6	0.6	44.9	25.6	74.1	105.4	113.6	88.5	37.5	7.3	0.4
1999	13.7	64.0	0.6	44.0	24.4	73.0	105.0	114.9	90.7	38.5	7.4	0.4
2000	13.9	65.3	0.6	43.2	23.3	72.3	106.6	116.7	94.6	40.2	7.9	0.4
2001	13.7	65.0	0.5	41.2	21.4	70.8	103.7	117.0	95.8	41.3	8.0	0.5
2002	13.5	64.8	0.5	39.4	20.5	68.0	101.6	117.4	95.5	42.4	8.2	0.5
2003	13.6	66.1	0.5	38.3	19.8	66.2	100.6	119.5	99.3	44.8	8.7	0.5
2004	13.5	66.1	0.5	37.7	19.5	65.0	99.2	118.6	99.1	46.4	8.9	0.5

Prenatal Care, Prematurity, and Low Birth Weight

Early prenatal care, which is defined as pregnancy-related care started during the first trimester (one to three months), can detect and often correct many potential health problems early in pregnancy. Regular visits to a physician or clinic usually give the mother-to-be information and

TABLE 1.1

Crude birth rates, fertility rates, and birth rates, by age of mother, according to race and Hispanic origin, selected years 1950–2008

[CONTINUED]

Race, Hispanic origin, and year	Crude birth rate[a]	Fertility rate[b]	10–14 years	15–19 years Total	15–17 years	18–19 years	20–24 years	25–29 years	30–34 years	35–39 years	40–44 years	45–54 years[c]
							Live births per 1,000 women					
2005	13.4	66.3	0.5	37.0	18.9	64.7	99.2	118.3	99.3	47.3	9.0	0.6
2006	13.7	68.0	0.5	38.2	19.4	67.5	102.5	119.1	100.9	48.2	9.2	0.6
2007	13.7	68.8	0.5	38.8	19.7	68.1	102.8	119.4	102.7	48.1	9.4	0.6
2008	13.4	67.8	0.4	37.8	19.3	65.0	99.2	116.6	101.8	47.2	9.7	0.6
Race of child:[d] Black or African American												
1960	31.9	153.5	4.3	156.1	—	—	295.4	218.6	137.1	73.9	21.9	1.1
1970	25.3	115.4	5.2	140.7	101.4	204.9	202.7	136.3	79.6	41.9	12.5	1.0
1980	22.1	88.1	4.3	100.0	73.6	138.8	146.3	109.1	62.9	24.5	5.8	0.3
Race of mother:[e] Black or African American												
1980	21.3	84.7	4.3	97.8	72.5	135.1	140.0	103.9	59.9	23.5	5.6	0.3
1981	20.8	82.0	4.0	94.5	69.3	131.0	136.5	102.3	57.4	23.1	5.4	0.3
1982	20.7	80.9	4.0	94.3	69.7	128.9	135.4	101.3	57.5	23.3	5.1	0.4
1983	20.2	78.7	4.1	93.9	69.6	127.1	131.9	98.4	56.2	23.3	5.1	0.3
1984	20.1	78.1	4.4	94.1	69.2	128.1	132.2	98.4	56.7	23.3	4.8	0.2
1985	20.4	78.8	4.5	95.4	69.3	132.4	135.0	100.2	57.9	23.9	4.6	0.3
1986	20.5	78.9	4.7	95.8	69.3	135.1	137.3	101.1	59.3	23.8	4.8	0.3
1987	20.8	80.1	4.8	97.6	72.1	135.8	142.7	104.3	60.6	24.6	4.8	0.2
1988	21.5	82.6	4.9	102.7	75.7	142.7	149.7	108.2	63.1	25.6	5.1	0.3
1989	22.3	86.2	5.1	111.5	81.9	151.9	156.8	114.4	66.3	26.7	5.4	0.3
1990	22.4	86.8	4.9	112.8	82.3	152.9	160.2	115.5	68.7	28.1	5.5	0.3
1991	21.8	84.8	4.7	114.8	83.5	157.6	159.7	112.0	67.3	28.2	5.5	0.2
1992	21.1	82.4	4.6	111.3	80.5	156.3	156.2	109.7	67.0	28.6	5.6	0.2
1993	20.2	79.6	4.5	107.3	78.9	150.2	150.2	106.4	66.6	29.0	5.9	0.3
1994	19.1	75.9	4.5	102.9	75.1	146.2	142.9	101.5	65.0	28.7	5.9	0.3
1995	17.8	71.0	4.1	94.4	68.5	135.0	133.7	95.6	63.0	28.4	6.0	0.3
1996	17.3	69.2	3.5	89.6	63.3	130.5	133.2	94.3	62.0	28.7	6.1	0.3
1997	17.1	69.0	3.1	86.3	59.3	127.7	135.2	95.0	62.6	29.3	6.5	0.3
1998	17.1	69.4	2.8	83.5	55.4	124.8	138.4	97.5	63.2	30.0	6.6	0.3
1999	16.8	68.5	2.5	79.1	50.5	120.6	137.9	97.3	62.7	30.2	6.5	0.3
2000	17.0	70.0	2.3	77.4	49.0	118.8	141.3	100.3	65.4	31.5	7.2	0.4
2001	16.3	67.6	2.0	71.8	43.9	114.0	133.2	99.2	64.8	31.6	7.2	0.4
2002	15.7	65.8	1.8	66.6	40.0	107.6	127.1	99.0	64.4	31.5	7.4	0.4
2003	15.7	66.3	1.6	63.8	38.2	103.7	126.1	100.4	66.5	33.2	7.7	0.5
2004	16.0	67.6	1.6	63.3	37.2	104.4	127.7	103.6	67.9	34.0	7.9	0.5
2005	16.2	69.0	1.7	62.0	35.5	104.9	129.9	105.9	70.3	35.3	8.5	0.5
2006	16.8	72.1	1.5	64.6	36.6	110.2	135.8	109.4	74.0	36.6	8.5	0.5
2007	16.9	72.7	1.5	64.9	36.1	110.7	135.9	109.6	75.4	36.9	8.8	0.6
2008	16.6	71.9	1.4	63.4	35.2	105.6	132.3	107.2	75.6	37.0	8.9	0.6
American Indian or Alaska Native mothers[e]												
1980	20.7	82.7	1.9	82.2	51.5	129.5	143.7	106.6	61.8	28.1	8.2	*
1985	19.8	78.6	1.7	79.2	47.7	124.1	139.1	109.6	62.6	27.4	6.0	*
1990	18.9	76.2	1.6	81.1	48.5	129.3	148.7	110.3	61.5	27.5	5.9	*
1991	18.3	73.9	1.6	84.1	51.9	134.2	143.8	105.6	60.8	26.4	5.8	0.4
1992	17.9	73.1	1.6	82.4	52.3	130.5	142.3	107.0	61.0	26.7	5.9	*
1993	17.0	69.7	1.4	79.8	51.5	126.3	134.2	103.5	59.5	25.5	5.6	*
1994	16.0	65.8	1.8	76.4	48.4	123.7	126.5	98.2	56.6	24.8	5.4	0.3
1995	15.3	63.0	1.6	72.9	44.6	122.2	123.1	91.6	56.5	24.3	5.5	*
1996	14.9	61.8	1.6	68.2	42.7	113.3	123.5	91.1	56.5	24.4	5.5	*
1997	14.7	60.8	1.5	65.2	41.0	107.1	122.5	91.6	56.0	24.4	5.4	0.3
1998	14.8	61.3	1.5	64.7	39.7	106.9	125.1	92.0	56.8	24.6	5.3	*
1999	14.2	59.0	1.4	59.9	36.5	98.0	120.7	90.6	53.8	24.3	5.7	0.3
2000	14.0	58.7	1.1	58.3	34.1	97.1	117.2	91.8	55.5	24.6	5.7	0.3
2001	13.7	58.1	1.0	56.3	31.4	94.8	115.0	90.4	55.9	24.7	5.7	0.3
2002	13.8	58.0	0.9	53.8	30.7	89.2	112.6	91.8	56.4	25.4	5.8	0.3
2003	13.8	58.4	1.0	53.1	30.6	87.3	110.0	93.5	57.4	25.4	5.5	0.4
2004	14.0	58.9	0.9	52.5	30.0	87.0	109.7	92.8	58.0	26.8	6.0	0.2
2005	14.2	59.9	0.9	52.7	30.5	87.6	109.2	93.8	60.1	27.0	6.0	0.3
2006	14.9	63.1	0.9	55.0	30.7	93.0	115.4	97.8	61.8	28.4	6.1	0.4
2007	15.3	64.9	0.9	59.3	31.8	101.6	116.8	96.4	64.0	29.5	6.1	0.3
2008	14.5	64.6	0.9	58.4	32.5	96.6	115.6	94.4	63.8	28.8	6.4	0.4

encouragement about eating properly, exercising regularly, taking prenatal vitamins, and avoiding harmful substances such as alcohol, drugs, and tobacco. The benefits of these preventive measures can literally make a lifetime of difference for a newborn.

Sophisticated diagnostic medical procedures, such as obstetric ultrasound scans and amniocentesis, can be performed to detect possible birth defects and other prenatal problems. Ultrasound uses high-frequency sound waves to compose a picture of the fetus and is used to detect and

TABLE 1.1

Crude birth rates, fertility rates, and birth rates, by age of mother, according to race and Hispanic origin, selected years 1950–2008
[CONTINUED]

Race, Hispanic origin, and year	Crude birth rate[a]	Fertility rate[b]	10–14 years	Total	15–19 years 15–17 years	15–19 years 18–19 years	Age of mother 20–24 years	Age of mother 25–29 years	Age of mother 30–34 years	Age of mother 35–39 years	Age of mother 40–44 years	Age of mother 45–54 years[c]
Asian or Pacific Islander mothers[e]					Live births per 1,000 women							
1980	19.9	73.2	0.3	26.2	12.0	46.2	93.3	127.4	96.0	38.3	8.5	0.7
1985	18.7	68.4	0.4	23.8	12.5	40.8	83.6	123.0	93.6	42.7	8.7	1.2
1990	19.0	69.6	0.7	26.4	16.0	40.2	79.2	126.3	106.5	49.6	10.7	1.1
1991	18.3	67.1	0.8	27.3	16.3	42.2	73.8	118.9	103.3	49.2	11.2	1.1
1992	17.9	66.1	0.7	26.5	15.4	41.9	71.7	114.6	102.7	50.7	11.1	0.9
1993	17.3	64.3	0.7	26.5	16.1	41.2	68.1	110.3	101.2	49.4	11.2	0.9
1994	17.1	63.9	0.7	26.6	16.3	41.3	66.4	108.0	102.2	50.4	11.5	1.0
1995	16.7	62.6	0.7	25.5	15.6	40.1	64.2	103.7	102.3	50.1	11.8	0.8
1996	16.5	62.3	0.6	23.5	14.7	36.8	63.5	102.8	104.1	50.2	11.9	0.8
1997	16.2	61.3	0.5	22.3	14.0	34.9	61.2	101.6	102.5	51.0	11.5	0.9
1998	15.9	60.1	0.5	22.2	13.8	34.5	59.2	98.7	101.6	51.4	11.8	0.9
1999	15.9	60.9	0.4	21.4	12.4	33.9	58.9	100.8	104.3	52.9	11.3	0.9
2000	17.1	65.8	0.3	20.5	11.6	32.6	60.3	108.4	116.5	59.0	12.6	0.8
2001	16.4	64.2	0.2	19.8	10.3	32.8	59.1	106.4	112.6	56.7	12.3	0.9
2002	16.5	64.1	0.3	18.3	9.0	31.5	60.4	105.4	109.6	56.5	12.5	0.9
2003	16.8	66.3	0.2	17.4	8.8	29.8	59.6	108.5	114.6	59.9	13.5	0.9
2004	16.8	67.1	0.2	17.3	8.9	29.6	59.8	108.6	116.9	62.1	13.6	1.0
2005	16.5	66.6	0.2	17.0	8.2	30.1	61.1	107.9	115.0	61.8	13.8	1.0
2006	16.6	67.5	0.2	17.0	8.8	29.5	63.2	108.4	116.9	63.0	14.1	1.0
2007	17.2	71.3	0.2	16.9	8.2	29.9	65.5	118.0	125.4	66.3	14.4	1.1
2008	16.8	71.3	0.2	16.2	7.9	28.4	64.4	120.1	126.8	66.8	15.2	1.2
Hispanic or Latina mothers[e, f]												
1980	23.5	95.4	1.7	82.2	52.1	126.9	156.4	132.1	83.2	39.9	10.6	0.7
1990	26.7	107.7	2.4	100.3	65.9	147.7	181.0	153.0	98.3	45.3	10.9	0.7
1991	26.5	106.9	2.4	104.6	69.2	155.5	184.6	150.0	95.1	44.7	10.7	0.6
1992	26.1	106.1	2.5	103.3	68.9	153.9	185.2	148.8	94.8	45.3	11.0	0.6
1993	25.4	103.3	2.6	101.8	68.5	151.1	180.0	146.0	93.2	44.1	10.6	0.6
1994	24.7	100.7	2.6	101.3	69.9	147.5	175.7	142.4	91.1	43.4	10.7	0.6
1995	24.1	98.8	2.6	99.3	68.3	145.4	171.9	140.4	90.5	43.7	10.7	0.6
1996	23.8	97.5	2.4	94.6	64.2	140.0	170.2	140.7	91.3	43.9	10.7	0.6
1997	23.0	94.2	2.1	89.6	61.1	132.4	162.6	137.5	89.6	43.4	10.7	0.6
1998	22.7	93.2	1.9	87.9	58.5	131.5	159.3	136.1	90.5	43.4	10.8	0.6
1999	22.5	93.0	1.9	86.8	56.9	129.5	157.3	135.8	92.3	44.5	10.6	0.6
2000	23.1	95.9	1.7	87.3	55.5	132.6	161.3	139.9	97.1	46.6	11.5	0.6
2001	23.0	96.0	1.6	86.4	52.8	135.5	163.5	140.4	97.6	47.9	11.6	0.7
2002	22.6	94.4	1.4	83.4	50.7	133.0	164.3	139.4	95.1	47.8	11.5	0.7
2003	22.9	96.9	1.3	82.3	49.7	132.0	163.4	144.4	102.0	50.8	12.2	0.7
2004	22.9	97.8	1.3	82.6	49.7	133.5	165.3	145.6	104.1	52.9	12.4	0.7
2005	23.1	99.4	1.3	81.7	48.5	134.6	170.0	149.2	106.8	54.2	13.0	0.8
2006	23.4	101.5	1.3	83.0	47.9	139.7	177.0	152.4	108.5	55.6	13.3	0.8
2007	23.4	102.2	1.2	81.8	47.9	137.2	178.6	155.7	111.0	56.5	13.4	0.8
2008	22.2	98.8	1.2	77.5	46.1	127.2	170.7	152.6	109.6	56.1	13.7	0.9
White, not Hispanic or Latina mothers[e, f]												
1980	14.2	62.4	0.4	41.2	22.4	67.7	105.5	110.6	59.9	17.7	3.0	0.1
1990	14.4	62.8	0.5	42.5	23.2	66.6	97.5	115.3	79.4	30.0	4.7	0.2
1991	13.9	60.9	0.5	43.4	23.6	70.6	95.7	112.1	77.7	30.2	4.7	0.2
1992	13.4	60.0	0.5	41.7	22.7	69.8	93.9	110.6	78.3	30.4	5.1	0.2
1993	13.1	58.9	0.5	40.7	22.7	67.7	92.2	108.2	79.0	31.0	5.4	0.2
1994	12.8	58.2	0.5	40.4	22.7	67.6	90.9	106.6	80.2	32.0	5.7	0.2
1995	12.5	57.5	0.4	39.3	22.0	66.2	90.2	105.1	81.5	32.8	5.9	0.3
1996	12.3	57.1	0.4	37.6	20.6	64.0	90.1	104.9	82.8	33.9	6.2	0.3
1997	12.2	56.8	0.4	36.0	19.3	62.1	90.0	104.8	84.3	34.8	6.5	0.3
1998	12.2	57.6	0.3	35.3	18.3	60.9	91.2	107.4	87.2	36.4	6.8	0.4
1999	12.1	57.7	0.3	34.1	17.1	59.4	90.6	108.6	89.5	37.3	6.9	0.4
2000	12.2	58.5	0.3	32.6	15.8	57.5	91.2	109.4	93.2	38.8	7.3	0.4
2001	11.8	57.7	0.3	30.3	14.0	54.8	87.1	108.9	94.3	39.8	7.5	0.4
2002	11.7	57.4	0.2	28.5	13.1	51.9	84.3	109.3	94.4	40.9	7.6	0.5
2003	11.8	58.5	0.2	27.4	12.4	50.0	83.5	110.8	97.6	43.2	8.1	0.5

assess fetal development and malformations in the fetus. During amniocentesis, a physician inserts a needle through the abdominal wall into the uterus to obtain a small sample of the amniotic fluid surrounding the fetus. When tested in a laboratory, this fluid can reveal chromosomal abnormalities, metabolic disorders, and physical abnormalities.

Pregnant women older than age 35 are generally advised to undergo amniocentesis and other diagnostic testing, because they are at greater risk than younger women of giving birth to babies with chromosomal abnormalities such as Down syndrome (also called Down's syndrome). Instead of the normal 46 chromosomes, newborns with Down syndrome

TABLE 1.1

Crude birth rates, fertility rates, and birth rates, by age of mother, according to race and Hispanic origin, selected years 1950–2008 [CONTINUED]

Race, Hispanic origin, and year	Crude birth rate[a]	Fertility rate[b]	10–14 years	Total	15–19 years 15–17 years	15–19 years 18–19 years	Age of mother 20–24 years	25–29 years	30–34 years	35–39 years	40–44 years	45–54 years[c]
							Live births per 1,000 women					
2004	11.6	58.4	0.2	26.7	12.0	48.7	81.9	110.0	97.1	44.8	8.2	0.5
2005	11.5	58.3	0.2	25.9	11.5	48.0	81.4	109.1	96.9	45.6	8.3	0.5
2006	11.6	59.5	0.2	26.6	11.8	49.3	83.4	109.1	98.1	46.3	8.4	0.6
2007	11.6	60.1	0.2	27.2	11.8	50.4	83.2	108.6	99.5	45.8	8.6	0.6
2008	11.3	59.4	0.2	26.7	11.5	48.5	80.7	106.0	98.7	44.7	8.8	0.6
Black or African American, not Hispanic or Latina mothers[e, f]												
1980	22.9	90.7	4.6	105.1	77.2	146.5	152.2	111.7	65.2	25.8	5.8	0.3
1990	23.0	89.0	5.0	116.2	84.9	157.5	165.1	118.4	70.2	28.7	5.6	0.3
1991	22.4	87.0	4.9	118.2	86.1	162.2	164.8	115.1	68.9	28.7	5.6	0.2
1992	21.6	84.5	4.8	114.7	82.9	161.1	160.8	112.8	68.4	29.1	5.7	0.2
1993	20.7	81.5	4.6	110.5	81.1	154.6	154.5	109.2	68.1	29.4	5.9	0.3
1994	19.5	77.5	4.6	105.7	77.0	150.4	146.8	104.1	66.3	29.1	6.0	0.3
1995	18.2	72.8	4.2	97.2	70.4	139.2	137.8	98.5	64.4	28.8	6.1	0.3
1996	17.6	70.7	3.6	91.9	64.8	134.1	137.0	96.7	63.2	29.1	6.2	0.3
1997	17.4	70.3	3.2	88.3	60.7	131.0	138.8	97.2	63.6	29.6	6.5	0.3
1998	17.5	70.9	2.9	85.7	56.8	128.2	142.5	99.9	64.4	30.4	6.7	0.3
1999	17.1	69.9	2.6	81.0	51.7	123.9	142.1	99.8	63.9	30.6	6.5	0.3
2000	17.3	71.4	2.4	79.2	50.1	121.9	145.4	102.8	66.5	31.8	7.2	0.4
2001	16.6	69.1	2.1	73.5	44.9	116.7	137.2	102.1	66.2	32.1	7.3	0.4
2002	16.1	67.4	1.9	68.3	41.0	110.3	131.0	102.1	66.1	32.1	7.5	0.4
2003	15.9	67.1	1.6	64.7	38.7	105.3	128.1	102.1	67.4	33.4	7.7	0.5
2004	15.8	67.0	1.6	63.1	37.1	103.9	126.9	103.0	67.4	33.7	7.8	0.5
2005	15.7	67.2	1.7	60.9	34.9	103.0	126.8	103.0	68.4	34.3	8.2	0.5
2006	16.5	70.6	1.6	63.7	36.2	108.4	133.2	107.1	72.6	36.0	8.3	0.5
2007	16.6	71.6	1.5	64.2	35.8	109.3	133.6	107.5	74.3	36.4	8.6	0.6
2008	16.4	71.1	1.4	62.8	34.8	104.6	130.6	105.7	74.9	36.7	8.8	0.6

—Data not available.

*Rates based on fewer than 20 births are considered unreliable and are not shown.

[a]Live births per 1,000 population.

[b]Total number of live births regardless of age of mother per 1,000 women 15–44 years of age.

[c]Prior to 1997, data are for live births to mothers 45–49 years of age per 1,000 women 45–49 years of age. In subsequent years, rates were computed by relating the number of births to women age 45 years and over to the population of women age 45–49 years. Population of women age 45–49 years.

[d]Live births are tabulated by race of child.

[e]Live births are tabulated by race and/or Hispanic origin of mother.

[f]Prior to 1993, data from states lacking an Hispanic-origin item on the birth certificate were excluded. Rates in 1985 were not calculated because estimates for the Hispanic and non-Hispanic populations were not available.

Notes: Data are based on births adjusted for underregistration for 1950 and on registered births for all other years. Starting with 1970 data, births to persons who were not residents of the 50 states and the District of Columbia are excluded. Starting with Health, United States, 2003, rates for 1991–1999 were revised using intercensal population estimates based on the 2000 census. Rates for 2000 were computed using the 2000 census counts and starting in 2001 rates were computed using 2000-based postcensal estimates. The race groups, white, black, American Indian or Alaska Native, and Asian or Pacific Islander, include persons of Hispanic and non-Hispanic origin. Persons of Hispanic origin may be of any race. Starting with 2003 data, some states reported multiple-race data. The multiple-race data for these states were bridged to the single-race categories of the 1977 Office of Management and Budget standards for comparability with other states. Interpretation of trend data should take into consideration expansion of reporting areas and immigration.

SOURCE: "Table 3. Crude Birth Rates, Fertility Rates, and Birth Rates, by Age, Race, and Hispanic Origin of Mother: United States, Selected Years 1950–2008," in *Health, United States, 2010: With Special Feature on Death and Dying*, Centers for Disease Control and Prevention, National Center for Health Statistics, 2011, http://www.cdc.gov/nchs/data/hus/2010/003.pdf (accessed December 14, 2011)

have an extra copy of chromosome 21, giving them a total of 47 chromosomes. These children have varying degrees of mental retardation, and, according to the Cincinnati Children's Hospital Medical Center, in "Down Syndrome (Trisomy 21)" (2011, http://www.cincinnatichildrens.org/health/heart-encyclopedia/disease/syndrome/down.htm), up to 50% have congenital heart diseases. Mikyong Shin et al. estimate in "Prevalence of Down Syndrome among Children and Adolescents in 10 Regions of the United States" (*Pediatrics*, vol. 124, no. 6, December 1, 2009) that the average prevalence of children born with Down syndrome is one out 800 births, or 5,400 infants in the United States each year.

Ideally, every woman should receive prenatal care, and according to the National Center for Health Statistics (NCHS), the United States is capable of delivering prenatal care to nearly all pregnant women during the first trimester of pregnancy. However, not all mothers-to-be seek or receive early or adequate prenatal care. The Adequacy of Prenatal Care Utilization Index explains that adequate/adequate plus prenatal care is defined as pregnancy-related care beginning during the first four months of pregnancy with the appropriate number of visits for gestational age. The March of Dimes Foundation, a national voluntary organization that seeks to improve infant health by preventing birth defects, notes in "Distribution of Prenatal Care

Adequacy Categories: US, 2002" (2012, https://www.marchofdimes.com/peristats/level1.aspx?dv=ms&reg=99&top=5&stop=33&lev=1&slev=1&obj=3) that 74.7% of expectant mothers received adequate/adequate plus prenatal care in 2002 (the most recent year for which the March of Dimes reported prenatal care data). That same year 14% of women received intermediate prenatal care and 11.3% received inadequate care. The U.S. target, as stated in Healthy People 2020, for expectant mothers receiving adequate prenatal care is 77.6%.

The percentage of expectant mothers receiving prenatal care beginning during the first trimester increased from 68% in 1970 to 70.7% in 2008 in the states that reported these data. (See Table 1.2.) More Asian or Pacific Islander (77.4%) and white (72.2%) women received early prenatal care than did Hispanic (64.7%), African-American (59.1%), or Native American or Alaskan Native (55.8%) women in 2008. The percentage of expectant mothers who received inadequate prenatal care (care beginning during the third trimester or no prenatal care at all) declined from 7.9% in

TABLE 1.2

Prenatal care, by selected characteristics, in selected states and selected years 1970–2008

[Data are based on birth certificates]

Prenatal care, race, and Hispanic origin of mother	1970	1980	1990	2000	28 reporting areas (1989 revision)		18 reporting areas (2003 revision)		
					2006[a]	2007[a]	2006[b]	2007[b]	2008
Prenatal care began during 1st trimester					Percent of live births[c]				
All races	68.0	76.3	75.8	83.2	82.4	82.0	69.0	67.5	70.7
White	72.3	79.2	79.2	85.0	84.4	84.0	70.9	69.5	72.2
Black or African American	44.2	62.4	60.6	74.3	75.6	75.0	58.3	57.0	59.1
American Indian or Alaska Native	38.2	55.8	57.9	69.3	68.9	68.3	54.3	53.2	55.8
Asian or Pacific Islander[d]	—	73.7	75.1	84.0	82.0	82.6	71.4	69.8	77.4
Hispanic or Latina[e]	—	60.2	60.2	74.4	72.3	72.4	57.7	56.1	64.7
Mexican	—	59.6	57.8	72.9	70.5	70.7	53.4	51.5	63.7
Puerto Rican	—	55.1	63.5	78.5	78.7	78.3	68.1	66.1	67.2
Cuban	—	82.7	84.8	91.7	83.3	83.6	80.4	78.9	81.6
Central and South American	—	58.8	61.5	77.6	71.8	71.7	61.0	59.0	65.9
Other and unknown Hispanic or Latina	—	66.4	66.4	75.8	78.3	79.0	63.5	63.7	66.2
Not Hispanic or Latina:[e]									
White	—	81.2	83.3	88.5	88.0	87.7	76.2	74.9	76.1
Black or African American	—	60.8	60.7	74.3	75.7	75.0	58.4	57.1	59.1
Prenatal care began during 3rd trimester or no prenatal care									
All races	7.9	5.1	6.1	3.9	3.9	3.9	7.9	8.4	7.0
White	6.3	4.3	4.9	3.3	3.3	3.2	7.2	7.6	6.4
Black or African American	16.6	8.9	11.3	6.7	5.8	6.0	11.8	12.6	11.5
American Indian or Alaska Native	28.9	15.2	12.9	8.6	8.2	8.5	13.2	14.0	12.4
Asian or Pacific Islander[d]	—	6.5	5.8	3.3	3.9	3.6	7.1	7.7	5.1
Hispanic or Latina[e]	—	12.0	12.0	6.3	6.4	6.2	12.2	12.9	9.1
Mexican	—	11.8	13.2	6.9	6.8	6.5	14.2	15.1	9.6
Puerto Rican	—	16.2	10.6	4.5	4.1	3.9	6.7	7.8	7.3
Cuban	—	3.9	2.8	1.4	3.7	3.2	3.1	3.4	3.1
Central and South American	—	13.1	10.9	5.4	6.9	6.7	10.1	11.0	8.8
Other and unknown Hispanic or Latina	—	9.2	8.5	5.9	4.9	5.0	9.5	9.4	8.3
Not Hispanic or Latina:[e]									
White	—	3.5	3.4	2.3	2.3	2.3	5.2	5.5	5.0
Black or African American	—	9.7	11.2	6.7	5.8	6.0	11.8	12.6	11.6

—Data not available.

[a]Data are for the 28 reporting areas that used the 1989 Revision of the U.S. Standard Certificate of Live Birth for data on prenatal care in 2006 and 2007. Reporting areas that have implemented the 2003 Revision of the U.S. Standard Certificate of Live Birth are excluded because prenatal care data based on the 2003 revision are not comparable with data based on the 1989 and earlier revisions of the U.S. Standard Certificate of Live Birth.

[b]Data are for the 18 reporting areas that used the 2003 Revision of the U.S. Standard Certificate of Live Birth for data on prenatal care in 2006 and 2007. Reporting areas that used the 1989 Revision of the U.S. Standard Certificate of Live Birth are excluded because prenatal care data based on the 2003 revision are not comparable with data based on the 1989 or earlier revisions.

[c]Excludes live births where trimester when prenatal care began is unknown.

[d]Starting with 2003 data, estimates are not available for Asian or Pacific Islander subgroups during the transition from single-race to multiple-race reporting.

[e]Prior to 1993, data from states lacking an Hispanic-origin item on the birth certificate were excluded. Data for non-Hispanic white and non-Hispanic black women for years prior to 1989 are not nationally representative and are provided for comparison with Hispanic data.

Notes: Prior to 2003, all data are based on the 1989 and earlier revisions of the U.S. Standard Certificate of Live Birth. Data for 1970 and 1975 exclude births that occurred in states not reporting prenatal care. Starting in 2003 some states have implemented the 2003 Revision of the U.S. Standard Certificate of Live Birth on a voluntary basis. Data are not shown for 2006 and 2007 for the six states that implemented the 2003 revision mid-year 2006 or during 2007. California implemented a partial revision of the 2003 Revision of the U.S. Standard Certificate of Live Birth in 2006 but continued to use the 1989 revision format for data on prenatal care. The race groups white, black, American Indian or Alaska Native, and Asian or Pacific Islander include persons of Hispanic and non-Hispanic origin. Persons of Hispanic origin may be of any race. Starting with 2003 data, some states reported multiple-race data. The multiple-race data for these states were bridged to the single-race categories of the 1977 Office of Management and Budget standards for comparability with other states. Interpretation of trend data should take into consideration changes in reporting areas and immigration. Data for additional years are available.

SOURCE: Adapted from "Table 8. Prenatal Care for Live Births, by Detailed Race and Hispanic Origin of Mother: United States, Selected Years 1970–2000 and Selected States 2006–2007," in *Health, United States, 2010: With Special Feature on Death and Dying,* Centers for Disease Control and Prevention, National Center for Health Statistics, 2011, http://www.cdc.gov/nchs/data/hus/hus10.pdf#listtables (accessed December 14, 2011)

1970 to 7% in 2008. (See Table 1.2.) In 2008 more Native American or Alaskan Native (12.4%), African-American (11.5%), and Hispanic (9.1%) women failed to receive adequate prenatal care than did white (6.4%) or Asian or Pacific Islander (5.1%) women.

The March of Dimes cites the lack of health insurance, transportation, and child care; inconvenient health care provider service hours; unplanned pregnancies; and cultural and personal factors as obstacles that prevent expectant mothers from receiving prenatal care.

Early prenatal care can prevent or reduce the risk of low birth weight (LBW). Infants who weigh less than 5 pounds, 8 ounces (2,500 g) at birth are considered to be of LBW. Those born weighing less than 3 pounds, 4 ounces (1,500 g) are called very low birth weight (VLBW). LBW may result from premature birth (infants born before 37 weeks of pregnancy are considered premature), poor maternal nutrition, teen pregnancy, drug and alcohol use, smoking, or sexually transmitted diseases.

Infants who are premature or have an LBW are at greater risk of death and disability than infants of normal weight. About 80% of women at risk for delivering an LBW infant can be identified during the first prenatal visit, and interventions can be made to try to prevent problems. Between 1990 and 2008 the proportion of newborn babies weighing less than 5 pounds, 8 ounces increased by 18%. (See Table 1.3.) The NCHS notes in *Health, United States, 2010* (2011, http://www.cdc.gov/nchs/data/hus/hus10.pdf) that between 2007 and 2008 the percentage of LBW births was unchanged—between 8.1% and 8.2%.

As with access to prenatal care, the percentage of LBW live births varies by geography, race, and ethnicity. Among non-Hispanic African-Americans, 13.7% of live births in 2008 weighed less than 5 pounds, 8 ounces, compared with 8.2% of Asian or Pacific Islander births, 7.4% of Native American or Alaskan Native births, 7.2% of non-Hispanic white births, and 7% of Hispanic births. (See Table 1.3.) In 2006–08 over 15% of live births to non-Hispanic African-American mothers in Alabama, Colorado, Kentucky, Louisiana, Mississippi, Oklahoma, and West Virginia were LBW, compared with 5.5% of LBW live births to non-Hispanic white mothers in Alaska and 5.9% in Oregon. (See Table 1.4.)

The usual length of pregnancy is 40 weeks from the first day of the woman's last menstrual period. Infants born prematurely do not have fully formed organ systems. If, however, the premature infant is born with a birth weight that is comparable to a full-term baby and has organ systems that are only slightly undeveloped, the chances of survival are great. Premature infants of VLBW are susceptible to many risks and are less likely to survive than full-term infants. If they survive, they may suffer from mental retardation, developmental disabilities, and other abnormalities of the nervous system.

A severe medical condition called hyaline membrane disease (or respiratory distress syndrome) commonly affects premature infants. It is caused by the inability of immature lungs to function properly. Occurring immediately after birth, the disease may cause infant death within hours. Intensive care of affected infants includes the use of a mechanical ventilator to facilitate breathing. Also, premature infants' immature gastrointestinal systems preclude them from taking in nourishment properly. Unable to suck and swallow, they must be fed through a nasogastric feeding tube (nutrient-rich formula enters through a tube inserted into the stomach via the nose).

LBW and VLBW are major predictors of infant morbidity (illness or disease) and mortality. Hamilton, Martin, and Ventura explain that for LBW infants, the risk of dying during the first year of life is more than five times that of normal-weight infants; the risk for VLBW infants is nearly 100 times higher. The risk of delivering an LBW infant is greatest among the youngest and oldest mothers; however, many of the LBW births among older mothers are attributable to their higher rates of multiple births. Even though older mothers and multiples account for many LBW infants, between 1990 and 2006 there was an increase in LBW singletons. However, the percentage of LBW singletons has declined slowly since 2006. (See Table 1.5.)

Birth Weight Influences the Risk of Infant Death and Future Disease

Even though the precise mechanisms of the relationship between birth weight and the development of disease in adulthood have not yet been completely described, and researchers do not yet know exactly how or why birth weight can predict health and illness in adulthood, there is ample evidence that lower- and higher-than-average birth weight are associated with health in later life. LBW infants are more likely than normal-weight infants to develop disease as they age and male LBW infants—who gain weight rapidly before their first birthday—are disproportionately affected and seem to be at the highest risk for future health problems. Researchers conjecture that LBW infants have fewer muscle cells at birth and that rapid weight gain during the first year of life may lead to different ratios of fat to muscle and above-average body mass. LBW infants who later develop above-average body mass are at higher risk of developing diseases such as type 2 diabetes, hypertension (high blood pressure), and cardiovascular disease (heart disease and stroke) than normal-weight infants who do not gain weight rapidly during their first year of life.

LBW is not only an important predictor of infant health risks but is also a leading cause of infant deaths. T. J. Mathews and Marian F. MacDorman of the CDC report in "Infant Mortality Statistics from the 2007 Period Linked Birth/Infant Death Data Set" (*National Vital Statistics Report*, vol. 59, no. 6, June 29, 2011) that in 2007 the

TABLE 1.3

Low birthweight live birth, by selected characteristics, selected years, 1970–2008

[Dates are based on birth certificates]

Birthweight, race and Hispanic origin of mother, and smoking status of mother	1970	1975	1980	1985	1990	1995	2000	2005	2006	2007	2008
Low birthweight (less than 2,500 grams)					Percent of live births[a]						
All races	7.93	7.38	6.84	6.75	6.97	7.32	7.57	8.19	8.26	8.22	8.18
White	6.85	6.27	5.72	5.65	5.70	6.22	6.55	7.16	7.21	7.16	7.13
Black or African American	13.90	13.19	12.69	12.65	13.25	13.13	12.99	13.59	13.59	13.55	13.39
American Indian or Alaska Native	7.97	6.41	6.44	5.86	6.11	6.61	6.76	7.36	7.52	7.46	7.40
Asian or Pacific Islander[b]	—	—	6.68	6.16	6.45	6.90	7.31	7.98	8.12	8.10	8.18
Hispanic or Latina[c]	—	—	6.12	6.16	6.06	6.29	6.41	6.88	6.99	6.93	6.96
Mexican	—	—	5.62	5.77	5.55	5.81	6.01	6.49	6.58	6.50	6.49
Puerto Rican	—	—	8.95	8.69	8.99	9.41	9.30	9.92	10.14	9.83	9.86
Cuban	—	—	5.62	6.02	5.67	6.50	6.49	7.64	7.14	7.66	7.83
Central and South American	—	—	5.76	5.68	5.84	6.20	6.34	6.78	6.81	6.71	6.70
Other and unknown Hispanic or Latina	—	—	6.96	6.83	6.87	7.55	7.84	8.27	8.54	8.61	8.24
Not Hispanic or Latina:[c]											
White	—	—	5.69	5.61	5.61	6.20	6.60	7.29	7.32	7.28	7.22
Black or African American	—	—	12.71	12.62	13.32	13.21	13.13	14.02	13.97	13.90	13.71
									21 reporting areas		
Cigarette smoker[d]	—	—	—	—	ψ	ψ	ψ	ψ	12.02	11.85	11.85
Nonsmoker[d]	—	—	—	—	ψ	ψ	ψ	ψ	7.69	7.36	7.32
Very low birthweight (less than 1,500 grams)											
All races	1.17	1.16	1.15	1.21	1.27	1.35	1.43	1.49	1.49	1.49	1.46
White	0.95	0.92	0.90	0.94	0.95	1.06	1.14	1.20	1.20	1.19	1.18
Black or African American	2.40	2.40	2.48	2.71	2.92	2.97	3.07	3.15	3.05	3.11	2.93
American Indian or Alaska Native	0.98	0.95	0.92	1.01	1.01	1.10	1.16	1.17	1.28	1.27	1.28
Asian or Pacific Islander[b]	—	—	0.92	0.85	0.87	0.91	1.05	1.14	1.12	1.14	1.16
Hispanic or Latina[c]	—	—	0.98	1.01	1.03	1.11	1.14	1.20	1.19	1.21	1.20
Mexican	—	—	0.92	0.97	0.92	1.01	1.03	1.12	1.12	1.13	1.11
Puerto Rican	—	—	1.29	1.30	1.62	1.79	1.93	1.87	1.91	1.89	1.93
Cuban	—	—	1.02	1.18	1.20	1.19	1.21	1.50	1.28	1.27	1.43
Central and South American	—	—	0.99	1.01	1.05	1.13	1.20	1.19	1.13	1.15	1.13
Other and unknown Hispanic or Latina	—	—	1.01	0.96	1.09	1.28	1.42	1.36	1.36	1.44	1.34
Not Hispanic or Latina:[c]											
White	—	—	0.87	0.91	0.93	1.04	1.14	1.21	1.20	1.19	1.18
Black or African American	—	—	2.47	2.67	2.93	2.98	3.10	3.27	3.15	3.20	3.01
									21 reporting areas		
Cigarette smoker[d]	—	—	—	—	ψ	ψ	ψ	ψ	1.73	1.80	1.79
Nonsmoker[d]	—	—	—	—	ψ	ψ	ψ	ψ	1.41	1.32	1.29

— = Data not available.

ψ = Data not shown. Due to a change in reporting, data are not comparable to other years. See footnote d.

[a]Excludes live births with unknown birthweight. Percent based on live births with known birthweight.

[b]Starting with 2003 data, estimates are not available for Asian or Pacific Islander subgroups during the transition from single-race to multiple-race reporting.

[c]Prior to 1993, data from states lacking an Hispanic-origin item on the birth certificate were excluded.

Data for non-Hispanic white and non-Hispanic black women for years prior to 1989 are not nationally representative and are provided for comparison with Hispanic data.

[d]Percent based on live births with known smoking status of mother and known birthweight. Only reporting areas that have implemented the 2003 Revision of the U.S. Standard Certificate of Live Birth are shown because maternal tobacco use data based on the 2003 revision are not comparable with data based on the 1989 or earlier revisions to the U.S. Standard Certificate of Live Birth.

Notes: Data are for the 21 reporting areas that used the 2003 Revision of the U.S. Standard Certificate of Live Birth for data on smoking in 2007 and 2008. The race groups, white, black, American Indian or Alaska Native, and Asian or Pacific Islander, include persons of Hispanic and non-Hispanic origin. Persons of Hispanic origin may be of any race. Starting with 2003 data, some states reported multiple-race data.

The multiple-race data for these states were bridged to the single-race categories of the 1977 Office of Management and Budget standards for comparability with other states.

Interpretation of trend data should take into consideration expansion of reporting areas and immigration.

SOURCE: "Table 9. Low Birthweight Live Births, by Detailed Race, Hispanic Origin and Smoking Status of Mother, United States, Selected Years 1970–2008," in *Health, United States, 2010: With Special Feature on Death and Dying*, Centers for Disease Control and Prevention, National Center for Health Statistics, 2011, http://www.cdc.gov/nchs/data/hus/hus10.pdf#listtables (accessed December 14, 2011)

---

mortality rate was about 25 times higher for LBW infants (56.1 per 1,000 live births) than for infants with birth weights of at least 5 pounds, 8 ounces (2.3 per 1,000 live births). (See Table 1.6.) The mortality rate for VLBW infants (240.9 per 1,000 live births) was more than 100 times the rate for infants with birth weights of at least 5 pounds, 8 ounces.

Magnus Kaijser et al. find in "Perinatal Risk Factors for Ischemic Heart Disease: Disentangling the Roles of Birth Weight and Preterm Birth" (*Circulation*, vol. 117, no. 3, January 22, 2008) that LBW is associated with an increased risk of developing heart disease. Based on a review of 6,425 subjects born with LBW, Kaijser et al. determine that this association reflects the length of

TABLE 1.4

Low-birthweight births by race, ethnicity, and state, 2000–08

[Data are based on birth certificates]

State	All races			Not Hispanic or Latina					
				White			Black or African American		
	2000–2002	2003–2005	2006–2008	2000–2002	2003–2005	2006–2008	2000–2002	2003–2005	2006–2008
	Percent of live births weighing less than 2,500 grams[a]								
United States	7.69	8.07	8.22	6.75	7.18	7.27	13.19	13.77	13.86
Alabama	9.75	10.35	10.49	7.77	8.46	8.45	14.10	15.02	15.58
Alaska	5.71	6.02	5.86	4.84	5.34	5.52	10.70	11.74	10.97
Arizona	6.91	7.05	7.09	6.78	7.01	6.88	13.16	12.38	12.53
Arkansas	8.64	9.04	9.18	7.48	7.83	7.97	13.81	14.86	14.93
California	6.29	6.71	6.84	5.86	6.30	6.40	11.66	12.46	12.00
Colorado	8.60	9.04	8.96	8.24	8.81	8.64	14.59	15.20	15.11
Connecticut	7.52	7.74	8.07	6.48	6.60	6.91	12.28	12.88	12.79
Delaware	9.29	9.31	9.01	7.80	7.62	7.33	14.08	14.32	13.74
District of Columbia	11.85	11.06	11.02	6.35	6.28	6.76	14.60	13.96	14.28
Florida	8.18	8.59	8.72	6.98	7.38	7.48	12.58	13.28	13.48
Georgia	8.79	9.27	9.57	6.92	7.44	7.54	12.98	13.81	14.19
Hawaii	7.98	8.23	8.05	6.17	6.42	5.97	11.01	*7.03	*9.71
Idaho	6.41	6.65	6.65	6.29	6.60	6.59	*	*	*
Illinois	8.04	8.40	8.50	6.74	7.22	7.34	14.04	14.70	14.23
Indiana	7.54	8.10	8.36	6.95	7.54	7.69	12.89	13.46	14.12
Iowa	6.39	6.92	6.81	6.19	6.72	6.58	11.77	12.22	11.49
Kansas	6.96	7.28	7.14	6.66	6.97	6.81	12.37	13.42	12.68
Kentucky	8.38	8.86	9.20	7.84	8.50	8.72	13.84	13.52	15.02
Louisiana	10.40	11.02	11.15	7.56	8.12	8.34	14.44	15.33	15.70
Maine	6.12	6.58	6.61	6.13	6.57	6.51	*9.47	8.47	9.01
Maryland	8.88	9.17	9.24	6.79	7.19	7.27	13.00	13.13	13.14
Massachusetts	7.26	7.77	7.85	6.56	7.15	7.22	11.54	11.82	11.32
Michigan	7.94	8.28	8.44	6.55	7.00	7.17	14.24	14.43	14.09
Minnesota	6.23	6.43	6.54	5.80	5.93	5.98	10.54	10.71	10.66
Mississippi	10.82	11.62	12.16	7.97	8.67	8.84	14.48	15.60	16.39
Missouri	7.74	8.12	8.01	6.79	7.18	7.09	13.27	13.90	13.44
Montana	6.65	7.02	7.29	6.60	6.81	7.11	*	*15.58	*
Nebraska	6.88	6.97	7.06	6.52	6.76	6.54	13.07	12.16	13.37
Nevada	7.44	8.11	8.20	7.19	7.78	8.07	13.40	13.98	13.89
New Hampshire	6.40	6.65	6.57	6.24	6.59	6.51	10.58	10.85	8.95
New Jersey	7.89	8.19	8.51	6.59	7.11	7.43	13.20	13.48	13.52
New Mexico	7.99	8.38	8.71	7.89	8.33	8.55	13.88	15.01	14.08
New York	7.76	8.11	8.22	6.48	6.82	6.94	12.02	12.78	12.66
North Carolina	8.90	9.07	9.13	7.49	7.73	7.73	13.83	14.33	14.39
North Dakota	6.28	6.49	6.60	6.13	6.37	6.52	*9.02	*9.43	*5.94
Ohio	8.07	8.51	8.71	7.08	7.53	7.55	13.45	13.83	14.36
Oklahoma	7.75	7.92	8.27	7.35	7.63	7.87	13.57	13.62	15.06
Oregon	5.65	6.09	6.08	5.44	6.02	5.91	10.32	11.16	9.74
Pennsylvania	7.93	8.20	8.41	6.78	7.06	7.21	13.79	13.67	13.76
Rhode Island	7.47	8.12	7.98	6.75	7.39	7.35	12.32	11.22	11.18
South Carolina	9.74	10.15	10.04	7.40	7.82	7.78	14.29	15.19	14.96
South Dakota	6.58	6.71	6.82	6.37	6.62	6.54	*11.51	*7.27	10.61
Tennessee	9.20	9.35	9.41	7.95	8.26	8.30	14.23	14.51	14.44
Texas	7.54	8.07	8.43	6.81	7.43	7.66	12.82	13.91	14.17
Utah	6.48	6.68	6.79	6.28	6.45	6.52	13.09	12.05	11.64
Vermont	6.15	6.57	6.67	6.12	6.55	6.58	*	*	*10.15
Virginia	7.90	8.23	8.38	6.54	7.01	7.10	12.56	12.83	13.22
Washington	5.75	6.13	6.38	5.43	5.63	5.98	10.34	10.63	9.81
West Virginia	8.60	9.16	9.58	8.39	9.03	9.42	13.81	13.15	15.22
Wisconsin	6.58	6.93	6.96	5.83	6.18	6.19	13.25	13.59	13.28
Wyoming	8.35	8.71	8.77	8.12	8.74	8.80	*13.29	*	*14.06

pregnancy and problems in pregnancy such as maternal malnutrition that might limit the growth of the unborn child.

In "Low Birth Weight and Increased Cardiovascular Risk: Fetal Programming" (*International Journal of Cardiology*, vol. 144, no. 1, September 24, 2010), Mustafa Mucahit Balci, Sadik Acikel, and Ramazan Akdemir posit that LBW infants may have hyper-responsive immune systems that predispose them to inflammatory conditions such as certain forms of heart disease, diabetes, arthritis, and asthma.

Evidence also indicates that birth weight is related to a risk of developing breast cancer. Xiaohui Xu et al. reviewed relevant medical literature to determine whether studies conducted between 1996 and 2008 confirm that birth weight influences the risk of developing breast cancer in adulthood. The results of this meta-analysis were published in "Birth Weight as a Risk Factor for Breast Cancer: A Meta-analysis

TABLE 1.4

Low-birthweight births by race, ethnicity, and state, 2000–08 [CONTINUED]

[Data are based on birth certificates]

State	Hispanic or Latina[b]			American Indian or Alaska Native[c]			Asian or Pacific Islander[c]		
	2000–2002	2003–2005	2006–2008	2000–2002	2003–2005	2006–2008	2000–2002	2003–2005	2006–2008
	Percent of live births weighing less than 2,500 grams[a]								
United States	6.48	6.79	6.96	7.11	7.39	7.46	7.54	7.89	8.13
Alabama	6.95	6.92	6.66	9.68	10.53	*6.77	7.38	8.02	8.31
Alaska	6.07	5.31	6.50	5.81	5.86	5.59	7.33	6.57	6.30
Arizona	6.56	6.69	6.73	6.85	7.11	6.98	7.95	7.92	8.30
Arkansas	5.79	6.54	6.65	8.11	8.86	8.54	7.73	6.74	7.85
California	5.66	6.10	6.22	6.21	6.49	7.01	7.15	7.42	7.73
Colorado	8.33	8.53	8.49	9.05	9.45	9.78	10.17	10.26	10.60
Connecticut	8.25	8.49	8.38	10.06	7.45	9.05	8.07	7.83	8.60
Delaware	6.81	7.03	7.14	*	*	*	9.89	9.33	7.73
District of Columbia	8.04	7.46	6.91	*	*	*	*7.00	8.97	8.47
Florida	6.61	6.98	7.13	7.11	7.38	7.16	8.35	8.73	8.21
Georgia	5.77	5.96	6.31	9.29	9.00	8.40	8.18	8.35	7.94
Hawaii	8.00	8.34	7.92	*4.99	*	*	8.45	8.84	8.80
Idaho	6.95	6.67	6.62	6.15	8.31	7.59	7.38	6.67	7.91
Illinois	6.31	6.60	6.86	8.60	9.46	8.24	8.49	8.28	8.72
Indiana	6.09	6.33	6.88	*7.74	*10.00	*6.37	7.41	7.87	7.81
Iowa	6.01	6.12	6.40	7.23	9.15	7.09	7.13	7.71	8.07
Kansas	5.93	6.09	5.79	6.20	7.09	7.66	6.69	7.34	8.58
Kentucky	7.73	6.85	6.80	*7.17	*8.54	*	7.75	7.56	8.57
Louisiana	6.56	7.62	6.89	9.06	10.11	10.26	7.89	8.46	8.77
Maine	*6.03	*4.74	8.18	*	*	*6.29	*5.46	8.69	7.25
Maryland	6.73	7.18	7.02	9.74	10.87	*8.43	7.42	7.93	7.97
Massachusetts	8.37	8.41	8.27	*7.11	*7.62	10.51	7.57	7.63	8.30
Michigan	6.26	6.46	6.98	7.26	6.98	7.45	7.46	8.33	8.36
Minnesota	6.02	5.70	5.85	7.10	6.87	6.38	7.28	7.43	7.77
Mississippi	6.61	6.42	6.94	7.30	6.24	7.48	6.83	8.06	9.29
Missouri	6.18	6.33	5.88	8.67	7.63	6.59	7.34	7.61	7.94
Montana	7.44	8.63	7.65	7.14	7.80	7.86	*5.95	*8.70	*10.77
Nebraska	6.30	6.20	6.66	7.27	6.78	6.88	8.05	7.61	7.85
Nevada	6.34	6.74	6.71	6.80	7.58	7.18	7.56	10.35	9.96
New Hampshire	4.84	6.55	7.60	*	*	*	5.95	7.75	7.16
New Jersey	7.15	7.27	7.55	11.09	9.83	9.93	7.57	8.10	8.50
New Mexico	8.13	8.45	8.82	6.88	7.32	7.59	7.67	8.60	9.15
New York	7.38	7.59	7.85	7.81	7.31	6.41	7.33	7.89	7.86
North Carolina	6.13	6.27	6.30	10.30	11.01	10.61	8.20	7.77	8.88
North Dakota	*8.10	*5.84	7.69	6.62	6.78	6.81	*	*8.39	*6.20
Ohio	7.20	7.13	7.67	8.86	10.22	10.54	7.86	8.27	8.64
Oklahoma	6.41	6.46	6.47	6.48	6.69	7.37	7.87	6.82	6.88
Oregon	5.54	5.43	5.86	7.23	7.34	6.34	6.78	7.00	7.40
Pennsylvania	8.97	9.00	8.78	9.15	10.95	10.80	7.48	7.99	8.29
Rhode Island	7.20	8.61	7.99	*10.32	13.66	13.40	9.31	10.11	8.85
South Carolina	6.87	6.66	6.49	10.22	10.75	8.26	8.02	8.13	8.30
South Dakota	6.89	5.94	7.88	6.84	7.04	7.29	*11.39	*9.50	*8.28
Tennessee	6.28	6.04	6.36	*7.11	*6.63	5.70	8.60	7.76	8.43
Texas	6.88	7.23	7.60	6.67	7.33	8.32	7.78	8.33	8.93
Utah	7.20	7.26	7.41	6.37	7.46	7.75	7.23	8.20	8.21
Vermont	*	*	*	*	*	*	*	*8.08	*7.67
Virginia	6.07	6.28	6.31	*10.73	*9.20	*6.13	7.50	7.71	7.87
Washington	5.31	5.93	6.00	7.08	7.31	7.78	6.37	6.90	7.50
West Virginia	*	*6.06	*5.71	*	*	*	*9.16	*9.51	*6.65
Wisconsin	6.13	6.34	6.29	6.12	6.04	7.12	6.97	7.50	6.98
Wyoming	8.81	8.43	7.73	9.55	8.39	9.77	*12.04	*	*12.24

*Percents preceded by an asterisk are based on fewer than 50 births. Percents not shown are based on fewer than 20 births.
[a]Excludes live births with unknown birthweight.
[b]Persons of Hispanic origin may be of any race.
[c]Includes persons of Hispanic and non-Hispanic origin.
Notes: Starting with 2003 data, some states reported multiple-race data. The multiple-race data for these states were bridged to the single-race categories of the 1977 Office of Management and Budget standards for comparability with other states.

SOURCE: "Table 11. Low Birthweight Live Births, by Race and Hispanic Origin of Mother, and State: United States, 2000–2002, 2003–2005, and 2006–2008," in *Health, United States, 2010: With Special Feature on Death and Dying,* Centers for Disease Control and Prevention, National Center for Health Statistics, 2011, http://www.cdc.gov/nchs/data/hus/hus10.pdf#listtables (accessed December 14, 2011)

of 18 Epidemiological Studies" (*Journal of Women's Health,* vol. 18, no. 8, August 2009). By examining 18 studies and 16,424 cases of breast cancer, the researchers determine that size at birth was associated with breast cancer risk. Risk was higher among women who weighed more than 8 pounds, 13 ounces (4,000 g).

TABLE 1.5

Singleton very low and low birthweight, by selected characteristics, selected years 1990–2009

Year	Very low birthweight[a]	Low birthweight[b]
All races[c]		
2009	1.10	6.36
2008	1.11	6.40
2007	1.14	6.45
2006	1.14	6.49
2005	1.14	6.41
2000	1.11	6.00
1995	1.08	6.05
1990	1.05	5.90
Non-Hispanic white[d]		
2009	0.81	5.23
2008	0.82	5.26
2007	0.83	5.32
2006	0.85	5.37
2005	0.84	5.32
2000	0.80	4.88
1995	0.78	4.87
1990	0.73	4.56
Non-Hispanic black[d]		
2009	2.51	11.44
2008	2.49	11.60
2007	2.65	11.78
2006	2.61	11.85
2005	2.71	11.90
2000	2.62	11.28
1995	2.55	11.66
1990	2.54	11.92
Hispanic[e]		
2009	0.96	5.72
2008	0.96	5.74
2007	0.97	5.74
2006	0.98	5.79
2005	0.97	5.69
2000	0.94	5.36
1995	0.93	5.36
1990[f]	0.87	5.23

[a]Less than 1,500 grams (3 lb. 4 oz.).
[b]Less than 2,500 grams (5 lb. 8 oz.).
[c]Includes races other than white and black and origin not stated.
[d]Race and Hispanic origin are reported separately on birth certificates. Persons of Hispanic origin may be of any race. Race categories are consistent with the 1977 Office of Management and Budget standards. Thirty-three states and the District of Columbia reported multiple race data for 2009. Multiple race data for these states were bridged to the single race categories of the 1977 Office of Management and Budget standards for comparability with other states. Multiple race reporting areas vary for 2003–2009.
[e]Includes all persons of Hispanic origin of any race.
[f]Data by Hispanic origin exclude New Hampshire and Oklahoma, which did not report Hispanic origin.

SOURCE: Joyce A. Martin et al., "Table G. Singleton Very Low and Low Birthweight, by Race and Hispanic Origin of Mother: United States, Selected Years 1990–2009," in "Births: Final Data for 2009," *National Vital Statistics Reports*, vol. 60, no. 1, November 2011, http://www.cdc.gov/nchs/data/nvsr/nvsr60/nvsr60_01.pdf (accessed December 15, 2011).

In "Birth Weight and the Risk of Testicular Cancer: A Meta-analysis" (*International Journal of Cancer*, vol. 121, no. 5, September 1, 2007), Athanasios Michos, Fei Xue, and Karin B. Michels indicate that both LBW and high birth weight (HBW; greater than 8 pounds, 13 ounces) increase the risk of testicular cancer in men. Men with LBW were 18% more likely and men with HBW were 12% more likely to develop testicular cancer than men of average birth weight.

Marilyn Rogers et al. report in "Aerobic Capacity, Strength, Flexibility, and Activity Level in Unimpaired Extremely Low Birth Weight ($\leq$800 g) Survivors at 17 Years of Age Compared with Term-Born Control Subjects" (*Pediatrics*, vol. 116, no. 1, July 2005) that infants born either prematurely or with a VLBW were significantly more likely to suffer lower levels of fitness later in life—including less strength, endurance, and flexibility—and had a greater risk of health problems as adults. When compared with normal-birth-weight teens, the VLBW teens had lower aerobic capacity, grip strength, leg power, and vertical jump. They were unable to perform as many pushups, had less abdominal strength as measured by curl-ups, had less lower-back flexibility, and had tighter hamstrings. The VLBW teens reported less previous and current sports participation, lower physical activity levels, and poorer coordination compared with full-term-born control subjects. VLBW teens also had more trouble maintaining rhythm and tempo than their normal-birth-weight peers.

The only action able to alter the birth weight of an infant is to modify weight gain by the mother during pregnancy. In 2012 health professionals concurred that for normal-weight women the ideal weight gain during pregnancy ranges from 25 to 35 pounds (11.3 to 15.9 kg) of fat and lean mass. Furthermore, research published in 2003 revealed that a newborn's birth weight and a mother's postpregnancy weight are influenced not only by how much weight is gained during pregnancy but also by the source of the excess weight. In the landmark study "Composition of Gestational Weight Gain Impacts Maternal Fat Retention and Infant Birth Weight" (*American Journal of Obstetrics and Gynecology*, vol. 189, no. 5, November 2003), Nancy F. Butte et al. of the Children's Nutrition Research Center in Houston, Texas, conducted body scans of 63 women before, during, and after their pregnancies and recorded changes in the women's weight from water, protein, fat, and potassium—a marker for changes in muscle tissue, which is one component of lean mass. The researchers find that only increases in lean mass, and not fat mass, appeared to influence infant size. Independent of how much fat was gained by women during pregnancy, only lean body mass increased the birth weight of the infant, with women who gained more lean body mass giving birth to larger infants.

Women with a higher prepregnancy weight and those who gain large amounts of weight during pregnancy are more likely to give birth to heavier infants. In "Maternal Pre-pregnant Body Mass Index, Maternal Weight Change and Offspring Birthweight" (*Acta Obstetricia et Gynecologica Scandinavica*, vol. 91, no. 2, February 2012), Unni Mette Stamnes Koepp et al. analyze the association between prepregnancy weight and the infant's birth weight and determine that prepregnancy weight is an important predictor of birth weight. The researchers conclude that overweight and obese women should be encouraged to attain a healthy weight before becoming pregnant and should aim for moderate weight gain during pregnancy.

TABLE 1.6

Infant mortality rates, by selected characteristics including birthweight, 2007

Characteristic	All races	Race of mother			
		White	Black	American Indian or Alaska Native	Asian or Pacific Islander
		Infant mortality rates per 1,000 live births in specified group			
Total	6.75	5.62	12.92	9.22	4.78
Age at death					
Total neonatal	4.42	3.67	8.51	4.55	3.38
Early neonatal (less than 7 days)	3.51	2.90	6.80	3.36	2.75
Late neonatal (7–27 days)	0.92	0.77	1.71	1.19	0.62
Postneonatal	2.33	1.94	4.42	4.67	1.40
Sex					
Male	7.37	6.15	14.07	10.13	5.19
Female	6.11	5.06	11.74	8.28	4.33
Plurality					
Single births	5.93	4.92	11.43	8.59	4.16
Plural births	30.33	25.78	51.69	35.10	25.76
Birthweight					
Less than 2,500 grams	56.12	51.23	71.99	63.41	40.87
Less than 1,500 grams	240.88	230.05	261.95	273.16	229.73
1,500–2,499 grams	14.62	15.02	14.55	20.20	9.53
2,500 grams or more	2.29	2.08	3.54	4.81	1.56
Period of gestation					
Less than 32 weeks	178.36	165.13	207.75	156.99	173.30
32–33 weeks	16.12	15.88	16.40	28.51	14.84
34–36 weeks	7.42	6.93	9.27	14.27	5.59
37–41 weeks	2.43	2.21	3.73	4.59	1.67
37–38 weeks	3.09	2.86	4.37	6.14	2.12
39–41 weeks	2.07	1.87	3.33	3.79	1.43
42 weeks or more	2.62	2.36	4.26	*	1.69
Age of mother					
Under 20 years	9 80	8.32	13.59	11.46	11.89
20–24 years	7.67	6.31	13.02	9.57	5.41
25–29 years	5.97	5.01	11.93	7.97	4.22
30–34 years	5.37	4.53	12.35	8.48	3.96
35–39 years	6.20	5.23	14.26	7.62	4.85
40–54 years	8.57	7.28	16.84	*	8.10
Live-birth order					
1	6.75	5.68	13.07	8.05	4.60
2	5.96	5.00	11.88	8.33	4.34
3	6.62	5.50	11.92	11.78	5.81
4	7.79	6.50	13.44	8.56	5.11
5 or more	10.06	7.98	16.62	11.66	7.14
Marital status					
Married	5.16	4.67	11.27	6.93	4.39
Unmarried	9.17	7.39	13.59	10.44	6.76
Mother's place of birth					
Born in the 50 states or D.C	7.15	5.75	13.37	9.49	6.32
Born elsewhere	5.10	4.84	8.70	*	4.25

*Figure does not meet standards of reliability or precision; based on fewer than 20 deaths in the numerator.
Notes: Infant deaths are weighted, so numbers may not exactly add to totals due to rounding. "Not stated" responses were included in totals but not distributed among groups for rate computations. Race and Hispanic origin are reported separately on birth certificates. Race categories are consistent with 1977 Office of Management and Budget standards. In this table, all women, including Hispanic women, are classified only according to their race.

SOURCE: T. J. Mathews and Marian F. MacDorman, "Table 1. Infant Mortality Rates, Live Births, and Infant Deaths, by Selected Characteristics and Race of Mother: United States, 2007 Linked File," in "Infant Mortality Statistics from the 2007 Period Linked Birth/Infant Death Data Set," *National Vital Statistics Report*, vol. 59, no. 6, June 29, 2011, http://www.cdc.gov/nchs/data/nvsr/nvsr59/nvsr59_06.pdf (accessed December 15, 2011)

Kathleen M. Rasmussen et al. report in *Weight Gain during Pregnancy: Reexamining the Guidelines* (May 28, 2009, http://www.iom.edu/) that in 2009 the Institute of Medicine and the National Research Council issued new recommendations for pregnancy weight gain. (See Table 1.7.) The updated guidelines caution that obese expectant mothers (with a body mass index [BMI; a measure of body fat based on weight and height] of 30 or higher) should limit weight gain to between 11 and 20 pounds (5 and 9.1 kg). This recommendation replaces the 1990 guideline, which advised obese expectant mothers to gain no less than 15 pounds (6.8 kg). The updated

TABLE 1.7

Updated recommendations for weight gain during pregnancy by prepregnancy body mass index (BMI), 2009

Prepregnancy BMI	BMI (kg/m²)	Total weight gain (lbs)	Rates of weight gain 2nd and 3rd trimester (lbs/week)
Underweight	<18.5	28–40	1 (1–1.3)
Normal weight	18.5–24.9	25–35	1 (0.8–1)
Overweight	25.0–29.9	15–25	0.6 (0.5–0.7)
Obese (includes all classes)	≥30.0	11–20	0.5 (0.4–0.6)

Notes: To calculate BMI go to www.nhlbisupport.com/bmi. Calculations assume a 0.5 = 2 kg (1.1–4.4 lbs) weight gain in the first trimester (based on Siega-Riz et al., 1994; Abrams et al., 1995; Carmichael et al., 1997)

SOURCE: Kathleen M. Rasmussen et al., "Table 1. New Recommendations for Total and Rate of Weight Gain during Pregnancy, by Prepregnancy BMI," in *Weight Gain during Pregnancy: Reexamining the Guidelines*, Institute of Medicine of the National Academies, May 28, 2009, http://www.iom.edu/~/media/Files/Report%20Files/2009/Weight-Gain-During-Pregnancy-Reexamining-the-Guidelines/Resource%20Page%20-%20Weight%20Gain%20During%20Pregnancy.ashx (accessed December 15, 2011). Copyright © 2009 by the National Academy of Sciences. All rights reserved.

guidelines are based on the findings that the offspring of overweight or obese women face increased risk for preterm birth or being larger than normal at delivery, with extra fat. Large babies may suffer stuck shoulders and broken collar bones during birth and are at greater risk of becoming overweight, obese, and diabetic in adulthood.

Birth Defects

In "Birth Defects" (February 24, 2011, http://www.cdc.gov/ncbddd/bd/default.htm), the CDC states that birth defects affect one out of 33 babies and that birth defects account for more than 20% of all infant deaths. A birth defect may be a structural defect, a deficiency of function, or a disease that an infant has at birth (congenital). Some common birth defects are genetic—inherited abnormalities such as Tay-Sachs disease (a fatal disease that generally affects children of east European Jewish ancestry) or chromosomal irregularities such as Down syndrome. Other birth defects result from environmental factors—infections during pregnancy, such as rubella (German measles), or drugs used by the pregnant woman. Even though the specific causes of some birth defects are unknown, scientists believe that many result from a combination of genetic and environmental factors.

NEURAL TUBE DEFECTS. Neural tube defects (NTDs) are abnormalities of the brain and spinal cord resulting from the failure of the neural tube to develop properly during early pregnancy. The neural tube is the embryonic nerve tissue that eventually develops into the brain and the spinal cord. The two most common NTDs are anencephaly and spina bifida.

ANENCEPHALY. According to the National Institutes of Health, in "Anencephaly" (February 7, 2012, http://www.nlm.nih.gov/medlineplus/ency/article/001580.htm), anencephaly (the absence of a major part of the brain, skull, and scalp) occurs in about one out of 10,000 births. The exact number is unknown because many of these pregnancies end in miscarriage. Infants with anencephaly either die before birth (in utero or stillborn) or shortly thereafter.

T. J. Mathews of the CDC notes in *Trends in Spina Bifida and Anencephalus in the United States, 1991–2006* (April 2009, http://www.cdc.gov/nchs/data/hestat/spine_anen/spine_anen.pdf) that the incidence of anencephaly decreased significantly between 1991 and 2001. In 1991, 18.4 infants per 100,000 live births were reported with the condition; this number dropped to 9.4 infants per 100,000 live births in 2001. However, between 2003 and 2006 the rate rose to around 11 infants per 100,000 live births, which was higher than the rate of 10 infants per 100,000 live births reported between 1998 and 2002.

SPINA BIFIDA. Spina bifida, which literally means "divided spine," is caused by the failure of the vertebrae (backbone) to completely cover the spinal cord early in fetal development, leaving the spinal cord exposed. Depending on the amount of nerve tissue exposed, spina bifida defects range from minor developmental disabilities to paralysis. The March of Dimes reports in "Spina Bifida" (2011, http://www.marchofdimes.com/professionals/14332_1224.asp) that spina bifida occurs in about 1,500 infants per year.

Mathews indicates that after an increase in the spina bifida rates between 1992 and 1995, there was a significant decline between 1995 and 1999. Between 1999 and 2002 the rates did not change much, but they were much lower than in 1997. (See Figure 1.2.) The rate of spina bifida decreased from 20.1 infants per 100,000 live births in 2002 to 18 infants per 100,000 live births in 2006. The 2006 rate was nearly identical to the rate for 2005, which was the lowest ever reported, at 17.9 infants per 100,000 live births.

PREVENTION. Scientists now know that daily consumption of 400 micrograms of the B vitamin folic acid by women before and during the first trimester of pregnancy greatly reduces the risk of spina bifida and other birth defects. Because half of all pregnancies in the United States are unplanned or incorrectly timed and because NTDs occur during the first month of pregnancy—before most women know they are pregnant—the U.S. Public Health Service began recommending in 1992 that all women of childbearing age consume 400 micrograms of folic acid daily. To comply with a mandate from the U.S. Food and Drug Administration, as of January 1998 all enriched cereal grain products must be fortified with folic acid. According to the March of Dimes, in "Perinatal Data Snapshots" (October 2011, https://www.marchofdimes.com/peristats/pdflib/999/pds_99_4.pdf), the occurrence of NTDs can be reduced by up to 70% if women consume the recommended amount of folic acid before conception and throughout the first month of pregnancy.

FIGURE 1.2

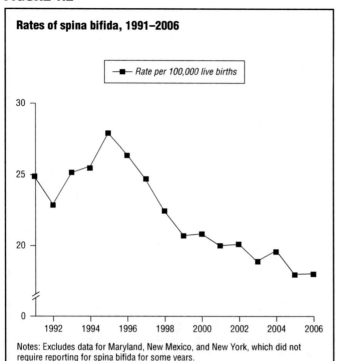

Rates of spina bifida, 1991–2006

— Rate per 100,000 live births

Notes: Excludes data for Maryland, New Mexico, and New York, which did not require reporting for spina bifida for some years.

SOURCE: T. J. Mathews, "Figure 1. Spina Bifida Rates, 1991–2006," in *Trends in Spina Bifida and Anencephalus in the United States, 1991–2006*, NCHS Health E-Stats, Centers for Disease Control and Prevention, National Center for Health Statistics, April 2009, http://www.cdc.gov/nchs/data/hestat/spine_anen/spine_anen.htm (accessed December 15, 2011)

In "Spina Bifida: Data and Statistics" (March 18, 2011, http://www.cdc.gov/ncbddd/spinabifida/data.html), the CDC notes that the prevalence of spina bifida decreased by 31%, from 5 per 10,000 births in 1995–96, the period preceding the fortification of grain products, to 3.5 per 10,000 births in 1998–2006, the period after the mandatory fortification of grain products. This decline is an indicator of the successful efforts to prevent birth defects by increasing folic acid consumption and folate levels among women of childbearing age. Figure 1.3 shows the declining prevalence of spina bifida after the mandatory fortification of cereal grains.

LEGISLATION TO PREVENT BIRTH DEFECTS. In April 1998 President Bill Clinton (1946–) signed into law the Birth Defects Prevention Act, which authorized a nationwide network of birth defects research and prevention programs and called for a nationwide information clearinghouse on birth defects.

In December 2003 the Birth Defects and Development Disabilities Prevention Act was passed into law. This bill revises and extends the Birth Defects Prevention Act to expand and adjust research and reporting requirements. According to the CDC, in "Fiscal Year 2012: Proposed Budget Consolidation" (August 8, 2011, http://www.cdc.gov/ncbddd/AboutUs/budget/FY2012.html), the budget for activities related to the Birth Defects and Developmental Disabilities Program included $143.9 million for fiscal year 2012.

INFANT MORTALITY

Since 1958 infant mortality has declined or remained unchanged, except for a slight increase in 2002. In 2008

FIGURE 1.3

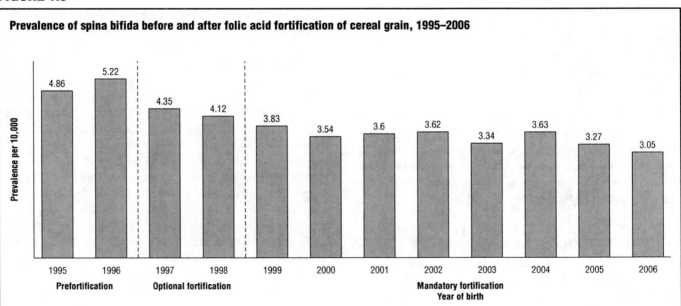

Prevalence of spina bifida before and after folic acid fortification of cereal grain, 1995–2006

SOURCE: "Prevalence of Spina Bifida," in *Spina Bifida Data and Statistics*, Centers for Disease Control and Prevention, National Center on Birth Defects and Developmental Disabilities, March 18, 2011, http://www.cdc.gov/ncbddd/spinabifida/data.html (accessed December 15, 2011)

FIGURE 1.4

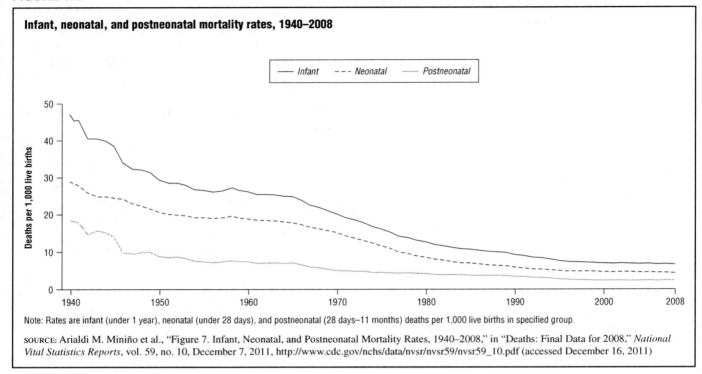

Infant, neonatal, and postneonatal mortality rates, 1940–2008

Note: Rates are infant (under 1 year), neonatal (under 28 days), and postneonatal (28 days–11 months) deaths per 1,000 live births in specified group.

SOURCE: Arialdi M. Miniño et al., "Figure 7. Infant, Neonatal, and Postneonatal Mortality Rates, 1940–2008," in "Deaths: Final Data for 2008," *National Vital Statistics Reports*, vol. 59, no. 10, December 7, 2011, http://www.cdc.gov/nchs/data/nvsr/nvsr59/nvsr59_10.pdf (accessed December 16, 2011)

there were 6.6 deaths per 1,000 live births, down 2.1% from 2007. (See Figure 1.4.)

Advances in neonatology (the medical subspecialty that is concerned with the care of newborns, especially those at risk) have contributed to the huge decline in infant death rates. Infants born prematurely or with LBWs, who were once likely to die, can survive life-threatening conditions due to the development of neonatal intensive care units. Improved access to health care has also contributed to the decline, as have public health initiatives such as education about how to prevent sudden infant death syndrome—specifically the Back to Sleep campaign, which teaches caregivers to place sleeping infants on their back.

Table 1.8 shows the U.S. infant mortality rate compared with those of other industrialized nations. In 2007 the United States had a higher infant mortality rate than 27 other countries and at least twice the rate of infant deaths as Austria, France, Greece, Japan, Norway, Portugal, South Korea (Republic of Korea), Spain, and Sweden.

LIFE EXPECTANCY

Along with infant mortality, life expectancy rates are an important measure of the health of the population. Life expectancy at birth is strongly influenced by infant and child mortality. Life expectancy in adulthood reflects death rates at or beyond specified ages and is independent of the effect of mortality at younger ages.

Kenneth D. Kochanek et al. of the CDC report in "Deaths: Preliminary Data for 2009" (*National Vital Statistics Reports*, vol. 59, no. 4, March 16, 2011) that overall (male and female) life expectancy increased from 78 years in 2008 to 78.2 years in 2009. Table 1.9 shows increasing life expectancy at every age.

Figure 1.5 shows the upward trend between 1980 and 2007 in U.S. life expectancy for males and females at birth. In *Health, United States, 2010*, the NCHS indicates that life expectancy increased throughout the latter part of the 20th century, from 70 years in 1980 to 75.4 years in 2007 for males and from 77.4 years in 1980 to 80.4 years in 2007 for females. Even though racial disparities in life expectancy at birth were still evident in 2007, the gap has narrowed since 1990. Similarly, life expectancy at age 65 also increased during the 20th century. Unlike life expectancy at birth, which rose early in the 20th century, much of the rise in life expectancy at age 65 occurred after 1950, in response to improved access to health care, advances in medicine, healthier current lifestyles, and better health throughout the life span. (See Table 1.10.) Nonetheless, the United States does not boast the longest life expectancy. Table 1.11 shows that in 2007 life expectancy at birth for both males and females was longer in Australia, Austria, Belgium, Denmark, Finland, France, Germany, Greece, Iceland, Ireland, Japan, Luxembourg, Netherlands, New Zealand, Norway, South Korea (Republic of Korea), Spain, Sweden, and Switzerland.

Specific segments of the U.S. population have even lower life expectancy. For example, African-American men continue to trail in terms of life expectancy. Several

TABLE 1.8

Infant mortality rates and international rankings by selected countries, selected years 1960–2007

Country[b]	1960	1970	1980	1990	2000	2005	2007	International rankings[a] 1960	International rankings[a] 2007
				Infant[c] deaths per 1,000 live births					
Australia	20.2	17.9	10.7	8.2	5.2	5.0	4.2	6	21
Austria	37.5	25.9	14.3	7.8	4.8	4.2	3.7	20	13
Belgium	31.4	21.1	12.1	8.0	4.8	3.7	3.9	18	15
Canada	27.3	18.8	10.4	6.8	5.3	5.4	5.1	13	24
Chile	120.3	79.3	33.0	16.0	8.9	7.9	8.3	28	29
Czech Republic	20.0	20.2	16.9	10.8	4.1	3.4	3.1	5	5
Denmark	21.5	14.2	8.4	7.5	5.3	4.4	4.0	9	19
Finland	21.0	13.2	7.6	5.6	3.8	3.0	2.7	7	4
France	27.7	18.2	10.0	7.3	4.5	3.8	3.8	14	14
Germany	35.0	22.5	12.4	7.0	4.4	3.9	3.9	19	15
Greece	40.1	29.6	17.9	9.7	5.9	3.8	3.5	21	9
Hungary	47.6	35.9	23.2	14.8	9.2	6.2	5.9	24	25
Iceland	13.0	13.2	7.7	5.9	3.0	2.3	2.0	1	1
Ireland	29.3	19.5	11.1	8.2	6.2	4.0	3.1	16	5
Israel	—	—	15.6	9.9	5.5	4.4	3.9	—	15
Italy	43.9	29.6	14.6	8.1	4.3	3.8	3.5	23	9
Japan	30.7	13.1	7.5	4.6	3.2	2.8	2.6	17	3
Mexico	92.3	80.9	52.6	39.2	19.4	16.8	15.7	27	30
Netherlands	16.5	12.7	8.6	7.1	5.1	4.9	4.1	3	20
New Zealand	22.6	16.7	13.0	8.4	6.3	5.0	4.8	11	22
Norway	16.0	11.3	8.1	6.9	3.8	3.1	3.1	2	5
Poland	54.8	36.7	25.5	19.3	8.1	6.4	6.0	25	26
Portugal	77.5	55.5	24.3	10.9	5.5	3.5	3.4	26	8
Republic of Korea	—	45.0	—	—	—	4.7	3.6	—	12
Slovak Republic	28.6	25.7	20.9	12.0	8.6	7.2	6.1	15	27
Spain	43.7	28.1	12.3	7.6	4.4	3.8	3.5	22	9
Sweden	16.6	11.0	6.9	6.0	3.4	2.4	2.5	4	2
Switzerland	21.1	15.1	9.1	6.8	4.9	4.2	3.9	8	15
Turkey	189.5	145.0	117.5	^51.5	31.6	18.4	15.9	29	31
United Kingdom	22.5	18.5	12.1	7.9	5.6	*5.1	4.8	10	22
United States	26.0	20.0	12.6	9.2	6.9	6.9	6.8	12	28

—Data not available.
*Data are estimated.
^Break in series.
[a]Rankings are from lowest to highest infant mortality rates (IMR). Countries with the same IMR receive the same rank. The country with the next highest IMR is assigned the rank it would have received had the lower-ranked countries not been tied, i.e., skip a rank.
[b]Refers to countries, territories, cities, or geographic areas with at least 2.5 million population and with complete counts of live births and infant deaths according to the United Nations Demographic Yearbook.
[c]Under 1 year of age.
Notes: Some rates for selected countries and selected years were revised and differ from previous editions of *Health, United States*. Data for additional years are available.

SOURCE: "Table 20. Infant Mortality Rates and International Rankings: Organisation for Economic Co-operation and Development (OECD) Countries, Selected Years 1960–2007," in *Health, United States, 2010: With Special Feature on Death and Dying*, Centers for Disease Control and Prevention, National Center for Health Statistics, 2011, http://www.cdc.gov/nchs/data/hus/hus10.pdf#listtables (accessed December 14, 2011). Data from The Organisation for Economic Co-operation and Development (OECD) Health Data 2009.

factors contribute to this group's significantly lower life expectancy. Besides issues of access to health care, some observers suggest that African-American men must deal with greater social, economic, and psychological stress than other men, leaving African-American men more susceptible to various diseases. Among African-American males in 2007, the NCHS indicates in *Health, United States 2010* that the observed number of deaths resulting from homicides, the human immunodeficiency virus (HIV; the virus that produces the acquired immunodeficiency syndrome), and cardiovascular disease was much higher than would be expected based on their proportion in the overall population.

Over time, the causes of death and threats to longevity have changed. As deaths from infectious diseases declined, mortality from chronic diseases, such as heart disease, cancer, and diabetes, increased. Table 1.12 displays the 10 leading causes of death in the United States in 1980 and 2007. Being overweight or obese is considered to be a contributing factor to at least four of the 10 leading causes of death in 2007: diseases of the heart, malignant neoplasms (cancer), cerebrovascular diseases (diseases affecting the supply of blood to the brain), and diabetes mellitus. Obesity may also be implicated in another leading cause of death: nephritis, nephrotic syndrome, and nephrosis (kidney disease or chronic renal failure). Table 1.12 also reveals the rise of diabetes as a cause of death. In 1980 it was the seventh-leading cause of death, claiming 34,851 lives. In 2007 it was still the seventh-leading cause of death; however, it claimed more lives: 71,382. Epidemiologists and medical researchers believe the increasing prevalence of diabetes in the U.S. population and the resultant rise in

TABLE 1.9

Expectation of life, by age, race and sex, 2008 and 2009

[Data are based on a continuous file of records from the states. Calculation of life expectancy employ populations estimated as of July 1 for 2009 and 2008.]

Age (years) and race	Both sexes 2009	Both sexes 2008[a]	Male 2009	Male 2008[a]	Female 2009	Female 2008[a]
All races[b]						
0	78.2	78.0	75.7	75.5	80.6	80.5
1	77.7	77.6	75.3	75.1	80.0	80.0
5	73.8	73.7	71.4	71.2	76.1	76.1
10	68.8	68.7	66.4	66.2	71.2	71.1
15	63.9	63.8	61.5	61.3	66.2	66.1
20	59.0	58.9	56.7	56.5	61.3	61.2
25	54.3	54.2	52.0	51.9	56.4	56.4
30	49.5	49.4	47.3	47.2	51.6	51.5
35	44.8	44.7	42.7	42.6	46.8	46.7
40	40.1	40.0	38.0	37.9	42.0	41.9
45	35.5	35.4	33.5	33.4	37.3	37.2
50	31.1	31.0	29.1	29.0	32.8	32.7
55	26.8	26.7	25.0	24.9	28.4	28.3
60	22.7	22.6	21.1	20.9	24.1	24.0
65	18.8	18.7	17.3	17.2	20.0	19.9
70	15.1	15.0	13.8	13.7	16.1	16.0
75	11.7	11.7	10.7	10.6	12.5	12.5
80	8.8	8.8	8.0	7.9	9.4	9.4
85	6.4	6.5	5.8	5.8	6.8	6.8
90	4.6	4.6	4.1	4.1	4.8	4.8
95	3.2	3.2	2.9	2.9	3.3	3.3
100	2.2	2.3	2.0	2.1	2.2	2.3
White						
0	78.6	78.4	76.2	75.9	80.9	80.8
1	78.0	77.8	75.6	75.4	80.3	80.2
5	74.1	73.9	71.7	71.5	76.3	76.3
10	69.1	68.9	66.8	66.5	71.4	71.3
15	64.1	64.0	61.8	61.6	66.4	66.3
20	59.3	59.2	57.0	56.8	61.5	61.4
25	54.5	54.4	52.3	52.2	56.6	56.6
30	49.8	49.6	47.6	47.5	51.8	51.7
35	45.0	44.9	43.0	42.8	47.0	46.9
40	40.3	40.2	38.3	38.1	42.2	42.1
45	35.7	35.6	33.8	33.6	37.5	37.4
50	31.2	31.1	29.4	29.2	32.9	32.8
55	26.9	26.8	25.2	25.0	28.5	28.3
60	22.8	22.6	21.2	21.0	24.1	24.0
65	18.8	18.7	17.4	17.3	20.0	19.9
70	15.1	15.0	13.9	13.7	16.1	16.0
75	11.7	11.6	10.6	10.6	12.5	12.4
80	8.8	8.8	7.9	7.9	9.3	9.3
85	6.4	6.4	5.7	5.7	6.7	6.8
90	4.5	4.5	4.1	4.1	4.7	4.8
95	3.1	3.2	2.8	2.9	3.2	3.3
100	2.2	2.2	2.0	2.0	2.2	2.2

[a]Life expectancies have been updated and may differ from those previously published.
[b]Includes races other than white and black.

Notes: "Race categories are consistent with 1977 Office of Management and Budget (OMB) standards. Multiple-race data were reported by 34 states and the District of Columbia in 2009 and 2008." Multiple-race data for these states were bridged to single-race categories of the 1977 OMB standards for comparability with other states. Data are subject to sampling or random variation.

SOURCE: Kenneth D. Kochanek et al., "Table 6. Expectation of Life, by Age, Race, and Sex: United States, Preliminary 2008 and 2009," in "Deaths: Preliminary Data for 2009," *National Vital Statistics Reports*, vol. 59, no. 4, March 16, 2011, http://www.cdc.gov/nchs/data/nvsr/nvsr59/nvsr59_04.pdf (accessed December 16, 2011)

deaths that are attributable to diabetes are direct consequences of the obesity epidemic in the United States.

Recent research suggests that the steady increase in life expectancy that the U.S. population has experienced over the past two centuries is likely to end in the coming years and that U.S. life expectancy may actually decline. In "Forecasting the Effects of Obesity and Smoking on U.S. Life Expectancy" (*New England Journal of Medicine*, vol. 361, no. 23, December 3, 2009), Susan T. Stewart, David M. Cutler, and Allison B. Rosen of the National Bureau of Economic Research in Cambridge, Massachusetts, use obesity prevalence data to predict that nearly half the U.S. population will be obese by 2020. When the researchers combine these data with past trends in smoking to project life expectancy, they find

FIGURE 1.5

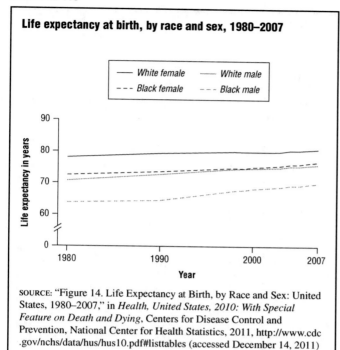

Life expectancy at birth, by race and sex, 1980–2007

SOURCE: "Figure 14. Life Expectancy at Birth, by Race and Sex: United States, 1980–2007," in *Health, United States, 2010: With Special Feature on Death and Dying,* Centers for Disease Control and Prevention, National Center for Health Statistics, 2011, http://www.cdc.gov/nchs/data/hus/hus10.pdf#listtables (accessed December 14, 2011)

that the negative effects of obesity, as measured by BMI, far outweigh the positive effects of declines in smoking in terms of life expectancy. Stewart, Cutler, and Rosen conclude that "if past obesity trends continue unchecked, the negative effects on the health of the U.S. population will increasingly outweigh the positive effects gained from declining smoking rates. Failure to address continued increases in obesity could result in an erosion of the pattern of steady gains in health observed since early in the 20th century."

MORTALITY

Years of Potential Life Lost

Years of potential life lost (YPLL) is a term used by medical and public health professionals to describe the number of years deceased people might have lived if they had not died prematurely (before their life expectancy). In 2007 most YPLL resulted from heart disease, malignant neoplasms, and unintentional injuries (accidents). (See Table 1.13.)

The increase in life expectancy during the 20th and 21st centuries has meant a decrease in the YPLL rate. In 1980 a total of 10,448.4 years per 100,000 population were lost to people younger than the age of 75 years; by 2007 this number had declined to 7,083.5 total years lost. (See Table 1.13.) Even though heart disease remains the number-one killer in the United States (see Table 1.12), it has been responsible for a smaller proportion of YPLL since 1980 (2,238.7 in 1980 and 1,042.4 in 2007). Similarly, the years lost to cerebrovascular diseases (e.g., strokes), liver diseases, influenza and pneumonia, and motor vehicle accidents have also declined since 1980. Similarly, the

years lost to HIV infection steadily decreased between 1996 and 2007. However, YPLL rates for diabetes increased over this same period, dropping slightly between 2005 and 2007, and chronic lower respiratory diseases remained roughly the same between 2006 and 2007.

Except for suicide, the YPLL due to all causes for African-Americans was significantly higher than for whites. In 2007, for all causes, African-Americans lost 11,259.8 years per 100,000 population, compared with 6,614.2 years for whites. (See Table 1.13.) African-Americans lost considerably more years of life to heart disease, cerebrovascular diseases, cancers, HIV, and homicide than did whites.

RACIAL AND GENDER DIFFERENCES. In *Health, United States, 2010,* the NCHS notes that significant racial and ethnic variations exist in the 10 leading causes of death. In 2007 chronic liver disease and cirrhosis were not listed as leading causes of death for all Americans; they were, however, listed as leading causes of death among Native Americans or Alaskan Natives and Hispanics. Homicide was a leading cause of death for African-American and Hispanic men; however, it was not among the top 10 causes of death for Native American or Alaskan Native men and Asian or Pacific Islander men. In 2007 homicide did not rank as a leading cause of death for women of any race or ethnicity.

AGE DIFFERENCES. The NCHS indicates in *Health, United States, 2010* that, as would be expected, death rates were highest for people aged 85 years and older (12,946.5 per 100,000 population) in 2007. From age 25 on, death rates doubled with each additional decade.

The 10 leading causes of death vary by age. In 2007 accidents (unintentional injuries) were the leading cause of death for children one to four years of age, followed by congenital malformations, homicide, and malignant neoplasms. (See Table 1.14.) Among children five to 14 years old, accidents were a leading cause of death, followed by cancer, congenital malformations, and homicide.

Accidents were the leading cause of death in 2007 for young people aged 15 to 24 years. (See Table 1.14.) Homicide was the second-leading cause of death, followed by suicide. Cancer was the fourth-leading cause of death among this age group.

Among adults aged 25 to 44 years in 2007, accidents were the most frequent cause of death, and cancer was second. (See Table 1.14.) Heart disease and suicide were the third- and fourth-leading causes of death, respectively, followed by homicide and HIV disease.

Among adults 45 to 64 years old, cancer and heart disease were ranked the first- and second-leading causes of death, respectively. (See Table 1.14.) Among those aged 65 years and older, these two categories were reversed.

SELF-ASSESSED HEALTH STATUS

The NCHS regularly asks respondents to the National Health Interview Survey to evaluate their health status.

TABLE 1.10

Life expectancy at birth and at age 65, by race and sex, selected years 1900–2007

[Data are based on death certificates]

Specified age and year	All races Both sexes	Male	Female	White Both sexes	Male	Female	Black or African American[a] Both sexes	Male	Female
				Remaining life expectancy in years					
At birth									
1900[b, c]	47.3	46.3	48.3	47.6	46.6	48.7	33.0	32.5	33.5
1950[c]	68.2	65.6	71.1	69.1	66.5	72.2	60.8	59.1	62.9
1960[c]	69.7	66.6	73.1	70.6	67.4	74.1	63.6	61.1	66.3
1970	70.8	67.1	74.7	71.7	68.0	75.6	64.1	60.0	68.3
1980	73.7	70.0	77.4	74.4	70.7	78.1	68.1	63.8	72.5
1990	75.4	71.8	78.8	76.1	72.7	79.4	69.1	64.5	73.6
1995	75.8	72.5	78.9	76.5	73.4	79.6	69.6	65.2	73.9
1999	76.7	73.9	79.4	77.3	74.6	79.9	71.4	67.8	74.7
2000	76.8	74.1	79.3	77.3	74.7	79.9	71.8	68.2	75.1
2001	76.9	74.2	79.4	77.4	74.8	79.9	72.0	68.4	75.2
2002	76.9	74.3	79.5	77.4	74.9	79.9	72.1	68.6	75.4
2003	77.1	74.5	79.6	77.6	75.0	80.0	72.3	68.8	75.6
2004	77.5	74.9	79.9	77.9	75.4	80.4	72.8	69.3	76.0
2005	77.4	74.9	79.9	77.9	75.4	80.4	72.8	69.3	76.1
2006	77.7	75.1	80.2	78.2	75.7	80.6	73.2	69.7	76.5
2007	77.9	75.4	80.4	78.4	75.9	80.8	73.6	70.0	76.8
At 65 years									
1950[c]	13.9	12.8	15.0	—	12.8	15.1	13.9	12.9	14.9
1960[c]	14.3	12.8	15.8	14.4	12.9	15.9	13.9	12.7	15.1
1970	15.2	13.1	17.0	15.2	13.1	17.1	14.2	12.5	15.7
1980	16.4	14.1	18.3	16.5	14.2	18.4	15.1	13.0	16.8
1990	17.2	15.1	18.9	17.3	15.2	19.1	15.4	13.2	17.2
1995	17.4	15.6	18.9	17.6	15.7	19.1	15.6	13.6	17.1
1999	17.7	16.1	19.1	17.8	16.1	19.2	16.0	14.3	17.3
2000	17.6	16.0	19.0	17.7	16.1	19.1	16.1	14.1	17.5
2001	17.7	16.2	19.0	17.8	16.3	19.1	16.2	14.2	17.6
2002	17.8	16.2	19.1	17.9	16.3	19.2	16.3	14.4	17.7
2003	17.9	16.4	19.2	18.0	16.5	19.3	16.4	14.5	17.9
2004	18.2	16.7	19.5	18.3	16.8	19.5	16.7	14.8	18.2
2005	18.2	16.8	19.5	18.3	16.9	19.5	16.8	14.9	18.2
2006	18.5	17.0	19.7	18.6	17.1	19.8	17.1	15.1	18.6
2007	18.6	17.2	19.9	18.7	17.3	19.9	17.2	15.2	18.7
At 75 years									
1980	10.4	8.8	11.5	10.4	8.8	11.5	9.7	8.3	10.7
1990	10.9	9.4	12.0	11.0	9.4	12.0	10.2	8.6	11.2
1995	11.0	9.7	11.9	11.1	9.7	12.0	10.2	8.8	11.1
1999	11.2	10.0	12.1	11.2	10.0	12.1	10.4	9.2	11.1
2000	11.0	9.8	11.8	11.0	9.8	11.9	10.4	9.0	11.3
2001	11.1	9.9	11.9	11.1	9.9	11.9	10.5	9.1	11.4
2002	11.0	9.9	11.9	11.1	9.9	11.9	10.5	9.2	11.4
2003	11.1	10.0	11.9	11.1	10.0	11.9	10.6	9.3	11.5
2004	11.4	10.3	12.2	11.4	10.3	12.2	10.8	9.5	11.7
2005	11.3	10.2	12.1	11.4	10.3	12.1	10.8	9.5	11.7
2006	11.6	10.5	12.3	11.5	10.5	12.3	11.1	9.8	12.0
2007	11.7	10.6	12.5	11.7	10.6	12.4	11.2	9.9	12.1

—Data not available.

[a]Data shown for 1900–1960 are for the nonwhite population.

[b]Death registration area only. The death registration area increased from 10 states and the District of Columbia (D.C.) in 1900 to the coterminous United States in 1933.

[c]Includes deaths of persons who were not residents of the 50 states and D.C.

Notes: Populations for computing life expectancy for 1991–1999 are 1990-based postcensal estimates of U.S. resident population. In 1997, life table methodology was revised to construct complete life tables by single years of age that extend to age 100 (Anderson RN. Method for constructing complete annual U.S. life tables. NCHS. Vital Health Stat 2(129). 1999). Previously, abridged life tables were constructed for 5-year age groups ending with 85 years and over. Life table values for 2000 and later years were computed using a slight modification of the new life table method due to a change in the age detail of populations received from the U.S. Census Bureau. Values for data years 2000–2007 are based on a newly revised methodology that uses vital statistics death rates for ages under 66 and modeled probabilities of death for ages 66 to 100 based on blended vital statistics and Medicare probabilities of dying and may differ from figures previously published. The revised methodology is similar to that developed for the 1999–2001 decennial life tables. Starting with 2003 data, some states allowed the reporting of more than one race on the death certificate. The multiple-race data for these states were bridged to the single-race categories of the 1977 Office of Management and Budget Standards for comparability with other states. Some data have been revised and differ from previous editions of Health, United States. Data for additional years are available.

SOURCE: "Table 22. Life Expectancy at Birth and at 65 Years of Age, and at 75 Years of Age, by Race and Sex: United States, 1970–2007," in *Health, United States, 2010*, Centers for Disease Control and Prevention, National Center for Health Statistics, 2011, http://www.cdc.gov/nchs/data/hus/hus10.pdf#listtables (accessed December 14, 2011)

Figure 1.6 shows that between 1997 and June 2011 the percentage of people who considered their health to be excellent or very good was relatively unchanged, ranging from a high of 69.1% in 1998 but hovering around 66% for most years. Between January and June 2011, 65.1% of respondents assessed their health as excellent or very good.

TABLE 1.11

Life expectancy at birth and at 65 years of age, by sex: selected countries, selected years 1980–2007

	Male						Female					
Country	1980	1990	1995	2000	2004	2007	1980	1990	1995	2000	2004	2007
At birth						Life expectancy in years						
Australia	71.0	73.9	75.0	76.6	78.1	79.0	78.1	80.1	80.8	82.0	83.0	83.7
Austria	69.0	72.2	73.3	75.1	76.4	77.3	76.1	78.8	79.9	81.1	82.1	82.9
Belgium	69.9	72.7	73.5	74.6	76.0	77.1	76.7	79.5	80.4	81.0	81.8	82.6
Canada	71.7	74.4	75.1	76.7	77.8	—	78.9	80.8	81.1	81.9	82.6	—
Czech Republic[a]	66.9	67.6	69.7	71.7	72.6	73.8	74.0	75.5	76.8	78.5	79.2	80.2
Denmark	71.2	72.0	72.7	74.5	75.4	76.2	77.3	77.8	77.9	79.2	80.2	80.6
Finland	69.3	71.0	72.9	74.2	75.4	76.0	78.0	79.0	80.4	81.2	82.5	83.1
France	70.2	72.8	73.8	75.3	76.7	77.5	78.4	80.9	81.9	82.8	83.8	84.4
Germany[b]	69.6	72.0	73.3	75.1	76.5	77.4	76.2	78.5	79.9	81.2	81.9	82.7
Greece	72.2	74.6	75.0	75.5	76.6	77.0	76.8	79.5	80.3	80.5	81.5	82.0
Hungary	65.5	65.1	65.3	67.4	68.6	69.2	72.7	73.7	74.5	75.9	76.9	77.3
Iceland	73.7	75.4	75.9	78.4	79.2	79.4	79.7	80.5	80.0	81.8	82.7	82.9
Ireland	70.1	72.1	72.8	74.0	76.5	77.4	75.6	77.7	78.3	79.2	81.4	82.1
Italy	70.6	73.8	75.0	76.9	77.9	—	77.4	80.3	81.5	82.8	83.8	—
Japan	73.4	75.9	76.4	77.7	78.6	79.2	78.8	81.9	82.9	84.6	85.6	86.0
Luxembourg	70.0	72.4	73.0	74.6	76.0	76.7	75.6	78.7	80.6	81.3	82.4	82.2
Mexico	64.1	67.7	69.7	71.3	72.1	72.6	70.2	73.5	75.2	76.5	77.0	77.4
Netherlands	72.5	73.8	74.6	75.5	76.9	78.0	79.2	80.1	80.4	80.5	81.4	82.3
New Zealand	70.1	72.5	74.1	75.9	77.3	78.2	76.2	78.4	79.5	80.8	81.8	82.2
Norway	72.4	73.5	74.8	76.0	77.6	78.3	79.3	79.9	80.9	81.5	82.6	82.9
Poland	66.0	66.2	67.6	69.7	70.7	71.0	74.4	75.2	76.4	78.0	79.2	79.7
Portugal	67.9	70.6	71.7	73.2	75.0	75.9	74.9	77.5	79.0	80.2	81.5	82.2
Republic of Korea	61.8	67.3	69.6	72.3	74.5	76.1	70.0	75.5	77.4	79.6	81.4	82.7
Slovak Republic[a]	66.8	66.6	68.4	69.1	70.3	70.5	74.3	75.4	76.3	77.4	77.8	78.1
Spain	72.3	73.4	74.4	75.8	76.9	77.8	78.5	80.6	81.8	82.9	83.7	84.3
Sweden	72.8	74.8	76.2	77.4	78.4	78.9	78.8	80.4	81.4	82.0	82.7	83.0
Switzerland	72.3	74.0	75.4	77.0	78.6	79.5	79.0	80.9	81.9	82.8	83.8	84.4
Turkey	55.8	65.4	67.2	69.0	70.5	71.1	60.3	69.5	71.3	73.1	74.6	75.6
United Kingdom	70.2	72.9	74.0	75.5	76.8	—	76.2	78.5	79.3	80.3	81.0	—
United States	70.0	71.8	72.5	74.1	74.9	75.4	77.4	78.8	78.9	79.3	79.9	80.4
At 65 years												
Australia	13.7	15.2	15.7	16.9	17.8	18.5	17.9	19.0	19.5	20.4	21.1	21.6
Austria	12.9	14.3	14.9	16.0	16.9	17.4	16.3	17.8	18.6	19.4	20.3	20.8
Belgium	12.9	14.3	14.8	15.6	16.4	17.3	16.8	18.8	19.3	19.8	20.2	21.0
Canada	14.5	15.7	16.0	16.8	17.7	—	18.9	19.9	20.0	20.4	21.0	—
Czech Republic[a]	11.2	11.7	12.7	13.8	14.2	15.1	14.4	15.3	16.2	17.3	17.6	18.5
Denmark	13.6	14.0	14.1	15.2	15.9	16.5	17.6	17.9	17.6	18.3	19.0	19.2
Finland	12.6	13.8	14.6	15.5	16.5	17.0	17.0	17.8	18.8	19.5	20.7	21.3
France	13.6	15.5	16.1	16.7	17.7	—	18.2	19.8	20.6	21.2	22.1	—
Germany[b]	12.8	14.0	14.8	15.8	16.7	17.4	16.3	17.7	18.7	19.6	20.1	20.7
Greece	14.6	15.7	16.1	16.2	17.0	17.4	16.8	18.0	18.4	18.3	19.2	19.6
Hungary	11.6	12.0	12.1	12.7	13.1	13.4	14.6	15.3	15.8	16.5	16.9	17.3
Iceland	15.8	16.2	16.2	18.1	17.9	18.3	19.1	19.5	19.0	19.7	20.5	20.6
Ireland	12.6	13.3	13.5	14.6	16.2	17.1	15.7	17.0	17.2	18.0	19.7	20.1
Italy	13.3	15.1	15.9	16.7	17.5	—	17.1	19.0	19.9	20.7	21.6	—
Japan	14.6	16.2	16.5	17.5	18.2	18.6	17.7	20.0	20.9	22.4	23.3	23.6
Luxembourg	12.6	14.3	14.8	15.5	16.5	16.4	16.5	18.5	19.7	20.1	20.5	20.3
Mexico	15.4	16.0	16.1	16.5	16.7	16.8	17.0	17.8	17.8	18.1	18.2	18.3
Netherlands	13.7	14.4	14.7	15.3	16.3	17.0	18.0	18.9	19.0	19.2	19.8	20.5
New Zealand	13.2	14.6	15.4	16.5	17.5	18.1	17.0	18.3	19.0	19.8	20.4	20.7
Norway	14.3	14.6	15.1	16.1	17.1	17.5	18.2	18.7	19.3	19.9	20.7	20.8
Poland	12.0	12.4	12.9	13.6	14.2	14.6	15.5	16.1	16.6	17.5	18.4	18.9
Portugal	13.1	14.0	14.7	15.4	16.3	16.8	16.1	17.1	18.1	18.9	19.7	20.2
Republic of Korea	10.5	12.4	13.3	14.3	15.5	16.3	15.1	16.3	17.0	18.2	19.4	20.5
Slovak Republic[a]	12.3	12.2	12.7	12.9	13.3	13.4	15.4	15.7	16.1	16.5	16.9	17.1
Spain	14.6	15.5	16.2	16.7	17.3	17.8	17.8	19.3	20.2	20.8	21.5	22.0
Sweden	14.3	15.3	16.0	16.7	17.4	17.8	17.9	19.0	19.6	20.0	20.6	20.7
Switzerland	14.3	15.3	16.2	17.0	18.2	18.6	18.2	19.7	20.4	20.9	21.6	22.2
Turkey	11.7	12.8	13.1	13.4	13.8	13.9	12.8	14.3	14.7	15.1	15.5	15.8

Overall, men were slightly more likely to rate their health as excellent. (See Figure 1.7.) However, for both men and women the percentage who considered their health as excellent or very good decreased with advancing age—82.4% for those younger than age 18, 63.2% for those aged 18 to 64 years, and 41.5% for those aged 65 years and older. (See Figure 1.8.) Compared with the 69.4% of non-Hispanic white survey respondents who assessed their health as excellent or very good, fewer non-Hispanic African-American (56.4%) and Hispanic (56.5%) survey respondents rated their health status as excellent or very good. (See Figure 1.9.)

TABLE 1.11

Life expectancy at birth and at 65 years of age, by sex: selected countries, selected years 1980–2007 [CONTINUED]

Country	Male						Female					
	1980	1990	1995	2000	2004	2007	1980	1990	1995	2000	2004	2007
United Kingdom	12.6	14.0	14.6	15.8	16.8	—	16.6	17.9	18.2	19.0	19.4	—
United States	14.1	15.1	15.6	16.0	16.7	17.2	18.3	18.9	18.9	19.0	19.5	19.9

—Data not available.

[a]In 1993, Czechoslovakia was divided into two nations, the Czech Republic and Slovakia. Data for years prior to 1993 are from the Czech and Slovak regions of Czechoslovakia.
[b]Until 1990, estimates refer to the Federal Republic of Germany; from 1995 onwards, data refer to Germany after reunification.
Notes: Since calculation of life expectancy (LE) estimates varies among countries, ranks are not presented; comparisons among countries and their interpretation should be made with caution. Some estimates for selected countries and selected years were revised and differ from the previous editions of *Health, United States.* Data for additional years are available.

SOURCE: Adapted from "Table 21. Life Expectancy at Birth and at 65 Years of Age, by Sex: Organisation for Economic Co-operation and Development (OECD) Countries, Selected Years 1980–2007," in *Health, United States, 2010: With Special Feature on Death and Dying*, Centers for Disease Control and Prevention, National Center for Health Statistics, 2011, http://www.cdc.gov/nchs/data/hus/hus10.pdf#listtables (accessed December 14, 2011). Non-government data from Organisation for Economic Co-operation and Development (OECD) Health Data 2009.

TABLE 1.12

Leading causes of death and numbers of deaths, by sex, race, and Hispanic origin, 1980 and 2007

[Data are based on death certificates]

Sex, race, Hispanic origin, and rank order	1980 Cause of death	Deaths	2007 Cause of death	Deaths
All persons				
Rank	All causes	1,989,841	All causes	2,423,712
1	Diseases of heart	761,085	Diseases of heart	616,067
2	Malignant neoplasms	416,509	Malignant neoplasms	562,875
3	Cerebrovascular diseases	170,225	Cerebrovascular diseases	135,952
4	Unintentional injuries	105,718	Chronic lower respiratory diseases	127,924
5	Chronic obstructive pulmonary diseases	56,050	Unintentional injuries	123,706
6	Pneumonia and influenza	54,619	Alzheimer's disease	74,632
7	Diabetes mellitus	34,851	Diabetes mellitus	71,382
8	Chronic liver disease and cirrhosis	30,583	Influenza and pneumonia	52,717
9	Atherosclerosis	29,449	Nephritis, nephrotic syndrome and nephrosis	46,448
10	Suicide	26,869	Septicemia	34,828
Male				
Rank	All causes	1,075,078	All causes	1,203,968
1	Diseases of heart	405,661	Diseases of heart	309,821
2	Malignant neoplasms	225,948	Malignant neoplasms	292,857
3	Unintentional injuries	74,180	Unintentional injuries	79,827
4	Cerebrovascular diseases	69,973	Chronic lower respiratory diseases	61,235
5	Chronic obstructive pulmonary diseases	38,625	Cerebrovascular diseases	54,111
6	Pneumonia and influenza	27,574	Diabetes mellitus	35,478
7	Suicide	20,505	Suicide	27,269
8	Chronic liver disease and cirrhosis	19,768	Influenza and pneumonia	24,071
9	Homicide	18,779	Nephritis, nephrotic syndrome and nephrosis	22,616
10	Diabetes mellitus	14,325	Alzheimer's disease	21,800
Female				
Rank	All causes	914,763	All causes	1,219,744
1	Diseases of heart	355,424	Diseases of heart	306,246
2	Malignant neoplasms	190,561	Malignant neoplasms	270,018
3	Cerebrovascular diseases	100,252	Cerebrovascular diseases	81,841
4	Unintentional injuries	31,538	Chronic lower respiratory diseases	66,689
5	Pneumonia and influenza	27,045	Alzheimer's disease	52,832
6	Diabetes mellitus	20,526	Unintentional injuries	43,879
7	Atherosclerosis	17,848	Diabetes mellitus	35,904
8	Chronic obstructive pulmonary diseases	17,425	Influenza and pneumonia	28,646
9	Chronic liver disease and cirrhosis	10,815	Nephritis, nephrotic syndrome and nephrosis	. 23,832
10	Certain conditions originating in the perinatal period	9,815	Septicemia	18,989
White				
Rank	All causes	1,738,607	All causes	2,074,151
1	Diseases of heart	683,347	Diseases of heart	531,636
2	Malignant neoplasms	368,162	Malignant neoplasms	483,939
3	Cerebrovascular diseases	148,734	Chronic lower respiratory diseases	118,081
4	Unintentional injuries	90,122	Cerebrovascular diseases	114,695
5	Chronic obstructive pulmonary diseases	52,375	Unintentional injuries	106,252
6	Pneumonia and influenza	48,369	Alzheimer's disease	68,933
7	Diabetes mellitus	28,868	Diabetes mellitus	56,390
8	Atherosclerosis	27,069	Influenza and pneumonia	45,947
9	Chronic liver disease and cirrhosis	25,240	Nephritis, nephrotic syndrome and nephrosis	36,871
10	Suicide	24,829	Suicide	31,348

TABLE 1.12

Leading causes of death and numbers of deaths, by sex, race, and Hispanic origin, 1980 and 2007 [CONTINUED]

[Data are based on death certificates]

Sex, race, Hispanic origin, and rank order	1980		2007	
	Cause of death	Deaths	Cause of death	Deaths
Black or African American				
	All causes	233,135	All causes	289,585
Rank	Diseases of heart	72,956	Diseases of heart	71,209
1	Malignant neoplasms	45,037	Malignant neoplasms	64,049
2	Cerebrovascular diseases	20,135	Cerebrovascular diseases	17,085
3	Unintentional injuries	13,480	Unintentional injuries	13,559
4	Homicide	10,172	Diabetes mellitus	12,459
5	Certain conditions originating in the perinatal period	6,961	Homicide	8,870
6	Pneumonia and influenza	5,648	Nephritis, nephrotic syndrome and nephrosis	8,392
7	Diabetes mellitus	5,544	Chronic lower respiratory diseases	7,901
8	Chronic liver disease and cirrhosis	4,790	Human immunodeficiency virus (HIV) disease	6,470
9	Nephritis, nephrotic syndrome, and nephrosis	3,416	Septicemia	6,297
10				

—Data not available.
Notes: Starting in 2006, the category essential (primary) hypertension and hypertensive renal disease was changed to essential hypertension and hypertensive renal disease to reflect the addition of secondary hypertension. Starting with 2003 data, some states allowed the reporting of more than one race on the death certificate. The multiple-race data for these states were bridged to the single-race categories of the 1977 Office of Management and Budget standards for comparability with other states. The race groups, white, black, Asian or Pacific Islander, and American Indian or Alaska Native, include persons of Hispanic and non-Hispanic origin. Persons of Hispanic origin may be of any race.

SOURCE: Adapted from "Table 26. Leading Causes of Death and Numbers of Deaths, by Sex, Race, and Hispanic Origin: United States, 1980 and 2007," in *Health, United States, 2010: With Special Feature on Death and Dying*, Centers for Disease Control and Prevention, National Center for Health Statistics, 2011, http://www.cdc.gov/nchs/data/hus/hus10.pdf#listtables (accessed December 14, 2011).

TABLE 1.13

Years of potential life lost before age 75 for selected causes of death, by sex and race, selected years 1980–2007

[Data are based on death certificates]

Sex, race, Hispanic origin, and cause of death[b]	Crude 2007[c]	Age-adjusted[a]					
		1980	1990	2000[c]	2005[c]	2006[c]	2007[c]
All persons		Years lost before age 75 per 100,000 population under 75 years of age					
All causes	7,366.2	10,448.4	9,085.5	7,578.1	7,299.8	7,214.3	7,083.5
Diseases of heart	1,112.6	2,238.7	1,617.7	1,253.0	1,110.4	1,077.8	1,042.4
Ischemic heart disease	694.0	1,729.3	1,153.6	841.8	701.8	675.5	642.1
Cerebrovascular diseases	195.4	357.5	259.6	223.3	193.3	190.2	184.5
Malignant neoplasms	1,574.0	2,108.8	2,003.8	1,674.1	1,525.2	1,490.5	1,461.4
Trachea, bronchus, and lung	402.9	548.5	561.4	443.1	392.9	378.7	366.8
Colorectal	136.8	190.0	164.7	141.9	124.7	126.1	126.7
Prostate[d]	55.4	84.9	96.8	63.6	55.1	54.8	53.5
Breast[e]	300.0	463.2	451.6	332.6	296.2	286.7	275.4
Chronic lower respiratory diseases	185.5	169.1	187.4	188.1	181.2	171.0	172.1
Influenza and pneumonia	74.5	160.2	141.5	87.1	83.6	76.4	71.6
Chronic liver disease and cirrhosis	167.0	300.3	196.9	164.1	152.6	149.9	157.6
Diabetes mellitus	181.9	134.4	155.9	178.4	179.9	176.5	170.1
Human immunodeficiency virus (HIV) disease	113.7	—	383.8	174.6	133.6	126.0	115.2
Unintentional injuries	1,155.5	1,543.5	1,162.1	1,026.5	1,132.7	1,167.5	1,159.5
Motor vehicle-related injuries	536.4	912.9	716.4	574.3	564.4	561.2	538.4
Poisoning	351.2	68.0	81.2	163.6	287.3	332.5	354.3
Suicide[f]	357.2	392.0	393.1	334.5	347.3	348.7	357.5
Homicide[f]	276.0	425.5	417.4	266.5	276.8	281.8	278.3
Male							
All causes	9,171.1	13,777.2	11,973.5	9,572.2	9,206.1	9,092.6	8,919.9
Diseases of heart	1,528.7	3,352.1	2,356.0	1,766.0	1,561.6	1,517.5	1,468.2
Ischemic heart disease	1,008.8	2,715.1	1,766.3	1,255.4	1,044.3	1,009.2	962.1
Cerebrovascular diseases	213.1	396.7	286.6	244.6	213.7	212.0	206.2
Malignant neoplasms	1,642.2	2,360.8	2,214.6	1,810.8	1,639.7	1,595.2	1,565.1
Trachea, bronchus, and lung	459.1	821.1	764.8	554.9	476.3	454.5	434.0
Colorectal	155.7	214.9	194.3	167.3	146.2	145.4	148.5
Prostate	55.4	84.9	96.8	63.6	55.1	54.8	53.5
Chronic lower respiratory diseases	194.0	235.1	224.8	206.0	195.8	182.4	187.5
Influenza and pneumonia	85.6	202.5	180.0	102.8	97.8	88.9	83.5
Chronic liver disease and cirrhosis	231.9	415.0	283.9	236.9	216.1	210.9	222.4
Diabetes mellitus	215.3	140.4	170.4	203.8	216.5	213.2	207.1
Human immunodeficiency virus (HIV) disease	158.5	—	686.2	258.9	192.0	178.3	161.0
Unintentional injuries	1,648.6	2,342.7	1,715.1	1,475.6	1,608.5	1,659.2	1,639.2
Motor vehicle-related injuries	774.0	1,359.7	1,018.4	796.4	795.9	790.9	766.5
Poisoning	479.2	96.4	123.6	242.1	395.6	461.6	480.7
Suicide[f]	564.1	605.6	634.8	539.1	548.0	549.0	561.5
Homicide[f]	444.2	675.0	658.0	410.5	439.0	447.1	439.4
Female							
All causes	5,560.6	7,350.3	6,333.1	5,644.6	5,425.7	5,364.7	5,274.2
Diseases of heart	696.4	1,246.0	948.5	774.6	682.6	660.6	637.9
Ischemic heart disease	379.2	852.1	600.3	457.6	379.0	360.6	339.7
Cerebrovascular diseases	177.7	324.0	235.9	203.9	174.4	169.8	164.3
Malignant neoplasms	1,505.7	1,896.8	1,826.6	1,555.3	1,424.3	1,398.6	1,370.3
Trachea, bronchus, and lung	346.8	310.4	382.2	342.1	316.9	309.7	305.6
Colorectal	117.9	168.7	138.7	118.7	104.9	108.4	106.6
Breast	300.0	463.2	451.6	332.6	296.2	286.7	275.4
Chronic lower respiratory diseases	177.0	114.0	155.9	172.3	168.2	160.5	158.0
Influenza and pneumonia	63.4	122.0	106.2	72.3	70.0	64.7	60.3
Chronic liver disease and cirrhosis	102.1	194.5	115.1	94.5	91.6	91.3	95.3
Diabetes mellitus	148.4	128.5	142.3	154.4	145.1	141.7	135.0
Human immunodeficiency virus (HIV) disease	68.8	—	87.8	92.0	76.2	74.5	70.1
Unintentional injuries	662.1	755.3	607.4	573.2	648.0	666.1	670.2
Motor vehicle-related injuries	298.8	470.4	411.6	348.5	327.1	325.4	304.5
Poisoning	223.1	40.2	39.1	85.0	177.2	201.0	225.3
Suicide[f]	150.4	184.2	153.3	129.1	144.1	145.7	150.8
Homicide[f]	107.7	181.3	174.3	118.9	108.7	110.4	111.2

TABLE 1.13

Years of potential life lost before age 75 for selected causes of death, by sex and race, selected years 1980–2007 [CONTINUED]

[Data are based on death certificates]

Sex, race, Hispanic origin, and cause of death[b]	Crude 2007[c]	Age-adjusted[a]					
		1980	1990	2000 [c]	2005[c]	2006[c]	2007[c]
		Years lost before age 75 per 100,000 population under 75 years of age					
White[g]							
All causes	6,985.7	9,554.1	8,159.5	6,949.5	6,775.6	6,713.1	6,614.2
Diseases of heart	1,052.9	2,100.8	1,490.3	1,149.4	1,011.7	985.9	952.2
Ischemic heart disease	693.0	1,682.7	1,113.4	805.3	672.0	648.2	617.1
Cerebrovascular diseases	168.4	300.7	213.1	187.1	160.4	158.1	154.0
Malignant neoplasms	1,593.8	2,035.9	1,929.3	1,627.8	1,485.9	1,456.6	1,428.3
Trachea, bronchus, and lung	419.1	529.9	544.2	436.3	389.4	374.8	364.8
Colorectal	133.9	186.8	157.8	134.1	117.3	118.9	119.6
Prostate[d]	50.6	74.8	86.6	54.3	47.0	47.3	46.2
Breast[e]	289.1	460.2	441.7	315.6	275.1	269.0	256.9
Chronic lower respiratory diseases	197.2	165.4	182.3	185.3	182.2	172.0	174.0
Influenza and pneumonia	69.2	130.8	116.9	77.7	76.3	70.4	65.2
Chronic liver disease and cirrhosis	177.9	257.3	175.8	162.7	156.7	155.3	163.6
Diabetes mellitus	163.7	115.7	133.7	155.6	156.3	152.8	147.7
Human immunodeficiency virus (HIV) disease	57.5	—	309.0	94.7	69.8	64.6	58.1
Unintentional injuries	1,193.3	1,520.4	1,139.7	1,031.8	1,170.9	1,209.8	1,208.5
Motor vehicle-related injuries	548.5	939.9	726.7	586.1	585.7	580.5	557.5
Poisoning	385.7	64.9	74.4	167.2	310.6	360.6	391.9
Suicide[f]	392.6	414.5	417.7	362.0	381.2	383.5	393.8
Homicide[f]	158.2	271.7	234.9	156.6	159.7	160.1	162.4
Black or African American[g]							
All causes	11,005.6	17,873.4	16,593.0	12,897.1	11,890.7	11,646.3	11,259.8
Diseases of heart	1,728.1	3,619.9	2,891.8	2,275.2	2,046.0	1,969.3	1,906.3
Ischemic heart disease	864.8	2,305.1	1,676.1	1,300.1	1,080.2	1,034.5	972.4
Cerebrovascular diseases	375.0	883.2	656.4	507.0	441.7	431.8	416.5
Malignant neoplasms	1,768.4	2,946.1	2,894.8	2,294.7	2,069.7	2,003.1	1,966.9
Trachea, bronchus, and lung	415.8	776.0	811.3	593.0	511.8	496.4	470.9
Colorectal	178.4	232.3	241.8	222.4	199.6	198.9	199.5
Prostate[d]	103.3	200.3	223.5	171.0	144.8	140.0	138.8
Breast[e]	422.8	524.2	592.9	500.0	485.7	450.1	445.3
Chronic lower respiratory diseases	175.8	203.7	240.6	232.7	211.0	197.6	192.7
Influenza and pneumonia	117.4	384.9	330.8	161.2	145.3	127.6	123.7
Chronic liver disease and cirrhosis	119.9	644.0	371.8	185.6	138.4	127.0	130.4
Diabetes mellitus	321.7	305.3	361.5	383.4	379.9	375.4	358.6
Human immunodeficiency virus (HIV) disease	483.2	—	1,014.7	763.3	594.4	566.8	522.1
Unintentional injuries	1,139.3	1,751.5	1,392.7	1,152.8	1,134.6	1,170.7	1,116.5
Motor vehicle-related injuries	539.4	750.2	699.5	580.8	532.3	541.6	521.4
Poisoning	250.7	99.4	144.3	196.6	253.8	296.1	263.5
Suicide[f]	190.0	238.0	261.4	208.7	194.0	187.3	187.3
Homicide[f]	1,031.8	1,580.8	1,612.9	941.6	967.8	998.6	967.7
American Indian or Alaska Native[g]							
All causes	8,164.2	13,390.9	9,506.2	7,758.2	8,624.4	8,517.6	8,463.6
Diseases of heart	885.5	1,819.9	1,391.0	1,030.1	1,010.2	1,008.6	985.4
Ischemic heart disease	514.5	1,208.2	901.8	709.3	625.2	614.2	587.1
Cerebrovascular diseases	148.7	269.3	223.3	198.1	209.4	178.2	170.0
Malignant neoplasms	881.4	1,101.3	1,141.1	995.7	1,084.3	983.9	991.1
Trachea, bronchus, and lung	190.1	181.1	268.1	227.8	268.2	225.3	226.3
Colorectal	89.2	78.8	82.4	93.8	109.7	88.1	100.5
Prostate[d]	26.6	66.7	42.0	44.5	37.6	38.8	33.5
Breast[e]	153.8	205.5	213.4	174.1	149.2	172.9	163.8
Chronic lower respiratory diseases	147.3	89.3	129.0	151.8	155.3	144.6	171.4
Influenza and pneumonia	103.3	307.9	206.3	124.0	113.6	101.6	110.9
Chronic liver disease and cirrhosis	529.3	1,190.3	535.1	519.4	498.9	479.2	576.3
Diabetes mellitus	253.0	305.5	292.3	305.6	347.3	324.8	292.6
Human immunodeficiency virus (HIV) disease	72.0	—	70.1	68.4	89.9	76.1	79.7

TABLE 1.13

Years of potential life lost before age 75 for selected causes of death, by sex and race, selected years 1980–2007 [CONTINUED]

[Data are based on death certificates]

Sex, race, Hispanic origin, and cause of death[b]	Crude 2007[c]	Age-adjusted[a]					
		1980	1990	2000[c]	2005[c]	2006[c]	2007[c]
		Years lost before age 75 per 100,000 population under 75 years of age					
Unintentional injuries	1,955.0	3,541.0	2,183.9	1,700.1	1,875.6	1,885.1	1,870.6
Motor vehicle-related injuries	1,009.1	2,102.4	1,301.5	1,032.2	1,004.9	1,021.7	930.5
Poisoning	421.9	92.9	119.5	180.1	333.8	358.5	416.7
Suicide[f]	514.3	515.0	495.9	403.1	498.6	487.8	470.6
Homicide[f]	305.3	628.9	434.2	278.5	337.5	328.3	283.3

—Data not available.

*Rates based on fewer than 20 deaths are considered unreliable and are not shown.

[a]Age-adjusted rates are calculated using the year 2000 standard population. Prior to 2003, age-adjusted rates were calculated using standard million proportions based on rounded population numbers. Starting with 2003 data, unrounded population numbers are used to calculate age-adjusted rates.

[b]Underlying cause of death was coded according to the 6th Revision of the *International Classification of Diseases* (ICD) in 1950, 7th Revision in 1960, 8th Revision in 1970, and 9th Revision in 1980–1998.

[c]Starting with 1999 data, cause of death is coded according to ICD-10

[d]Rate for male population only.

[e]Rate for female population only.

[f]Figures for 2001 include September 11-related deaths for which death certificates were filed as of October 24, 2002.

[g]The race groups, white, black, Asian or Pacific Islander, and American Indian or Alaska Native, include persons of Hispanic and non-Hispanic origin. Persons of Hispanic origin may be of any race. Death rates for the American Indian or Alaska Native and Asian or Pacific Islander populations are known to be underestimated.

Notes: Starting with *Health, United States, 2003*, rates for 1991–1999 were revised using intercensal population estimates based on the 2000 census. Rates for 2000 were revised based on 2000 census counts. Rates for 2001 and later years were computed using 2000-based postcensal estimates. Starting with 2003 data, some states allowed the reporting of more than one race on the death certificate. The multiple-race data for these states were bridged to the single-race categories of the 1977 Office of Management and Budget Standards for comparability with other states. Data for additional years are available.

SOURCE: Adapted from "Table 25. Years of Potential Life Lost before Age 75 for Selected Causes of Death, by Sex, Race, and Hispanic Origin: United States, Selected Years 1980–2007," in *Health, United States, 2010: With Special Feature on Death and Dying*, Centers for Disease Control and Prevention, National Center for Health Statistics, 2011, http://www.cdc.gov/nchs/data/hus/hus10.pdf#listtables (accessed December 14, 2011)

TABLE 1.14

Leading causes of death and numbers of deaths by age, 1980 and 2007

[Data are based on death certificates]

Age and rank order	1980 Cause of death	Deaths	2007 Cause of death	Deaths
Under 1 year				
Rank	All causes	45,526	All causes	29,138
1	Congenital anomalies	9,220	Congenital malformations, deformations and chromosomal abnormalities	5,785
2	Sudden infant death syndrome	5,510	Disorders related to short gestation and low birth weight, not elsewhere classified	4,857
3	Respiratory distress syndrome	4,989	Sudden infant death syndrome	2,453
4	Disorders relating to short gestation and unspecified low birthweight	3,648	Newborn affected by maternal complications of pregnancy	1,769
5	Newborn affected by maternal complications of pregnancy	1,572	Unintentional injuries	1,285
6	Intrauterine hypoxia and birth asphyxia	1,497	Newborn affected by complications of placenta, cord and membranes	1,135
7	Unintentional injuries	1,166	Bacterial sepsis of newborn	820
8	Birth trauma	1,058	Respiratory distress of newborn	789
9	Pneumonia and influenza	1,012	Diseases of circulatory system	624
10	Newborn affected by complications of placenta, cord, and membranes	985	Neonatal hemorrhage	597
1–4 years				
Rank	All causes	8,187	All causes	4,703
1	Unintentional injuries	3,313	Unintentional injuries	1,588
2	Congenital anomalies	1,026	Congenital malformations, deformations and chromosomal abnormalities	546
3	Malignant neoplasms	573	Homicide	398
4	Diseases of heart	338	Malignant neoplasms	364
5	Homicide	319	Diseases of heart	173
6	Pneumonia and influenza	267	Influenza and pneumonia	109
7	Meningitis	223	Septicemia	78
8	Meningococcal infection	110	Certain conditions originating in the perinatal period	70
9	Certain conditions originating in the perinatal period	84	In situ neoplasms, benign neoplasms and neoplasms of uncertain or unknown behavior	59
10	Septicemia	71	Chronic lower respiratory diseases	57
5–14 years				
Rank	All causes	10,689	All causes	6,147
1	Unintentional injuries	5,224	Unintentional injuries	2,194
2	Malignant neoplasms	1,497	Malignant neoplasms	959
3	Congenital anomalies	561	Congenital malformations, deformations and chromosomal abnormalities	374
4	Homicide	415	Homicide	346
5	Diseases of heart	330	Diseases of heart	241
6	Pneumonia and influenza	194	Suicide	184
7	Suicide	142	Chronic lower respiratory diseases	118
8	Benign neoplasms	104	Influenza and pneumonia	103
9	Cerebrovascular diseases	95	In situ neoplasms, benign neoplasms and neoplasms of uncertain or unknown behavior	84
10	Chronic obstructive pulmonary diseases	85	Cerebrovascular diseases	83
15–24 years				
Rank	All causes	49,027	All causes	33,982
1	Unintentional injuries	26,206	Unintentional injuries	15,897
2	Homicide	6,537	Homicide	5,551
3	Suicide	5,239	Suicide	4,140
4	Malignant neoplasms	2,683	Malignant neoplasms	1,653
5	Diseases of heart	1,223	Diseases of heart	1,084
6	Congenital anomalies	600	Congenital malformations, deformations and chromosomal abnormalities	402
7	Cerebrovascular diseases	418	Cerebrovascular diseases	195
8	Pneumonia and influenza	348	Diabetes mellitus	168
9	Chronic obstructive pulmonary diseases	141	Influenza and pneumonia	163
10	Anemias	133	Septicemia	160

TABLE 1.14

Leading causes of death and numbers of deaths by age, 1980 and 2007 [CONTINUED]

[Data are based on death certificates]

Age and rank order	1980 Cause of death	Deaths	2007 Cause of death	Deaths
25–44 years				
Rank	All causes	108,658	All causes	122,178
1	Unintentional injuries	26,722	Unintentional injuries	31,908
2	Malignant neoplasms	17,551	Malignant neoplasms	16,751
3	Diseases of heart	14,513	Diseases of heart	15,062
4	Homicide	10,983	Suicide	12,000
5	Suicide	9,855	Homicide	7,810
6	Chronic liver disease and cirrhosis	4,782	Human immunodeficiency virus (HIV) disease	4,663
7	Cerebrovascular diseases	3,154	Chronic liver disease and cirrhosis	2,954
8	Diabetes mellitus	1,472	Cerebrovascular diseases	2,638
9	Pneumonia and influenza	1,467	Diabetes mellitus	2,594
10	Congenital anomalies	817	Septicemia	1,207
45–64 years				
Rank	All causes	425,338	All causes	471,796
1	Diseases of heart	148,322	Malignant neoplasms	153,338
2	Malignant neoplasms	135,675	Diseases of heart	102,961
3	Cerebrovascular diseases	19,909	Unintentional injuries	32,508
4	Unintentional injuries	18,140	Diabetes mellitus	17,057
5	Chronic liver disease and cirrhosis	16,089	Chronic lower respiratory diseases	16,930
6	Chronic obstructive pulmonary diseases	11,514	Cerebrovascular diseases	16,885
7	Diabetes mellitus	7,977	Chronic liver disease and cirrhosis	16,216
8	Suicide	7,079	Suicide	12,847
9	Pneumonia and influenza	5,804	Nephritis, nephrotic syndrome and nephrosis	6,673
10	Homicide	4,019	Septicemia	6,662
65 years and over				
Rank	All causes	1,341,848	All causes	1,755,567
1	Diseases of heart	595,406	Diseases of heart	496,095
2	Malignant neoplasms	258,389	Malignant neoplasms	389,730
3	Cerebrovascular diseases	146,417	Cerebrovascular diseases	115,961
4	Pneumonia and influenza	45,512	Chronic lower respiratory diseases	109,562
5	Chronic obstructive pulmonary diseases	43,587	Alzheimer's disease	73,797
6	Atherosclerosis	28,081	Diabetes mellitus	51,528
7	Diabetes mellitus	25,216	Influenza and pneumonia	45,941
8	Unintentional injuries	24,844	Nephritis, nephrotic syndrome and nephrosis	38,484
9	Nephritis, nephrotic syndrome, and nephrosis	12,968	Unintentional injuries	38,292
10	Chronic liver disease and cirrhosis	9,519	Septicemia	26,362

SOURCE: "Table 26. Leading Causes of Death and Numbers of Deaths, by Age: United States, 1980 and 2007," in *Health, United States, 2010: With Special Feature on Death and Dying*, Centers for Disease Control and Prevention, National Center for Health Statistics, 2011, http://www.cdc.gov/nchs/data/hus/hus10.pdf#listtables (accessed December 14, 2011).

FIGURE 1.6

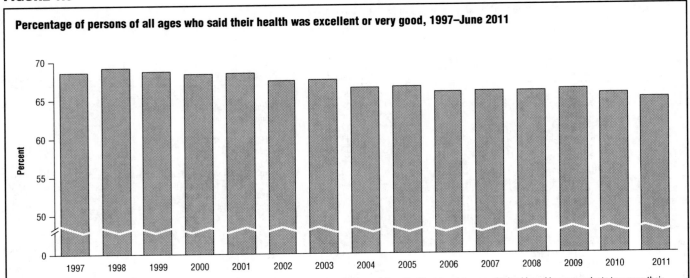

Percentage of persons of all ages who said their health was excellent or very good, 1997–June 2011

Notes: Data are based on household interviews of a sample of the civilian noninstitutionalized population. Health status data were obtained by asking respondents to assess their own health and that of family members living in the same household as excellent, very good, good, fair, or poor. The analyses excluded persons with unknown health status (about 0.2% of respondents each year).

SOURCE: "Figure 11.1. Percentage of Persons of All Ages Who Had Excellent or Very Good Health: United States, 1997–June 2011," in *Early Release of Selected Estimates Based on Data from the January–June 2011 National Health Interview Survey*, Centers for Disease Control and Prevention, National Center for Health Statistics, December 2011, http://www.cdc.gov/nchs/data/nhis/earlyrelease/201112_11.pdf (accessed December 17, 2011)

FIGURE 1.7

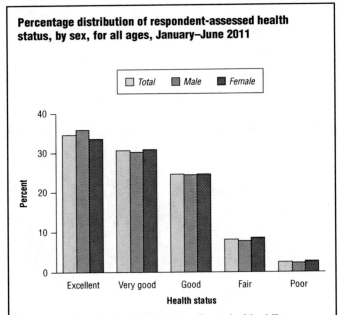

Percentage distribution of respondent-assessed health status, by sex, for all ages, January–June 2011

Notes: Data are based on household interviews of a sample of the civilian noninstitutionalized population. Health status data were obtained by asking respondents to assess their own health and that of family members living in the same household as excellent, very good, good, fair, or poor. The analyses excluded 0.1% of persons with unknown health status.

SOURCE: "Figure 11.2. Percent Distribution of Respondent-Assessed Health Status, by Sex, for All Ages: United States, January–June 2011," in *Early Release of Selected Estimates Based on Data from the January–June 2011 National Health Interview Survey*, Centers for Disease Control and Prevention, National Center for Health Statistics, December 2011, http://www.cdc.gov/nchs/data/nhis/earlyrelease/201112_11.pdf (accessed December 17, 2011)

FIGURE 1.8

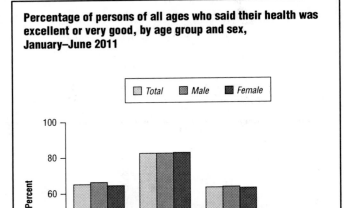

Percentage of persons of all ages who said their health was excellent or very good, by age group and sex, January–June 2011

Notes: Data are based on household interviews of a sample of the civilian noninstitutionalized population. Health status data were obtained by asking respondents to assess their own health and that of family members living in the same household as excellent, very good, good, fair, or poor. The analyses excluded 0.1% of persons with unknown health status.

SOURCE: "Figure 11.3. Percentage of Persons of All Ages Who Had Excellent or Very Good Health, by Age Group and Sex: United States, January–June 2011," in *Early Release of Selected Estimates Based on Data from the January–June 2011 National Health Interview Survey*, Centers for Disease Control and Prevention, National Center for Health Statistics, December 2011, http://www.cdc.gov/nchs/data/nhis/earlyrelease/201112_11.pdf (accessed December 17, 2011)

FIGURE 1.9

Age-sex-adjusted percentage of persons of all ages who said their health was excellent or very good, by race/ethnicity, January–June 2011

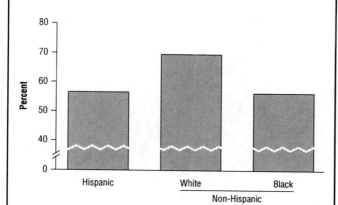

Notes: Data are based on household interviews of a sample of the civilian noninstitutionalized population. Health status data were obtained by asking respondents to assess their own health and that of family members living in the same household as excellent, very good, good, fair, or poor. The analyses excluded 0.1% of persons with unknown health status. Estimates are age-sex-adjusted using the projected 2000 U.S. population as the standard population and using three age groups: under 18, 18–64, and 65 and over.

SOURCE: "Figure 11.4. Age-Sex-Adjusted Percentage of Persons of All Ages Who Had Excellent or Very Good Health, by Race/Ethnicity: United States, January–June 2011," in *Early Release of Selected Estimates Based on Data from the January–June 2011 National Health Interview Survey*, Centers for Disease Control and Prevention, National Center for Health Statistics, December 2011, http://www.cdc.gov/nchs/data/nhis/earlyrelease/201112_11.pdf (accessed December 17, 2011)

CHAPTER 2
PREVENTION OF DISEASE

Prevention is better than cure.

—Desiderius Erasmus

Preventing disease involves a wide range of interrelated programs, actions, and activities. Some prevention measures are sweeping global policy initiatives, such as national and state government actions to reduce health risks by limiting air pollution and other toxic exposures or to increase standards to ensure the safety of food and water supplies. Others are focused efforts of public health professionals and agencies, such as the National Institutes of Health's Office of Disease Prevention, the Centers for Disease Control and Prevention (CDC), and the American Cancer Society (ACS), to reduce the incidence (occurrence of new cases) of specific diseases such as heart disease, diabetes, and lung cancer.

The effectiveness of local and global disease prevention programs largely depends on the extent to which individuals take personal responsibility for their own health by avoiding health risks such as tobacco use, substance abuse (misuse of alcohol and drugs), and unsafe sex. People who have a healthy diet; get adequate exercise and rest; wear seatbelts in automobiles and helmets on bicycles, motorcycles, and scooters; successfully manage stress; and maintain a positive outlook on life are on the front line of disease prevention. Similarly, individuals who effectively use health care resources by obtaining recommended immunizations, physical examinations, and health screenings are actively working to prevent disease and disability.

Prevention involves governments, professional organizations, public health professionals, health care practitioners (physicians, nurses, and allied health professionals), and individuals working at three levels to maintain and improve the health of communities. The first level, primary prevention, focuses on inhibiting the development of disease before it occurs. Secondary prevention, also called screening, refers to measures that detect disease before it is symptomatic. Tertiary prevention efforts focus on people

who are already affected by disease and attempt to reduce resultant disability and restore functionality.

PRIMARY PREVENTION

Primary prevention measures fall into two categories. The first category includes actions to protect against disease and disability, such as getting immunizations, ensuring the supply of safe drinking water, applying dental sealants to prevent tooth decay, and guarding against accidents. Examples of primary prevention of accidents include government and state requirements for workplace safety to prevent industrial injuries and equipping automobiles with air bags and antilock brakes. Examples of primary prevention of mental health problems include measures to strengthen family and community support systems as well as to teach children communication and interpersonal skills, conflict management, and other relationship and life skills that foster emotional resiliency.

General action to promote health is the other category of primary prevention measures. Health promotion includes the basic activities of a healthy lifestyle: good nutrition and hygiene, adequate exercise and rest, and avoidance of environmental and health risks. Limiting exposure to sunlight, using sunscreen, and wearing protective clothing are examples of primary prevention measures to reduce the risk of developing skin cancer.

Health promotion also includes education about the other interdependent dimensions of health known as wellness. Examples of health education programs that are aimed at wellness include stress management, parenting classes, preparation for retirement from the workforce, and cooking classes.

Historically, public health programs in developed countries have emphasized the primary prevention of infectious diseases (illnesses caused by microorganisms) by making environmental changes, such as improving the safety and purity of food and water supplies, and providing immunizations. Figure 2.1 shows the 2012 recommended schedule of immunization for people up to the age of six years, Figure 2.2 shows the 2012 recommended schedule of immunization for people aged seven to 18 years, and Figure 2.3 shows the 2012 recommended immunization schedule for adults aged 19 years and older. Immunization is a key primary prevention measure in the United States and other developed countries.

The most pressing health problems in developed countries in the 21st century are chronic diseases, such as heart disease, cancer, diabetes, and obesity. Primary prevention of chronic diseases is more challenging than primary prevention of infectious diseases because it requires changing health behaviors. Efforts to change

deeply rooted and often culturally influenced patterns of behaviors—such as diet, alcohol and tobacco use, and physical inactivity—generally have been less successful than environmental health and immunization programs.

Primary prevention programs are developed in response to actual and potential threats to community public health. Recent primary prevention programs have examined ways to prevent youth violence, smoking, and acts of bioterrorism (the use of biological or chemical weapons). In 2011 primary prevention programs included encouraging seasonal flu immunizations to reduce the spread and incidence of influenza and initiatives such as First Lady Michelle Obama's (1964–) Let's Move! (http://www.letsmove.gov/), which aims to prevent childhood obesity.

FIGURE 2.1

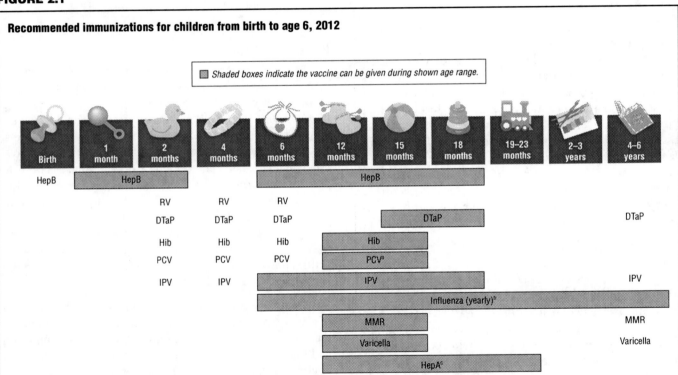

Recommended immunizations for children from birth to age 6, 2012

Note: If your child misses a shot, you don't need to start over, just go back to your child's doctor for the next shot. The doctor will keep your child up-to-date on vaccinations. Talk with your doctor if you have questions.
[a]Children 2 years old and older with certain medical conditions may need a dose of pneumococcal vaccine (PPSV) and meningococcal vaccine (MCV4).
[b]Two doses given at least four weeks apart are recommended for children aged 6 months through 8 years of age who are getting a flu vaccine for the first time. Children who only got one dose in their first year of vaccination should get two doses the following year.
[c]Two doses of HepA vaccine are needed for lasting protection. The first dose of HepA vaccine should be given between 12 months and 23 months of age. The second dose should be given 6 to 18 months later. HepA vaccination may be given to any child 12 months and older to protect against HepA. Children and adolescents who did not receive the HepA vaccine and are at high-risk, should be vaccinated against HepA.
HepB = Hepatitis B
RV = Rotavirus
DTaP = Diphtheria tetanus and pertusisis
Hib = Haemophilus influenzae type B
PCV = Pneumococcal conjugate vaccine
IPV = Polio vaccine
MMR = Measles, mumps and rubella
HepA = Hepatitis A

SOURCE: "2012 Recommended Immunizations for Children from Birth through 6 Years Old," in *2012 Child and Adolescent Immunization Schedules*, Centers for Disease Control and Prevention, February 6, 2012, http://www.cdc.gov/vaccines/spec-grps/infants/downloads/parent-ver-sch-0-6yrs.pdf (accessed March 24, 2012)

FIGURE 2.2

Recommended immunizations for children and teens from ages 7–18, 2012

□ These shaded boxes indicate when the vaccine is recommended for all children unless your doctor tells you that your child cannot safely receive the vaccine.

■ These shaded boxes indicate the vaccine should be given if a child is catching-up on missed vaccines.

■ These shaded boxes indicate the vaccine is recommended for children with certain health conditions that put them at high risk for serious diseases. Note that healthy children can get the HepA series[f].

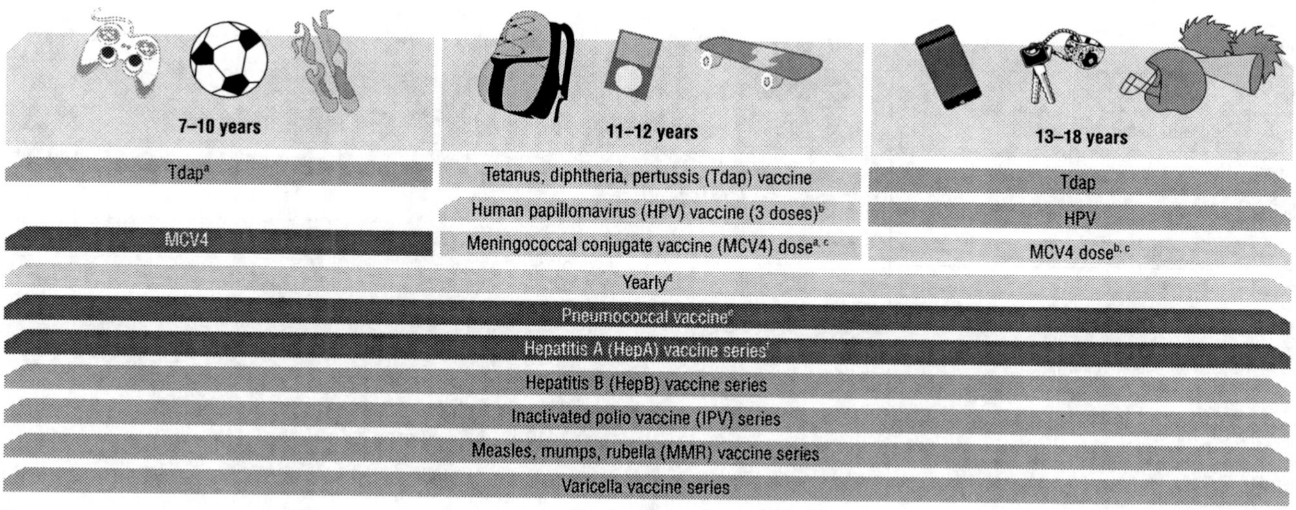

7–10 years	11–12 years	13–18 years
Tdap[a]	Tetanus, diphtheria, pertussis (Tdap) vaccine	Tdap
	Human papillomavirus (HPV) vaccine (3 doses)[b]	HPV
MCV4	Meningococcal conjugate vaccine (MCV4) dose[a, c]	MCV4 dose[b, c]
	Yearly[d]	
	Pneumococcal vaccine[e]	
	Hepatitis A (HepA) vaccine series[f]	
	Hepatitis B (HepB) vaccine series	
	Inactivated polio vaccine (IPV) series	
	Measles, mumps, rubella (MMR) vaccine series	
	Varicella vaccine series	

[a]Tdap vaccine is combination vaccine that is recommended at age 11 or 12 to protect against tetanus, diphtheria and pertussis. If your child has not received any or all of the DTaP vaccine series, or if you don't know if your child has received these shots, your child needs a single dose of Tdap when they are 7–10 years old. Talk to your child's health care provider to find out if they need additional catch-up vaccines.

[b]All 11 or 12 year olds—both girls and boys—should receive 3 doses of HPV vaccine to protect against HPV-related disease. Either HPV vaccine (Cervarix® or Gardisil®) can be given to girls and young women; only one HPV vaccine (Gardisil®) can be given to boys and young men.

[c]Meningococcal conjugate vaccine (MCV) is recommended at age 11 or 12. A booster shot is recommended at age 16. Teens who received MCV for the first time at age 13 through 15 years will need a one-time booster dose between the ages of 16 and 18 years. If your teenager missed getting the vaccine altogether, ask their health care provider about getting it now, especially if your teenager is about to move into a college dorm or military barracks.

[d]Everyone 6 months of age and older—including preteens and teens—should get a flu vaccine every year. Children under the age of 9 years may require more than one dose. Talk to your child's health care provider to find out if they need more than one dose.

[e]A single dose of Pneumococcal Conjugate Vaccine (PCV13) is recommended for children who are 6–18 years old with certain medical conditions that place them at high risk. Talk to your healthcare provider about pneumococcal vaccine and what factors may place your child at high risk for pneumococcal disease.

[f]Hepatitis A vaccination is recommended for older children with certain medical conditions that place them at high risk. HepA vaccine is licensed, safe, and effective for all children of all ages. Even if your child is not at high risk, you may decide you want your child protected against HepA. Talk to your healthcare provider about HepA vaccine and what factors may place your child at high risk for HepA.

SOURCE: "2012 Recommended Immunizations for Children from 7 through 18 Years Old," in *2012 Child and Adolescent Immunization Schedules*, Centers for Disease Control and Prevention, February 6, 2012, http://www.cdc.gov/vaccines/who/teens/downloads/parent-version-schedule-7-18yrs.pdf (accessed March 24, 2012)

Primary Prevention of Youth Violence

Violence on U.S. high school and college campuses has focused media attention on the problem of violence during childhood, adolescence, and young adulthood. Recent examples of school violence include three 15-year-old boys being accused of plotting a shooting at Lakeshore High School in Mandeville, Louisiana, in August 2011. Four months later, in December, two people were fatally shot on the Virginia Polytechnic Institute and State University campus, just five years after an April 2007 massacre claimed 33 lives on the same campus.

The CDC finds in "Trends in the Prevalence of Behaviors that Contribute to Violence on School Property National YRBS: 1991–2009" (May 2010, http://www.cdc.gov/healthyyouth/yrbs/pdf/us_violenceschool_trend_yrbs.pdf) that 5.6% of high school students interviewed in 2009 said they had carried a firearm at least once during the past month and 7.7% had threatened or injured someone with a weapon on school property one or more times during the 12 months preceding the survey. Table 2.1 shows that the percentage of students who carried a weapon on school property declined between 1993 and 2009, as did the reports of physical fights on school property. This decline may at least be in part attributable to the implementation of programs that aim to prevent school violence.

To develop programs that prevent violence and violent deaths among children and teens, the CDC follows a systematic public health approach that identifies and describes the problem, designs and evaluates measures to prevent the problem, and puts these measures in place in the community. The approach that public health

FIGURE 2.3

Adult immunization schedule, 2012

- For all persons in this category who meet the age requirements and who lack documentation of vaccination or have no evidence of previous infection
- Recommended if some other risk factor is present (e.g., on the basis of medical, occupational, lifestyle, or other indications)
- Tdap recommended for ≥65 if contact with <12 month old child. Either Td or Tdap can be used if no infant contact
- No recommendation

Vaccine ▼ / Age group ►	19–21 years	22–26 years	27–49 years	50–59 years	60–64 years	≥65 years
Influenza[a]	1 dose annually					
Tetanus, diphtheria, pertussis (Td/Tdap)[b, *]	Substitute 1-time dose of Tdap for Td booster; then boost with Td every 10 yrs					Td/Tdap
Varicella[c, *]	2 doses					
Human papillomavirus (HPV) female[d, *]	3 doses					
Human papillomavirus (HPV) male[d, *]	3 doses					
Zoster[e]					1 dose	
Measles, mumps, rubella (MMR)[f, *]	1 or 2 doses				1 dose	
Pneumococcal (polysaccharide)[g, h]			1 or 2 doses			1 dose
Meningococcal[i, *]	1 or more doses					
Hepatitis A[j, *]	2 doses					
Hepatitis B[k, *]	3 doses					

*Covered by the Vaccine Injury Compensation Program

professionals use to develop all prevention programs consists of the following steps, some of which may be conducted simultaneously:

- Surveillance—the first step is to collect and analyze data to determine the size and scope of the problem. To understand youth violence, researchers look at how many people were injured or killed as a result of youth violence. They look at the ages, attitudes, school performance, family histories, and other characteristics of the children and teens who committed violent acts. They also note when (day, night, weekends, summer, winter, spring, or fall) and where (school, home, or public parks) the violence occurred.

- Determine the cause—by analyzing the data collected in the surveillance process, researchers can identify the underlying causes of the problem. Once public health professionals know who is at risk for a particular problem and why a certain group is at risk, they are better able to design actions to prevent it.

- Develop and test preventive measures—using the results of the data analysis, public health professionals develop prevention programs called interventions. These interventions target specific populations and may be conducted at specific locations. Before recommending widespread use of interventions, health professionals test the programs to find out if

they work as effectively as hoped. Every intervention is evaluated to determine if it achieves its objectives.

- Implementation—during this phase the preventive measures found to be effective are communicated so they may be put into action. To communicate methods that prevent violence among children and teens, the CDC conducts training programs, publishes articles in journals for public health workers and health care practitioners, and oversees Striving to Reduce Youth Violence Everywhere (STRYVE; http://www.safeyouth.gov/Pages/AboutUs.aspx), a national initiative that aims to "prevent youth violence before it starts among young people ages 10 to 24."

- Evaluation—after preventive measures or interventions have been implemented, they are evaluated to see if they have effectively prevented the problem.

STRYVE provides communities with information and resources to launch effective youth violence prevention programs. The initiative offers:

- Online access to data and tools

- Effective evidence-based practices, policies, and programs

- Training and technical assistance

FIGURE 2.3

Adult immunization schedule, 2012 [CONTINUED]

- ▨ *For all persons in this category who meet the age requirements and who lack documentation of vaccination or have no evidence of previous infection*
- ▨ *Recommended if some other risk factor is present (e.g., on the basis of medical, occupational, lifestyle, or other indications)*
- ■ *Contraindicated*
- □ *No recommendation*

Indication ► / Vaccine ▼	Pregnancy	Immunocompromising conditions (excluding human immunodeficiency virus [HIV])[c, e, f, m]	HIV infection[c, f, l, m] CD4+ T lymphocyte count <200 cells/µL	HIV infection CD4+ T lymphocyte count ≥200 cells/µL	Men who have sex with men (MSM)	Heart disease, chronic lung disease, chronic alcoholism	Asplenia[i] (including elective splenectomy and persistent complement component deficiencies)	Chronic liver disease	Diabetes kidney failure, end-stage renal disease, receipt of hemodialysis	Health care personnel
Influenza[a]	1 dose TIV annually	1 dose TIV annually	1 dose TIV annually	1 dose TIV annually	1 dose TIV or LAIV annually	1 dose TIV annually	1 dose TIV annually	1 dose TIV annually	1 dose TIV annually	1 dose TIV or LAIV annually
Tetanus, diphtheria, pertussis (Td/Tdap)[b,*]	Substitute 1-time dose of Tdap for Td booster; then boost with Td every 10 yrs	Substitute 1-time dose of Tdap for Td booster; then boost with Td every 10 yrs	Substitute 1-time dose of Tdap for Td booster; then boost with Td every 10 yrs	Substitute 1-time dose of Tdap for Td booster; then boost with Td every 10 yrs	Substitute 1-time dose of Tdap for Td booster; then boost with Td every 10 yrs	Substitute 1-time dose of Tdap for Td booster; then boost with Td every 10 yrs	Substitute 1-time dose of Tdap for Td booster; then boost with Td every 10 yrs	Substitute 1-time dose of Tdap for Td booster; then boost with Td every 10 yrs	Substitute 1-time dose of Tdap for Td booster; then boost with Td every 10 yrs	Substitute 1-time dose of Tdap for Td booster; then boost with Td every 10 yrs
Varicella[c,*]	Contraindicated	Contraindicated	Contraindicated	2 doses	2 doses	2 doses	2 doses	2 doses	2 doses	2 doses
Human papillomavirus (HPV) female[d,*]		3 doses through age 26 yrs	3 doses through age 26 yrs	3 doses through age 26 yrs		3 doses through age 26 yrs	3 doses through age 26 yrs	3 doses through age 26 yrs	3 doses through age 26 yrs	3 doses through age 26 yrs
Human papillomavirus (HPV) male[d,*]		3 doses through age 26 yrs	3 doses through age 26 yrs	3 doses through age 26 yrs	3 doses through age 26 yrs	3 doses through age 21 yrs	3 doses through age 21 yrs	3 doses through age 21 yrs	3 doses through age 21 yrs	3 doses through age 21 yrs
Zoster[e]	Contraindicated	Contraindicated	Contraindicated		1 dose	1 dose	1 dose	1 dose	1 dose	1 dose
Measles, mumps, rubella (MMR)[f,*]	Contraindicated	Contraindicated	Contraindicated	1 or 2 doses	1 or 2 doses	1 or 2 doses	1 or 2 doses	1 or 2 doses	1 or 2 doses	1 or 2 doses
Pneumococcal (polysaccharide)[g, h]	1 or 2 doses	1 or 2 doses	1 or 2 doses	1 or 2 doses	1 or 2 doses	1 or 2 doses	1 or 2 doses	1 or 2 doses	1 or 2 doses	1 or 2 doses
Meningococcal[i,*]	1 or more doses	1 or more doses	1 or more doses	1 or more doses	1 or more doses	1 or more doses	1 or more doses	1 or more doses	1 or more doses	1 or more doses
Hepatitis A[j,*]	2 doses	2 doses	2 doses	2 doses	2 doses	2 doses	2 doses	2 doses	2 doses	2 doses
Hepatitis B[k,*]	3 doses	3 doses	3 doses	3 doses	3 doses	3 doses	3 doses	3 doses	3 doses	3 doses

*Covered by the Vaccine Injury Compensation Program

- Online community workspaces
- Connections to other communities

The CDC advocates several prevention strategies including:

- Family-based programs to improve family relations. These programs emphasize teaching parents about child development and helping them learn and practice communication skills so they can model problem solving that does not involve violence
- Teaching children how to handle tough social situations and how to resolve disagreements without using violence
- Mentoring programs that pair an adult, who serves as a positive role model, with a young person
- Modifications of the physical and social environment that help address the social and economic causes of violence

Another example of effective primary prevention of youth violence is described by David A. Wolfe et al. in "A School-Based Program to Prevent Adolescent Dating Violence: A Cluster Randomized Trial" (*Archives of Pediatric and Adolescent Medicine*, vol. 163, no. 8, August 2009). The program consisted of interactive lessons about healthy relationships, sexual health, and substance use that included information about preventing dating violence. The program was delivered to 1,722 students aged 14 to 15 years old and was intended to help students make decisions that favored safety in terms of their dating and other peer relationships. Over the course of two and a half years, students who participated in this primary prevention program reported fewer instances of physical dating violence, compared with a control group of students who did not receive this training.

SECONDARY PREVENTION

The goal of secondary prevention is to identify and detect disease in its earliest stages, before noticeable

FIGURE 2.3

Adult immunization schedule, 2012 [CONTINUED]

[a]**Influenza vaccination**
- Annual vaccination against influenza is recommended for all persons 6 months of age and older.
- Persons 6 months of age and older, including pregnant women, can receive the trivalent inactivated vaccine (TIV).
- Healthy, nonpregnant adults younger than age 50 years without high-risk medical conditions can receive either intranasally administered live, attenuated influenza vaccine (LAIV) (FluMist), or TIV. Health-care personnel who care for severely immunocompromised persons (i.e., those who require care in a protected environment) should receive TIV rather than LAIV. Other persons should receive TIV.
- The intramuscular or intradermal administered TIV are options for adults aged 18–64 years.
- Adults aged 65 years and older can receive the standard dose TIV or the high-dose TIV (Fluzone High-Dose).

[b]**Tetanus, diphtheria, and acellular pertussis (Td/Tdap) vaccination**
- Administer a one-time dose of Tdap to adults younger than age 65 years who have not received Tdap previously or for whom vaccine status is unknown to replace one of the 10-year Td boosters.
- Tdap is specifically recommended for the following persons:
  — pregnant women more than 20 weeks' gestation,
  — adults, regardless of age, who are close contacts of infants younger than age 12 months (e.g., parents, grandparents, or child care providers), and
  — health-care personnel.
- Tdap can be administered regardless of interval since the most recent tetanus or diphtheria-containing vaccine.
- Pregnant women not vaccinated during pregnancy should receive Tdap immediately postpartum.
- Adults 65 years and older may receive Tdap.
- Adults with unknown or incomplete history of completing a 3-dose primary vaccination series with Td-containing vaccines should begin or complete a primary vaccination series. Tdap should be substituted for a single dose of Td in the vaccination series with Tdap preferred as the first dose.
- For unvaccinated adults, administer the first 2 doses at least 4 weeks apart and the third dose 6–12 months after the second.
- If incompletely vaccinated (i.e., less than 3 doses), administer remaining doses.

[c]**Varicella vaccination**
- All adults without evidence of immunity to varicella (as defined below) should receive 2 doses of single-antigen varicella vaccine or a second dose if they have received only 1 dose.
- Special consideration for vaccination should be given to those who
  — have close contact with persons at high risk for severe disease (e.g., health-care personnel and family contacts of persons with immunocompromising conditions) or
  — are at high risk for exposure or transmission (e.g., teachers; child care employees; residents and staff members of institutional settings, including correctional institutions; college students; military personnel; adolescents and adults living in households with children; nonpregnant women of childbearing age; and international travelers).
- Pregnant women should be assessed for evidence of varicella immunity. Women who do not have evidence of immunity should receive the first dose of varicella vaccine upon completion or termination of pregnancy and before discharge from the health-care facility. The second dose should be administered 4–8 weeks after the first dose.
- Evidence of immunity to varicella in adults includes any of the following:
  — documentation of 2 doses of varicella vaccine at least 4 weeks apart;
  — U.S.-born before 1980 (although for health-care personnel and pregnant women, birth before 1980 should not be considered evidence of immunity);
  — history of varicella based on diagnosis or verification of varicella by a health-care provider (for a patient reporting a history of or having an atypical case, a mild case, or both, health-care providers should seek either an epidemiologic link to a typical varicella case or to a
  — laboratory-confirmed case or evidence of laboratory confirmation, if it was performed at the time of acute disease);
  — history of herpes zoster based on diagnosis or verification of herpes zoster by a health-care provider; or
  — laboratory evidence of immunity or laboratory confirmation of disease.

[d]**Human papillomavirus (HPV) vaccination**
- Two vaccines are licensed for use in females, bivalent HPV vaccine (HPV2) and quadrivalent HPV vaccine (HPV4), and one HPV vaccine for use in males (HPV4).
- For females, either HPV4 or HPV2 is recommended in a 3-dose series for routine vaccination at 11 or 12 years of age, and for those 13 through 26 years of age, if not previously vaccinated.
- For males, HPV4 is recommended in a 3-dose series for routine vaccination at 11 or 12 years of age, and for those 13 through 21 years of age, if not previously vaccinated. Males 22 through 26 years of age may be vaccinated.
- HPV vaccines are not live vaccines and can be administered to persons who are immunocompromised as a result of infection (including HIV infection), disease, or medications. Vaccine is recommended for immunocompromised persons through age 26 years who did not get any or all doses when they were younger. The immune response and vaccine efficacy might be less than that in immunocompetent persons.
- Men who have sex with men (MSM) might especially benefit from vaccination to prevent condyloma and anal cancer. HPV4 is recommended for MSM through age 26 years who did not get any or all doses when they were younger.
- Ideally, vaccine should be administered before potential exposure to HPV through sexual activity; however, persons who are sexually active should still be vaccinated consistent with age-based recommendations. HPV vaccine can be administered to persons with a history of genital warts, abnormal Papanicolaou test, or positive HPV DNA test.
- A complete series for either HPV4 or HPV2 consists of 3 doses. The second dose should be administered 1–2 months after the first dose; the third dose should be administered 6 months after the first dose (at least 24 weeks after the first dose).
- Although HPV vaccination is not specifically recommended for health-care personnel (HCP) based on their occupation, HCP should receive the HPV vaccine if they are in the recommended age group.

[e]**Zoster vaccination**
- A single dose of zoster vaccine is recommended for adults 60 years of age and older regardless of whether they report a prior episode of herpes zoster. Although the vaccine is licensed by the Food and Drug Administration (FDA) for use among and can be administered to persons 50 years and older, ACIP recommends that vaccination begins at 60 years of age.
- Persons with chronic medical conditions may be vaccinated unless their condition constitutes a contraindication, such as pregnancy or severe immunodeficiency.
- Although zoster vaccination is not specifically recommended for health-care personnel (HCP), HCP should receive the vaccine if they are in the recommended age group.

[f]**Measles, mumps, rubella (MMR) vaccination**
- Adults born before 1957 generally are considered immune to measles and mumps. All adults born in 1957 or later should have documentation of 1 or more doses of MMR vaccine unless they have a medical contraindication to the vaccine, laboratory evidence of immunity to each of the three diseases, or documentation of provider-diagnosed measles or mumps disease. For rubella, documentation of provider-diagnosed disease is not considered acceptable evidence of immunity.
Measles component:
- A routine second dose of MMR vaccine, administered a minimum of 28 days after the first dose, is recommended for adults who
  — are students in postsecondary educational institutions;
  — work in a health-care facility; or
  — plan to travel internationally.
- Persons who received inactivated (killed) measles vaccine or measles vaccine of unknown type from 1963 to 1967 should be revaccinated with 2 doses of MMR vaccine.

FIGURE 2.3

Adult immunization schedule, 2012 [CONTINUED]

Mumps component:
- A routine second dose of MMR vaccine, administered a minimum of 28 days after the first dose, is recommended for adults who
  — are students in postsecondary educational institutions;
  — work in a health-care facility; or
  — plan to travel internationally.
- Persons vaccinated before 1979 with either killed mumps vaccine or mumps vaccine of unknown type who are at high risk for mumps infection (e.g., persons who are working in a health-care facility) should be considered for revaccination with 2 doses of MMR vaccine.

Rubella component:
- For women of childbearing age, regardless of birth year, rubella immunity should be determined. If there is no evidence of immunity, women who are not pregnant should be vaccinated. Pregnant women who do not have evidence of immunity should receive MMR vaccine upon completion or termination of pregnancy and before discharge from the health-care facility.

Health-care personnel born before 1957:
- For unvaccinated health-care personnel born before 1957 who lack laboratory evidence of measles, mumps, and/or rubella immunity or laboratory confirmation of disease, health-care facilities should consider routinely vaccinating personnel with 2 doses of MMR vaccine at the appropriate interval for measles and mumps or 1 dose of MMR vaccine for rubella.

[g]Pneumococcal polysaccharide (PPSV) vaccination
- Vaccinate all persons with the following indications:
  — age 65 years and older without a history of PPSV vaccination;
  — adults younger than 65 years with chronic lung disease (including chronic obstructive pulmonary disease, emphysema, and asthma); chronic cardiovascular diseases; diabetes mellitus; chronic liver disease (including cirrhosis); alcoholism; cochlear implants; cerebrospinal fluid leaks; immunocompromising conditions; and functional or anatomic asplenia (e.g., sickle cell disease and other hemoglobinopathies, congenital or acquired asplenia, splenic dysfunction, or splenectomy [if elective splenectomy is planned, vaccinate at least 2 weeks before surgery]);
  — residents of nursing homes or long-term care facilities; and
  — adults who smoke cigarettes.
- Persons with asymptomatic or symptomatic HIV infection should be vaccinated as soon as possible after their diagnosis.
- When cancer chemotherapy or other immunosuppressive therapy is being considered, the interval between vaccination and initiation of immunosuppressive therapy should be at least 2 weeks. Vaccination during chemotherapy or radiation therapy should be avoided.
- Routine use of PPSV is not recommended for American Indians/Alaska Natives or other persons younger than 65 years of age unless they have underlying medical conditions that are PPSV indications. However, public health authorities may consider recommending PPSV for American Indians/Alaska Natives who are living in areas where the risk for invasive pneumococcal disease is increased.

[h]Revaccination with PPSV
- One-time revaccination 5 years after the first dose is recommended for persons 19 through 64 years of age with chronic renal failure or nephrotic syndrome; functional or anatomic asplenia (e.g., sickle cell disease or splenectomy); and for persons with immunocompromising conditions.
- Persons who received PPSV before age 65 years for any indication should receive another dose of the vaccine at age 65 years or later if at least 5 years have passed since their previous dose.
- No further doses are needed for persons vaccinated with PPSV at or after age 65 years.

[i]Meningococcal vaccination
- Administer 2 doses of meningococcal conjugate vaccine quadrivalent (MCV4) at least 2 months apart to adults with functional asplenia or persistent complement component deficiencies.
- HIV-infected persons who are vaccinated should also receive 2 doses.
- Administer a single dose of meningococcal vaccine to microbiologists routinely exposed to isolates of *Neisseria meningitidis*, military recruits, and persons who travel to or live in countries in which meningococcal disease is hyperendemic or epidemic.
- First-year college students up through age 21 years who are living in residence halls should be vaccinated if they have not received a dose on or after their 16th birthday.
- MCV4 is preferred for adults with any of the preceding indications who are 55 years old and younger; meningococcal polysaccharide vaccine (MPSV4) is preferred for adults 56 years and older.
- Revaccination with MCV4 every 5 years is recommended for adults previously vaccinated with MCV4 or MPSV4 who remain at increased risk for infection (e.g., adults with anatomic or functional asplenia or persistent complement component deficiencies).

[j]Hepatitis A vaccination
- Vaccinate any person seeking protection from hepatitis A virus (HAV) infection and persons with any of the following indications:
  — men who have sex with men and persons who use injection drugs;
  — persons working with HAV-infected primates or with HAV in a research laboratory setting;
  — persons with chronic liver disease and persons who receive clotting factor concentrates;
  — persons traveling to or working in countries that have high or intermediate endemicity of hepatitis A; and
  — unvaccinated persons who anticipate close personal contact (e.g., household or regular babysitting) with an international adoptee during the first 60 days after arrival in the United States from a country with high or intermediate endemicity. The first dose of the 2-dose hepatitis A vaccine series should be administered as soon as adoption is planned, ideally 2 or more weeks before the arrival of the adoptee.
- Single-antigen vaccine formulations should be administered in a 2-dose schedule at either 0 and 6–12 months (Havrix), or 0 and 6–18 months (Vaqta). If the combined hepatitis A and hepatitis B vaccine (Twinrix) is used, administer 3 doses at 0, 1, and 6 months; alternatively, a 4-dose schedule may be used, administered on days 0, 7, and 21–30 followed by a booster dose at month 12.

[k]Hepatitis B vaccination
- Vaccinate persons with any of the following indications and any person seeking protection from hepatitis B virus (HBV) infection:
  — sexually active persons who are not in a long-term, mutually monogamous relationship (e.g., persons with more than one sex partner during the previous 6 months); persons seeking evaluation or treatment for a sexually transmitted disease (STD); current or recent injection-drug users; and men who have sex with men;
  — health-care personnel and public-safety workers who are exposed to blood or other potentially infectious body fluids;
  — persons with diabetes younger than 60 years as soon as feasible after diagnosis; persons with diabetes who are 60 years or older at the discretion of the treating clinician based on increased need for assisted blood glucose monitoring in long-term care facilities, likelihood of acquiring hepatitis B infection, its complications or chronic sequelae, and likelihood of immune response to vaccination;
  — persons with end-stage renal disease, including patients receiving hemodialysis; persons with HIV infection; and persons with chronic liver disease;
  — household contacts and sex partners of persons with chronic HBV infection; clients and staff members of institutions for persons with developmental disabilities; and international travelers to countries with high or intermediate prevalence of chronic HBV infection; and
  — all adults in the following settings: STD treatment facilities; HIV testing and treatment facilities; facilities providing drug-abuse treatment and prevention services; health-care settings targeting services to injection-drug users or men who have sex with men; correctional facilities; end-stage renal disease programs and facilities for chronic hemodialysis patients; and institutions and nonresidential daycare facilities for persons with developmental disabilities.

FIGURE 2.3

Adult immunization schedule, 2012 [CONTINUED]

- Administer missing doses to complete a 3-dose series of hepatitis B vaccine to those persons not vaccinated or not completely vaccinated. The second dose should be administered 1 month after the first dose; the third dose should be given at least 2 months after the second dose (and at least 4 months after the first dose). If the combined hepatitis A and hepatitis B vaccine (Twinrix) is used, give 3 doses at 0, 1, and 6 months; alternatively, a 4-dose Twinrix schedule, administered on days 0, 7, and 21–30 followed by a booster dose at month 12 may be used.
- Adult patients receiving hemodialysis or with other immunocompromising conditions should receive 1 dose of 40 /μg/mL (Recombivax HB) administered on a 3-dose schedule or 2 doses of 20 μg/mL (Engerix-B) administered simultaneously on a 4-dose schedule at 0, 1, 2, and 6 months.

[l]**Selected conditions for which *Haemophilus influenzae* type b (Hib) vaccine may be used**
- 1 dose of Hib vaccine should be considered for persons who have sickle cell disease, leukemia, or HIV infection, or who have anatomic or functional asplenia if they have not previously received Hib vaccine.

[m]**Immunocompromising conditions**
- Inactivated vaccines generally are acceptable (e.g., pneumococcal, meningococcal, and influenza [inactivated influenza vaccine]), and live vaccines generally are avoided in persons with immune deficiencies or immunocompromising conditions.

SOURCE: "Recommended Adult Immunization Schedule, United States, 2012," in *2012 Adult Immunization Schedule*, Centers for Disease Control and Prevention, February 3, 2012, http://www.cdc.gov/vaccines/recs/schedules/downloads/adult/adult-schedule-bw.pdf (accessed March 26, 2012)

TABLE 2.1

Violent behaviors on school property, 1991–2009

	1991	1993	1995	1997	1999	2001	2003	2005	2007	2009	Changes from 1991–2009[a]	Change from 2007–2009[b]
Carried a weapon on school property on at least 1 day (for example, a gun, knife, or club during the 30 days before the survey)	NA[c]	11.8	9.8	8.5	6.9	6.4	6.1	6.5	5.9	5.6	Decreased, 1993–2003 No change, 2003–2009	No change
Did not go to school because they felt unsafe at school or on their way to or from school on at least 1 day (during the 30 days before the survey)	NA	4.4	4.5	4.0	5.2	6.6	5.4	6.0	5.5	5.0	Increased, 1993–2001 Decreased, 2001–2009	No change
Threatened or injured with a weapon on school property one or more times (for example, a gun, knife, or club during the 12 months before the survey)	NA	7.3	8.4	7.4	7.7	8.9	9.2	7.9	7.8	7.7	No change, 1993–2009	No change
In a physical fight on school property one or more times (during the 12 months before the survey)	NA	16.2	15.5	14.8	14.2	12.5	12.8	13.6	12.4	11.1	Decreased, 1993–2009	No change

[a]Based on trend analyses using a logistic regression model controlling for sex, race/ethnicity, and grade.
[b]Based on t-test analyses, $p < 0.05$.
[c]Not available.
Notes: The national Youth Risk Behavior Survey (YRBS) monitors priority health risk behaviors that contribute to the leading causes of death, disability, and social problems among youth and adults in the United States. The national YRBS is conducted every two years during the spring semester and provides data representative of 9th and 12th grade students in public and private schools throughout the United States.

SOURCE: "Trends in the Prevalence of Behaviors that Contribute to Violence on School Property National YRBS: 1991–2009," Centers for Disease Control and Prevention, National Center for Chronic Disease Prevention and Health Promotion, Division of Adolescent and School Health, November 3, 2011, http://www.cdc.gov/healthyyouth/yrbs/pdf/us_violenceschool_trend_yrbs.pdf (accessed December 17, 2011)

symptoms develop, when it is most likely to be treated successfully. With early detection and diagnosis, it may be possible to cure a disease, slow its progression, prevent or minimize complications, and limit disability.

Another goal of secondary prevention is to prevent the spread of communicable diseases (illnesses that can be transmitted from one person to another). In the community, early identification and treatment of people with communicable diseases, such as sexually transmitted diseases, provides not only secondary prevention for those who are infected but also primary prevention for people who come in contact with infected individuals.

Like primary prevention, individual health care practitioners and public health agencies and organizations perform secondary prevention. An example of secondary prevention that is conducted by many different professionals (physicians, nurses, and allied health professionals) in a variety of settings (medical offices, clinics, and health fairs) is blood pressure screening to identify people with hypertension (high blood pressure). An example of mental health secondary prevention is the effort to identify young children with behavior problems to intervene early and prevent development of, or progression to, more serious mental disorders.

The U.S. Preventive Services Task Force (USPSTF; 2012, http://www.uspreventiveservicestaskforce.org/adultrec.htm) was convened by the U.S. Public Health Service to "rigorously evaluate clinical research in order to assess the merits of preventive measures, including screening tests, counseling, immunizations, and preventive medications." Consisting of an independent panel of experts, the task force (2012, http://www.uspreventive servicestaskforce.org/) "conducts scientific evidence reviews of a broad range of clinical preventive health care services (such as screening, counseling, and preventive medications) and develops recommendations for primary care clinicians and health systems." It also stipulates the preventive measures that should be taken by healthy adult men, women, pregnant women, and children. Figure 2.4 shows the process the USPSTF uses as it researches, weighs the evidence, and develops recommendations. Table 2.2 lists the preventive services that are recommended by the USPSTF. The recommendations include screening to detect and identify a wide range of conditions, including high blood pressure, depression, obesity, and sexually transmitted diseases such as chlamydia and syphilis infection.

Secondary prevention plays an important role in diseases such as diabetes (a condition in which the body does not properly metabolize sugar), glaucoma (a disorder caused by too much fluid pressure inside the eyeball), breast cancer, and cancer of the cervix (the opening of the uterus). State and local health departments, voluntary health agencies, hospitals, medical clinics, schools, and physicians often conduct screenings for these conditions during which people with no signs or symptoms are tested to uncover these diseases in their earliest stages.

USPSTF Screening Guidelines for Heart Disease, Depression, Breast Cancer, and Osteoporosis

In 2009 the USPSTF presented new screening guidelines for heart disease, depression, and breast cancer. The recommendations for heart disease screening advise against using biomarkers, such as measuring high-sensitivity C-reactive protein or homocysteine levels in healthy adults, as a way to screen for heart disease. In "Using Nontraditional Risk Factors in Coronary Heart Disease Risk Assessment" (October 2009, http://www .ahrq.gov/clinic/uspstf/uspscoronaryhd.htm), the USPSTF evaluates the relevant research and medical evidence and concludes "that the evidence is insufficient to assess the balance of benefits and harms of using the nontraditional risk factors discussed in this statement to screen asymptomatic men and women with no history of CHD [coronary heart disease] to prevent CHD events."

In "Screening for Depression in Adults" (December 2009, http://www.ahrq.gov/clinic/uspstf/uspsaddepr.htm), the USPSTF updates the 2002 depression screening guidelines by recommending "screening adults for depression when staff-assisted depression care supports are in place to assure accurate diagnosis, effective treatment, and follow-up" and by advising against routine screening for depression when such supports are not available. Concerning

major depressive disorder in adolescents aged 12 to 18 years, the USPSTF puts forth in "Major Depressive Disorder in Children and Adolescents" (March 2009, http://www.ahrq.gov/clinic/uspstf/uspschdepr.htm) a similar recommendation by advising screening "when systems are in place to ensure accurate diagnosis, psychotherapy (cognitive-behavioral or interpersonal), and follow-up."

In November 2009 the USPSTF updated its breast cancer screening recommendations from doing annual mammography starting at the age of 40 to doing biennial (every two years) mammography starting at the age of 50. The new guidelines also advise against teaching breast self-examination. The USPSTF determined that the risks of this practice—in terms of unnecessary diagnostic tests and procedures such as fine-needle aspiration and biopsies (invasive procedures that remove some breast tissue cells for examination)—outweigh the benefits. Table 2.3 summarizes the USPSTF guidelines for the use of mammography and other screening tests in breast cancer screening by the age of the woman to be screened and describes the potential benefits, harms, and costs that are associated with screening.

In 2011 the USPSTF issued new guidelines for osteoporosis screening. In "Screening for Osteoporosis" (January 2011, http://www.uspreventiveservicestaskforce.org/uspstf10/osteoporosis/osteors.htm), the USPSTF advises screening for all women beginning at the age of 65 years. Women under the age of 65 years may also be screened if they have a family history of osteoporosis, low body weight, and drug and alcohol use.

BREAST CANCER SCREENING RECOMMENDATIONS GENERATE DEBATE. Many health practitioners, professional associations, and breast cancer survivors assert that women's health will be harmed by adherence to the new recommendations. Others question whether the new guidelines justify rationing preventive services. Still others flatly reject the new guidelines. For example, the ACS advises annual screening using mammography and clinical breast examination for all women beginning at the age of 40 years. In the press release "American Cancer Society Responds to Changes to USPSTF Mammography Guidelines" (November 16, 2009, http://pressroom.cancer.org/index.php?s=43&item=201), the ACS states, "Our experts make this recommendation having reviewed virtually all the same data reviewed by the USPSTF, but also additional data that the USPSTF did not consider. When recommendations are based on judgments about the balance of risks and benefits, reasonable experts can look at the same data and reach different conclusions."

According to the American College of Radiology/ American Roentgen Ray Society, in the press release "USPSTF Mammography Recommendations Will Result in Countless Unnecessary Breast Cancer Deaths Each Year"

FIGURE 2.4

How the USPSTF develops recommendations

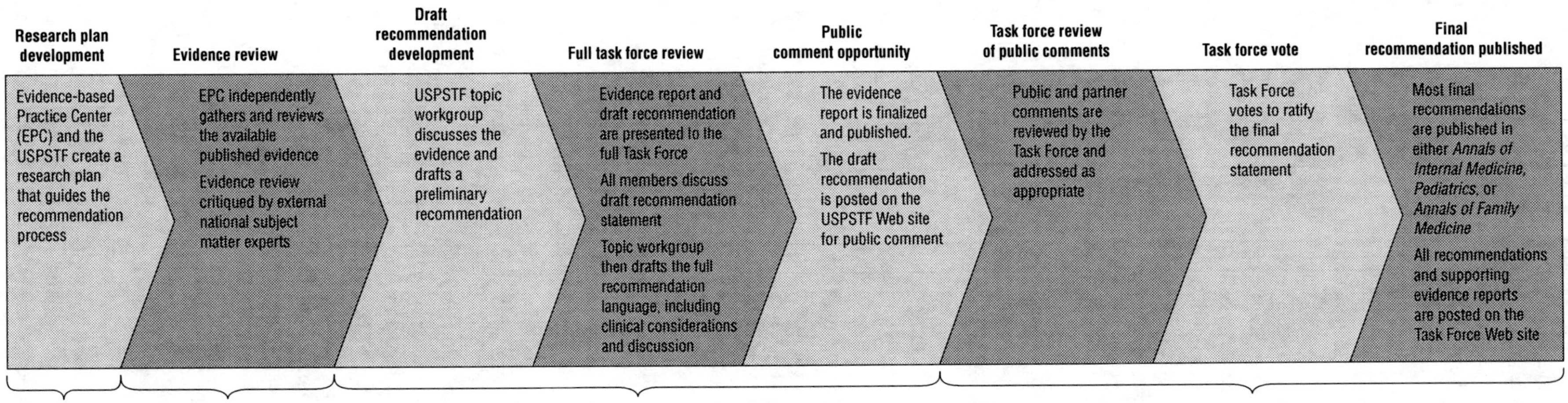

Research plan development	Evidence review	Draft recommendation development	Full task force review	Public comment opportunity	Task force review of public comments	Task force vote	Final recommendation published
Evidence-based Practice Center (EPC) and the USPSTF create a research plan that guides the recommendation process	EPC independently gathers and reviews the available published evidence Evidence review critiqued by external national subject matter experts	USPSTF topic workgroup discusses the evidence and drafts a preliminary recommendation	Evidence report and draft recommendation are presented to the full Task Force All members discuss draft recommendation statement Topic workgroup then drafts the full recommendation language, including clinical considerations and discussion	The evidence report is finalized and published. The draft recommendation is posted on the USPSTF Web site for public comment	Public and partner comments are reviewed by the Task Force and addressed as appropriate	Task Force votes to ratify the final recommendation statement	Most final recommendations are published in either *Annals of Internal Medicine, Pediatrics,* or *Annals of Family Medicine* All recommendations and supporting evidence reports are posted on the Task Force Web site

USPSTF = United States Preventive Services Task Force

SOURCE: "Stages of Development," in *Topics in Progress*, U.S. Preventive Services Task Force, December 2011, http://www.uspreventiveservicestaskforce.org/uspstf/topicsprog.htm (accessed December 17, 2011)

TABLE 2.2

Recommended preventive services, 2010–11

Recommendation	Adults		Special populations	
	Men	Women	Pregnant women	Children
Abdominal aortic aneurysm, screening[a]	X	—	—	—
Alcohol misuse screening and behavioral counseling interventions	X	X	X	—
Aspirin for the prevention of cardiovascular disease[b]	X	X	—	—
Asymptomatic bacteriuria in adults, screening[c]	—	—	X	—
Breast cancer, screening[d]	—	X	—	—
Breast and ovarian cancer susceptibility, genetic risk assessment and breast cancer (BRCA) mutation testing[e]	—	X	—	—
Breast feeding, primary care interventions to promote[f]	—	X	X	—
Cervical cancer, screening[g]	—	X	—	—
Chlamydial infection, screening[h]	—	X	X	—
Colorectal cancer, screening[i]	X	X	—	—
Congenital hypothyroidism, screening[j]	—	—	—	X
Depression (adults), screening[k]	X	X	—	—
Folic acid supplementation[l]	—	X	—	—
Gonorrhea, screening[m]	—	X	—	—
Gonorrhea, prophylactic medication[n]	—	—	—	X
Hearing loss in newborns, screening[o]	—	—	—	X
Hepatitis B virus infection, screening[p]	—	—	X	—
High blood pressure, screening	X	X	—	—
HIV, screening[q]	X	X	X	X
Iron deficiency anemia, prevention[r]	—	—	—	X
Iron deficiency anemia, screening[s]	—	—	X	—
Lipid disorders in adults, screening[t]	X	X	—	—
Major depressive disorder in children and adolescents, screening[u]	—	—	—	X
Obesity in adults, screening[v]	X	X	—	—
Obesity in children and adolescents, screening[w]	—	—	—	X
Osteoporosis, screening[x]	—	X	—	—
Phenylketonuria, screening[y]	—	—	—	X
Rh (D) incompatibility, screening[z]	—	—	X	—
Sexually transmitted infections, counseling[aa]	X	X	—	X
Sickle cell disease, screening[bb]	—	—	—	X
Syphilis infection, screening[cc]	X	X	X	—
Tobacco use and tobacco-caused disease, counseling and interventions[dd]	X	X	X	—
Type 2 diabetes mellitus in adults, screening[ee]	X	X	—	—
Visual impairment in children younger than age 5 years, screening[ff]	—	—	—	X

[a]One-time screening by ultrasonography in men aged 65 to 75 who have ever smoked.
[b]When the potential harm of an increase in gastrointestinal hemorrhage is outweighed by a potential benefit of a reduction in myocardial infarctions (men aged 45–79 years) or in ischemic strokes (women aged 55–79 years).
[c]Pregnant women at 12–16 weeks gestation or at first prenatal visit, if later.
[d]Biennial screening mammography for women aged 50 to 74 years.
[e]Refer women whose family history is associated with an increased risk for deleterious mutations in *BRCA1* or *BRCA2* genes for genetic counseling and evaluation for BRCA testing.
[f]Interventions during pregnancy and after birth to promote and support breast feeding.
[g]Women aged 21–65 who have been sexually active and have a cervix.
[h]Sexually active women 24 and younger and other asymptomatic women at increased risk for infection. Asymptomatic pregnant women 24 and younger and others at increased risk.
[i]Adults aged 50–75 using fecal occult blood testing, sigmoidoscopy, or colonoscopy.
[j]Newborns.
[k]When staff-assisted depression care supports are in place to assure accurate diagnosis, effective treatment, and follow-up.
[l]All women planning or capable of pregnancy take a daily supplement containing 0.4 to 0.8 mg (400 to 800 μg) of folic acid.
[m]Sexually active women, including pregnant women 25 and younger, or at increased risk for infection.
[n]Prophylactic ocular topical medication for all newborns against gonococcal ophthalmia neonatorum.
[o]Newborns.
[p]Pregnant women at first prenatal visit.
[q]All adolescents and adults at increased risk for HIV infection and all pregnant women.
[r]Routine iron supplementation for asymptomatic children aged 6 to 12 months who are at increased risk for iron deficiency anemia.
[s]Routine screening in asymptomatic pregnant women.
[t]Men aged 20–35 and women over age 20 who are at increased risk for coronary heart disease; all men aged 35 and older.
[u]Adolescents (age 12–18) when systems are in place to ensure accurate diagnosis, psychotherapy, and follow-up.
[v]Intensive counseling and behavioral interventions to promote sustained weight loss for obese adults.
[w]Screen children aged 6 years and older for obesity and offer them or refer them to comprehensive, intensive behavioral interventions to promote improvement in weight status.
[x]Women 65 and older and women 60 and older at increased risk for osteoporotic fractures.
[y]Newborns.
[z]Blood typing and antibody testing at first pregnancy-related visit. Repeated antibody testing for unsensitized Rh (D)-negative women at 24–28 weeks gestation unless biological father is known to be Rh (D) negative

(November 16, 2009, http://www.eurekalert.org/pub_releases/2009-11/acor-umr111609.php), Carol H. Lee, the chair of the American College of Radiology Breast Imaging Commission, assails the new guidelines by averring that they "ignore the valid scientific data and place a great many women at risk of dying unnecessarily from a disease that we have made significant headway against over the past 20 years. Mammography is not a perfect test, but it has unquestionably been shown to save lives.…These new recommendations seem to

TABLE 2.2

Recommended preventive services, 2010–11 [CONTINUED]

aaAll sexually active adolescents and adults at increased risk for STIs.
bbNewborns.
ccPersons at increased risk and all pregnant women.
ddAsk all adults about tobacco use and provide tobacco cessation interventions for those who use tobacco; provide augmented, pregnancy-tailored counseling for those pregnant women who smoke.
eeAsymptomatic adults with sustained blood pressure greater than 135/80 mg Hg.
ffTo detect amblyopia, strabismus, and defects in visual acuity.
USPSTF = United States Preventive Service Task Force.

SOURCE: "Section 1. Preventive Services Recommended by the USPSTF," in *Guide to Clinical Preventive Services, 2010–2011: Recommendations of the U.S. Preventive Services Task Force,* August 2010. Agency for Healthcare Research and Quality, Rockville, MD. http://www.ahrq.gov/clinic/pocketgd1011/gcp10s1.htm (accessed December 17, 2011)

reflect a conscious decision to ration care [and] could have deadly effects for American women."

In "Mammogram Math" (*New York Times*, December 10, 2009), John Allen Paulos observes that many people believe that because earlier and more frequent screening increases the odds of detecting cancer, it is always a good idea. However, he notes that the USPSTF guidelines are based on scientific evidence that the risks associated with more frequent mammography, including increased exposure to radiation, unnecessary biopsies, and aggressive treatment of slow-growing cancers that are unlikely to prove fatal, outweigh the benefits of more frequent screening.

TESTICULAR CANCER SCREENING RECOMMENDATIONS GENERATE NO DEBATE. In contrast to the fiery debate that was generated by the breast cancer screening recommendations, the USPSTF's recommendations advising against screening for testicular cancer went almost entirely unnoticed by the media in 2011. In "Screening for Testicular Cancer" (April 2011, http://www.uspreventiveservicestaskforce.org/uspstf10/testicular/testicuprs.htm), the USPSTF observes that testicular cancer is relatively rare—5.4 cases per 100,000 males—and that patients or their partners discover most cases. The USPSTF concludes that "there is inadequate evidence that screening by clinician examination or patient self-examination has a higher yield or greater accuracy for detecting testicular cancer at earlier (and more curable) stages.... Based on the low incidence of this condition and favorable outcomes of treatment, even in cases of advanced disease, there is adequate evidence that the benefits of screening for testicular cancer are small to none."

Screening and Early Detection of Breast and Cervical Cancers

The ACS estimates in *Breast Cancer Facts and Figures 2011–2012* (2011, http://www.cancer.org/acs/groups/content/@epidemiologysurveilance/documents/document/acspc-030975.pdf) that in 2011, 230,480 women were diagnosed with breast cancer and 39,520 died of the disease. In *Cancer Facts and Figures 2011* (2011, http://www.cancer.org/acs/groups/content/@epidemiologysurveilance/documents/document/acspc-029771.pdf), the ACS estimates that 12,710 new cases of cervical cancer were diagnosed in 2011 and that 4,290 women died of the disease. As with many other cancers, treatment for these types of cancer is most likely to be successful when the disease begins, before the cancer has metastasized (spread from its original site to other parts of the body).

In November 2009 the American College of Obstetrics and Gynecologists released new cervical cancer screening guidelines for the Papanicolaou test (also called Pap smear or Pap test). The Pap test is a screening examination for cancer of the cervix that can prevent practically all deaths from cervical cancer by detecting cervical cancer at an early stage, when it is most curable, or even preventing the disease if precancerous lesions found during the test are treated. The incidence of cervical cancer has decreased dramatically over the past 40 years largely due to screening and early treatment. The new guidelines indicate that women should have their first Pap test at age 21 and then should be screened every two years until age 30 as opposed to annually. Women aged 30 years and older should be screened every three years.

According to Saundra Young, in "New Cervical Cancer Screening Guidelines Released" (CNN.com, November 20, 2009), this change in cervical cancer screening frequency did not generate the kind of controversy that surrounded the new mammography screening guidelines because Pap tests detect precancers that can take from 10 to 20 years to develop into cancers. Furthermore, this change was welcomed by professional associations such as the ACS, which "supports the guidelines and said it is reviewing new data and updating its own recommendations."

Even though a vaccine to immunize women against contracting the strain of human papillomavirus (HPV) that causes cervical cancer has been available since 2006, it is only effective for females who have not yet become sexually active and contracted the virus. For this

TABLE 2.3

Recommended screening for breast cancer, 2009

Population	Women aged 40–49 years		Women aged 50–74 years	Women aged ≥75 years
Recommendation	Do not screen routinely. Individualize decision to begin biennial screening according to the patient's context and values.		Screen every 2 years.	No recommendation.
	Grade: C		Grade: B	Grade: I (insufficient evidence)
Risk assessment	This recommendation applies to women aged ≥40 years who are not at increased risk by virtue of a known genetic mutation or history of chest radiation. Increasing age is the most important risk factor for most women.			
Screening tests	Standardization of film mammography has led to improved quality. Refer patients to facilities certified under the Mammography Quality Standards Act (MQSA), listed at www.fda.gov/cdrh/mammmograph/certified.html.			
Timing of screening	Evidence indicates that biennial screening is optimal. A biennial schedule preserves most of the benefit of annual screening and cuts the harms nearly in half. A longer interval may reduce the benefit.			
Balance of harms and benefits	There is convincing evidence that screening with film mammography reduces breast cancer mortality, with a greater absolute reduction for women aged 50 to 74 years than for younger women.			
	Harms of screening include psychological harms, additional medical visits, imaging, and biopsies in women without cancer, inconvenience due to false-positive screening results, harms of unnecessary treatment, and radiation exposure. Harms seem moderate for each age group.			
	False-positive results are a greater concern for younger women; treatment of cancer that would not become clinically apparent during a woman's life (overdiagnosis) is an increasing problem as women age.			
Rationale for no recommendation (I statement)				Among women 75 years or older, evidence of benefit is lacking.
Relevant USPSTF recommendations	USPSTF recommendations on screening for genetic susceptibility for breast cancer and chemoprevention of breast cancer are available at www.preventiveservices.ahrq.gov.			

Population	Women aged ≥40 years			
Screening method	Digital mammography	Magnetic Resonance Imaging (MRI)	Clinical Breast Examination (CBE)	Breast Self-Examination (BSE)
Recommendation		Grade: I (insufficient evidence)		Grade: D
Rationale for no recommendation or negative recommendation	Evidence is lacking for benefits of digital mammography and MRI of the breast as substitutes for film mammography.		Evidence of CBE's additional benefit, beyond mammography, is inadequate.	Adequate evidence suggests that BSE does not reduce breast cancer mortality.
Considerations for practice				
Potential preventable burden	For younger women and women with dense breast tissue, overall detection is somewhat better with digital mammography.	Contrast-enhanced MRI has been shown to detect more cases of cancer in very high-risk populations than does mammography.	Indirect evidence suggests that when CBE is the only test available, it may detect a significant proportion of cancer cases.	
Potential harms	It is not certain whether overdiagnosis occurs more often with digital than with film mammography.	Contrast-enhanced MRI requires injection of contrast material. MRI yields many more false-positive results and potentially more overdiagnosis than mammography.	Harms of CBE include false-positive results, which lead to anxiety, unnecessary visits, imaging, and biopsies.	Harms of BSE include the same potential harms as for CBE and may be larger in magnitude.
Costs	Digital mammography is more expensive than film.	MRI is much more expensive than mammography.	Costs of CBE are primarily opportunity costs to clinicians.	Costs of BSE are primarily opportunity costs to clinicians.
Current practice	Some clinical practices are now switching to digital equipment.	MRI is not currently used to screen women of average risk.	No standard approach or reporting standards are in place.	The number of clinicians who teach BSE to patients is unknown; it is likely that few clinicians teach BSE to all women.

USPSTF = U.S. Preventive Services Task Forces

SOURCE: *Screening for Breast Cancer*, Topic Page, U.S. Preventive Services Task Force, July 2010, http://www.uspreventiveservicestaskforce.org/uspstf/uspsbrca.htm (accessed January 27, 2012)

reason, cervical cancer screening will continue to be important for several generations after widespread immunization has occurred.

Because immunization against HPV must be done before a young woman becomes sexually active, the vaccine is recommended for preteen girls aged 11 years and older. Some parents are uncomfortable with the idea of immunizing their daughters who are years away from risk of exposure. However, according to Richard Knox, in "HPV Vaccine: The Science behind the Controversy" (September 19, 2011, http://www.npr.org/2011/09/19/140543977/hpv-vaccine-the-science-behind-the-controversy), research reveals that before HPV vaccination, about 10%

of girls were infected with the virus by the age of 15 years. Nonetheless, the CDC and physicians' professional organizations, including the American Academy of Pediatrics and the American Academy of Family Physicians, strongly support vaccination and many communities and school districts require it.

In 1990 Congress passed the Breast and Cervical Cancer Mortality Prevention Act, establishing the CDC's National Breast and Cervical Cancer Early Detection Program (NBCCEDP). The NBCCEDP provides breast and pelvic examinations, screening mammography, and Pap tests to women who are at greater risk of death from breast or cervical cancer—racial and ethnic minorities, those who live below the poverty level, older women, and women with less than a high school education.

Between July 2006 and July 2010 the NBCCEDP (September 8, 2011, http://www.cdc.gov/cancer/nbccedp/data/summaries/national_aggregate.htm) had screened over 1.8 million women, and detected 16,076 breast cancers and 28,120 precancerous cervical lesions or cervical cancers. Figure 2.5 shows the number of women who were served by the NBCCEDP for each program year between July 2006 and July 2010. A significant component of the NBCCEDP effort is community education and outreach.

FIGURE 2.5

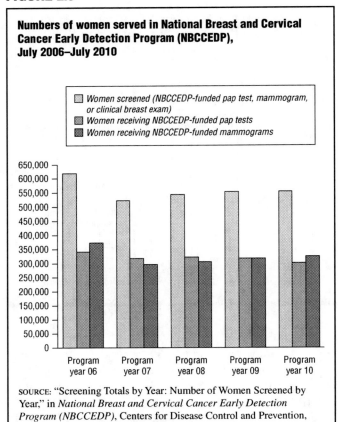

Numbers of women served in National Breast and Cervical Cancer Early Detection Program (NBCCEDP), July 2006–July 2010

☐ Women screened (NBCCEDP-funded pap test, mammogram, or clinical breast exam)
▨ Women receiving NBCCEDP-funded pap tests
▨ Women receiving NBCCEDP-funded mammograms

SOURCE: "Screening Totals by Year: Number of Women Screened by Year," in *National Breast and Cervical Cancer Early Detection Program (NBCCEDP)*, Centers for Disease Control and Prevention, September 8, 2011, http://www.cdc.gov/cancer/nbccedp/data/summaries/national_aggregate.htm (accessed December 17, 2011)

Health educators must not only communicate the life-saving benefits of screening and early identification of disease but also overcome barriers to access to care, such as the lack of transportation or child care.

The NBCCEDP also funds follow-up care for women who have abnormal screening results to enable them to receive needed services. These may include biopsy (surgical removal of a sample of cells for microscopic examination) to confirm the diagnosis and visits with surgeons and other medical specialists to receive timely treatment. The provision of follow-up care and treatment is a fundamental principle underlying screening programs.

Screening programs that do not provide facilities for diagnosis and treatment are unlikely to be effective, especially when they are serving populations that are unable to pay for medical care. Furthermore, many public health professionals believe it is unethical to offer screening without plans and provisions to care for diseases that have been identified through the screening process.

TERTIARY PREVENTION

Tertiary prevention programs aim to improve the quality of life for people with various diseases by limiting complications and disabilities, reducing the severity and progression of disease, and providing rehabilitation (therapy to restore functionality and self-sufficiency). Unlike primary and secondary prevention, tertiary prevention involves actual treatment for the disease and is conducted primarily by health care practitioners, rather than by public health agencies.

Tertiary prevention efforts demonstrate that it is possible to slow the natural course of some progressive diseases and prevent or delay many of the complications that are associated with chronic diseases such as arthritis (inflammation of the joints that causes pain, swelling, and stiffness), asthma (inflammation and obstruction of the airways that makes breathing difficult), heart disease, and diabetes.

Tertiary Prevention of Diabetes

Insulin is a hormone produced by the pancreas to control the amount of glucose (sugar) in the blood. Diabetes mellitus is a disease in which high blood glucose levels result from insufficient insulin production or action. When there is not enough insulin produced, the body is unable to metabolize (use, regulate, and store) glucose, and it remains in the blood.

Type 1 diabetes mellitus (also called insulin-dependent diabetes or juvenile-onset diabetes) occurs when pancreatic beta cells, the cells that make insulin, are destroyed by the body's own immune system. It usually develops in children and young adults. Because people with diabetes do not have enough insulin, they must be injected or inject themselves with insulin several times a day or receive insulin via a pump. In "National Diabetes Statistics, 2011" (February 2011, http://diabetes.niddk.nih.gov/dm/pubs/statistics/), the National Institute of Diabetes and Digestive and Kidney Diseases (NIDDK) states that about 5% to 10% of all diagnosed cases of diabetes are type 1.

Type 2 diabetes mellitus (also called noninsulin-dependent diabetes or adult-onset diabetes) occurs when the body becomes resistant to insulin. As a result of the cells being unable to use insulin effectively, the amount of glucose they can take up is sharply reduced and high levels of glucose accumulate in the blood. The NIDDK notes that approximately 90% to 95% of all diagnosed cases of diabetes are type 2 diabetes.

Many people with type 2 diabetes are able to control their blood sugar by losing excess weight, maintaining proper nutrition, and exercising regularly. Others require insulin injections or orally administered (taken by mouth) drugs to lower their blood sugar.

Other types of diabetes can occur as a result of pregnancy (gestational diabetes) or physiologic stress such as surgery, trauma, malnutrition, infections, and other illnesses. According to the NIDDK, these types of diabetes account for between 1% and 5% of all diagnosed cases of the disease.

The NIDDK reports that of the 8.3% (18.8 million people) of the U.S. population with diabetes, 37% (7 million people) are not aware that they have it. Table 2.4 shows diagnosed and undiagnosed cases of diabetes among people aged 20 years and older in 2010. Another 35% of adults have prediabetes, a condition in which blood sugar is high but not yet in the diabetic range.

COMPLICATIONS OF DIABETES. According to the NIDDK, in "National Diabetes Statistics, 2011," adults with diabetes suffer from heart disease at much higher rates—in fact, heart disease is the number-one cause of death among people with diabetes. Similarly, adults with diabetes have an increased risk for stroke (damage to the brain that occurs when its blood supply is cut off, frequently because of blockage in an artery that supplies the brain) and hypertension (67% of adults with diabetes have high blood pressure). Among people aged 65 years and older, heart disease accounts for 68% of deaths in people with diabetes, and stroke accounts for 16% of deaths. Other serious complications of this disease include:

- Diabetic retinopathy—this is a condition that can cause blindness

- Diabetic neuropathy—this condition causes damage to the nervous system that may produce pain or loss

TABLE 2.4

Diagnosed and undiagnosed diabetes among persons age 20 and older, 2010

Group	Number or percentage who have diabetes
Ages 20 years or older	25.6 million, or 11.3 percent, of all people in this age group
Ages 65 years or older	10.9 million, or 26.9 percent, of all people in this age group
Men	13.0 million, or 11.8 percent, of all men ages 20 years or older
Women	12.6 million, or 10.8 percent, of all women ages 20 years or older
Non-Hispanic whites	15.7 million, or 10.2 percent, of all non-Hispanic whites ages 20 years or older
Non-Hispanic blacks	4.9 million, or 18.7 percent, of all non-Hispanic blacks ages 20 years or older

Note: Sufficient data are not available to estimate the total prevalence of diabetes—diagnosed and undiagnosed—for other U.S. racial/ethnic minority populations.

SOURCE: "Diagnosed and Undiagnosed Diabetes among People Ages 20 Years or Older, United States, 2010," in *National Diabetes Statistics, 2011*, National Institutes of Health, National Institute of Diabetes and Digestive and Kidney Diseases, February 2011, http://diabetes.niddk.nih.gov/dm/pubs/statistics/#Diagnosed20 (accessed December 17, 2011)

of sensation in the hands or feet and other nerve problems

- Kidney disease—diabetes accounts for almost half of all new end-stage renal disease cases that require dialysis (mechanical cleansing of the blood of impurities) or kidney transplant

- Amputation—diabetes is responsible for 60% of all lower-limb amputations (surgical removal of toes, feet, and the leg below the knee) performed in the United States

- Dental disease—gum diseases are common among people with diabetes, and nearly one-third of all people with diabetes have severe periodontal (tooth and gum) diseases

- Problems with pregnancy—diabetes may cause birth defects, miscarriage (spontaneous abortion), and excessively large babies that may create additional health risks for expectant mothers

- Increased risk of infection—people with diabetes are more susceptible to infection and do not recover as quickly as people without diabetes

Furthermore, poorly controlled or uncontrolled diabetes may produce life-threatening medical emergencies, such as diabetic ketoacidosis (excessive ketones—chemicals in the blood resulting from insufficient insulin and an excessive amount of counterregulatory hormones such as glucagon) or hyperosmolar coma (extremely high blood glucose, leading to dehydration).

Achieving optimal control of blood glucose levels can prevent many of the complications of diabetes and decrease the risk of death that is associated with the disease. Optimal control involves aggressive treatment of diabetes with close attention to the roles of diet, exercise, weight management, and pharmacology (proper use of insulin and other medication) in the self-management of the disease.

PREVENTING COMPLICATIONS OF DIABETES. In "National Diabetes Statistics, 2011," the NIDDK explains that even modest improvement in controlling blood glucose acts to help prevent diabetic retinopathy, neuropathy, and kidney disease. Reducing blood pressure can decrease cardiovascular complications (heart disease and stroke) by as much as 50% and can reduce the risk of retinopathy, neuropathy, and kidney disease by 33%. Lowering blood cholesterol (a waxy substance produced by the body and found in animal products), low-density lipoproteins (LDL), and triglycerides also reduces, by as much as 50%, the cardiovascular complications of diabetes. (Cholesterol, LDL, and triglycerides are lipids that may be measured in the blood.)

The NIDDK reports that early detection and treatment of diabetic eye disease can reduce by 50% to 60% the possibility of blindness or serious loss of vision. Similarly, early detection and treatment of kidney disease sharply reduces the risk of developing kidney failure, and careful attention to foot care reduces the risk of amputation by as much as 85%.

To help increase early detection of diabetes (secondary prevention) and reduce the morbidity (illnesses) and mortality (deaths) associated with it (tertiary prevention), the CDC and the NIDDK launched the National Diabetes Education Program (NDEP) in 1997. The NDEP's objectives are to increase public awareness of diabetes, improve self-management of people with diabetes, enhance health care providers' knowledge and treatment of diabetes, and promote health policies that improve access, availability, and quality of diabetes care. To meet these educational objectives, the NDEP, in working with a variety of other health organizations, develops and distributes teaching tools and resources.

The NDEP enumerates in the fact sheet "Changing the Way Diabetes Is Treated" (July 2009, http://ndep.nih.gov/media/NDEP_FactSheet.pdf) the strategies it employs to achieve the NDEP goal of reducing illness and death caused by diabetes and its complications. These strategies are intended to:

- Create program partnerships with organizations concerned about diabetes and the health status of their members.
- Develop and implement ongoing diabetes awareness and education campaigns for health care professionals and people with or at risk for diabetes.

- Identify, develop, promote, and disseminate educational tools and resources for people with diabetes and those at risk, including materials that address the needs of special populations.
- Disseminate guiding principles that promote quality diabetes care to health care professionals, payers, purchasers, and policy makers.
- Promote policies and activities to improve the quality of and access to care for people with and at risk for diabetes.
- Address the economic case for quality diabetes care to inform health care payers, purchasers, and policy makers.

The NDEP partners with more than 200 public and private organizations that are concerned about diabetes. These organizations assist by:

- Disseminating the NDEP's messages within their organization and the communities they serve
- Customizing messages for target audiences
- Producing and promoting cooperative education programs and sharing resources with other partner organizations
- Using NDEP resources to improve quality of care and access the health care delivery system

EXEMPLARY MENTAL HEALTH PREVENTION PROGRAMS

This section presents a national mental health and suicide risk screening program for youth that is described in *Achieving the Promise: Transforming Mental Health Care in America* (July 2003) by the President's New Freedom Commission on Mental Health. It also offers recommendations and descriptions of interventions that are considered to be effective at preventing suicide from *Reducing Suicide: A National Imperative* (2002, http://www.nap.edu/books/0309083214/html/), which was edited by Sara K. Goldsmith et al.

Goldsmith et al. characterize current mental health prevention programs as rooted in the "universal, selective, and indicated prevention model." This model considers three defined populations: the entire population is included in universal programs, specific high-risk groups are targeted by selective programs, and indicated programs address specific high-risk individuals. Universal programming assumes a basically healthy population and generally aims at protection against developing a disorder by offering, for example, enhanced coping skills and resiliency training. Examples of universal programs are educational programs that heighten awareness of a problem and mass-media campaigns that are intended to increase understanding of and attitudes about a particular issue.

Population-based programs often produce greater gains than programs that target individuals because there are higher rates of program participation. For example, all the students in a given grade will be exposed to school-based drug prevention programs. Selective programs target subsets of populations that have been identified as at risk but are not yet diagnosed with a specific problem or disorder—people who have a greater-than-average likelihood of developing mental disorders, such as adolescents with truancy or suspected substance abuse problems. Indicated programs are aimed at specific high-risk individuals who have presented early signs or symptoms of mental disorders, such as children diagnosed with attention deficit/hyperactivity disorder, who may be at a greater risk of developing conduct disorders, or students who have engaged in disruptive or other disturbed behavior at school.

By recounting the histories, benefits, and scientific evaluation of mental health prevention programs, *Achieving the Promise* and *Reducing Suicide* offer a framework for developing and implementing mental health prevention programs and policies in a wide range of settings, including primary medical care practices and clinics, maternal and infant health and mental health programs, child care centers, school-based health centers, vocational training programs, social service agencies, parent education programs, and the media. Furthermore, these reports disseminate the methods and results of effective programs that have demonstrated efficacy, enabling mental health service providers and other stakeholders throughout the country to replicate these results in their local communities.

Adolescent Intervention Programs

One recommendation from *Achieving the Promise* is to "improve and expand school mental health programs." The commission cites research demonstrating that about 42% of students with serious emotional disturbances graduate from high school, compared with 57% of students with other disabilities. The commission believes this could be changed, because it finds ample evidence that school mental health programs improved academic achievement—with improved test scores, fewer absences, and less discipline problems—by detecting mental health problems early and providing timely referral to appropriate treatment.

The commission observes that the concerted effort needed to deliver quality mental health services in schools entails collaboration with parents and local providers of mental health care to support screening, assessment, and early intervention. It also asserts that mental health services must be integral parts of school health centers and that federal funds must be available to support the programs.

The commission lauds the Columbia University TeenScreen program as a model program of screening and early intervention. The program ensures mental health screening of all students before they leave high school and early identification of students who are at risk for suicide or those with symptoms of depression or other mental illness. A follow-up study found that the program is remarkably effective—of the students who were identified as at risk, more than 60% continued to have recurrent mental health problems or mental disorders four to six years later. Table 2.5 summarizes the goals, features,

TABLE 2.5

Columbia University teen mental health screening program

Program	Columbia University TeenScreen® Program
Goal	To ensure that all youth are offered a mental health check-up before graduating from high school. TeenScreen® identifies and refers for treatment those who are at risk for suicide or suffer from an untreated mental illness.
Features	All youngsters in a school, with parental consent, are given a computer-based questionnaire that screens them for mental illnesses and suicide risk. At no charge, the Columbia University TeenScreen® Program provides consultation, screening materials, software, training, and technical assistance to qualifying schools and communities. In return, TeenScreen® partners are expected to screen at least 200 youth per year and ensure that a licensed mental health professional is on-site to give immediate counseling and referral services for youth at greatest risk. The Columbia TeenScreen® Program is a not-for-profit organization funded solely by foundations. When the program identifies youth needing treatment, their care is paid for depending on the family's health coverage.
Outcomes	The computer-based questionnaire used by TeenScreen® is a valid and reliable screening instrument.[a] The vast majority of youth identified through the program as having already made a suicide attempt, or at risk for depression or suicidal thinking, are not in treatments.[b] A follow-up study found that screening in high school identified more than 60% of students who, four to six years later, continued to have long-term, recurrent problems with depression and suicidal attempts.[c]
Biggest challenge	To bridge the gap between schools and local providers of mental health services. Another challenge is to ensure, in times of fiscal austerity, that schools devote a health professional to screening and referral.
How other organizations can adopt	The Columbia University TeenScreen® program is pilot-testing a shorter questionnaire, which will be less costly and time-consuming for the school to administer. It is also trying to adapt the program to primary care settings.
Website	www.teenscreen.org
Sites where implemented	69 sites (mostly middle schools and high schools) in 27 states

[a]Shaffer, D., Fisher, P., Lucas, C. P., Dulcan, M. K., & Schwab-Stone, M. E. (2000). NIMH Diagnostic Interview Schedule for Children Version IV (NIMH DISC-IV): Description, differences from previous versions, and reliability of some common diagnoses. Journal of the American Academy of Child and Adolescent Psychiatry, 39, 28–38.
[b]Shaffer, D. & Craft, L. (1999). Methods of adolescent suicide prevention. Journal of Clinical Psychiatry, 60, Supplement 2, 70–74.
[c]Leslie McGuire, personal communication, June 24, 2003.

SOURCE: "Figure 4.2. Model Program: Screening Program for Youth," in *Achieving the Promise: Transforming Mental Health Care in America*, President's New Freedom Commission on Mental Health, 2003

outcomes, and principal challenges that were faced during implementation of the TeenScreen program.

Participants complete a 10-minute paper-and-pencil or computerized questionnaire. The questionnaire covers anxiety, depression, substance and alcohol abuse, and suicidal thoughts and behavior. The TeenScreen program does not recommend any particular type of treatment for the teens who are identified by the mental health screening. Parents of students who are identified as at possible risk are notified and offered information and referral to local mental health services where they can obtain further evaluation. No student is screened without parental consent, and the results of the screen are confidential. Screening occurs in a range of venues, including schools, clinics, physicians' offices, and juvenile justice facilities.

Screening increases the likelihood that students who are at risk for suicidal behavior will get into treatment. Madelyn S. Gould et al. indicate in "Service Use by At-Risk Youths after School-Based Suicide Screening" (*Journal of the American Academy of Child and Adolescent Psychiatry*, vol. 48, no. 12, December 2009) that school-based mental health assessments effectively identify adolescents who are at risk for suicidal behavior and help ensure high rates of follow-up treatment. The researchers indicate that nearly 70% of the adolescents who were identified by a school-based suicide screening effort followed through on referrals to treatment within one year. According to the TeenScreen National Center for Mental Health Checkups at Columbia University, in the press release "School-Based Mental Health Checkups Lead to High Rates of Follow-Up Care for Teens" (November 20, 2009, http://www.teenscreen.org/images/stories/PDF/Gould%20press%20release%2011%2018%2009%20FINAL.pdf), Laurie Flynn, the executive director of the TeenScreen National Center for Mental Health Checkups, said, "This study tells us adults, as parents and educators, that we are key players in improving our young peoples' access to care for mental illness. Dr. Gould's study affirms that mental health checkups are effective and that at-risk teens identified through school-based screenings are able to get help. As with any medical condition, the earlier you can identify illness and begin treatment, the better the outcome."

Countywide Primary Prevention to Reduce Substance Abuse and Improve Mental Health

In "A Primary Prevention Framework for Substance Abuse and Mental Health" (March 2009, http://www.preventioninstitute.org/component/jlibrary/article/id-53/127.html), the Prevention Institute describes a countywide effort by the Behavioral Health and Recovery Services of the San Mateo County Health System to promote mental health and emotional resilience and well-being. According to the Prevention Institute, the comprehensive program aims to "help prevent certain conditions, reduce or delay onset and severity of symptoms, and promote positive well-being for all." The Behavioral Health and Recovery Services developed the following strategies to achieve these aims:

- Improve and enhance the places where people live, work, play, attend school, worship, and socialize to support emotional and psychological health, reduce substance abuse, and decrease exposure to violence. This strategy involves actions that reduce access to and availability of alcohol and drugs; ensure availability of housing; enhance safety; and cultivate physical environments that promote and support social connections.

- Strengthen social connections to reduce isolation, substance abuse, and exposure to violence. This strategy entails the development of programs that support people of all ages to develop and maintain social connections and be involved in their community.

- Reduce stigma for people with mental illness and those who are at risk for mental illness and substance abuse. This strategy involves developing economic opportunities for those who are at risk to support and maintain financial self-sufficiency.

- Engage all stakeholders as partners in the effort to foster "prosperity to improve emotional health, promote mental well-being, reduce substance abuse, and decrease exposure to violence." This strategy involves participation of multiple sectors including the local government, the business community, and community members—consumers, clients of mental health and substance abuse services, and family members.

PREVENTING SUICIDE

In the landmark report *Mental Health: A Report of the Surgeon General* (1999, http://www.surgeongeneral.gov/library/mentalhealth/home.html), the Office of the Surgeon General states that suicide is a serious public health problem and recommends a three-pronged national strategy to prevent suicide, which includes programs that educate, heighten understanding, intervene, and advance the science of suicide prevention. Table 2.6 shows the components of AIM (awareness, intervention, and methodology)—the national strategy for suicide prevention—as well as the risk factors and protective factors for suicide.

According to the National Institutes of Health, in "Suicide Facts at a Glance" (Summer 2009, http://www.cdc.gov/violenceprevention/pdf/Suicide-DataSheet-a.pdf), in 2006 more than 33,000 suicides occurred. There was one suicide for every 25 attempted suicides. In 2007, 14.5% of high school students (grades nine to 12) said

TABLE 2.6

Suicide risk factors, protective factors, and national prevention strategy

- National Strategy for Suicide Prevention: AIM
  - Awareness: promote public awareness of suicide as a public health problem
  - Intervention: enhance services and programs
  - Methodology: advance the science of suicide prevention
- Risk factors
  - Male gender
  - Mental disorders, particularly depression and substance abuse
  - Prior suicide attempts
  - Unwillingness to seek help because of stigma
  - Barriers to accessing mental health treatment
  - Stressful life event/loss
  - Easy access to lethal methods such as guns
- Protective factors
  - Effective and appropriate clinical care for underlying disorders
  - Easy access to care
  - Support from family, community, and health and mental health care staff

SOURCE: Adapted from "Figure 4-1. Surgeon General's Call to Action to Prevent Suicide—1999," in *Mental Health: A Report of the Surgeon General*, U.S. Department of Health and Human Services, Substance Abuse and Mental Health Services Administration, Center for Mental Health Services, with the National Institute of Mental Health, 1999, http://www.surgeongeneral.gov/library/mentalhealth/toc.html#chapter4 (accessed December 18, 2011)

they had seriously considered suicide in the previous 12 months, 6.9% of students reported trying to commit suicide at least once in the previous 12 months, and 2% of students had tried to commit suicide that resulted in an injury, poisoning, or overdose that required medical attention.

The CDC describes in "Preventing Suicide: Program Activities Guide" (October 2010, http://www.cdc.gov/violenceprevention/pdf/PreventingSuicide-a.pdf) activities in key prevention areas, including surveillance, research, capacity building, communication, partnership, and leadership. The CDC's violence prevention activities emphasize primary prevention by advancing the science of prevention, translating scientific advances into practical applications, and building on existing efforts to address community needs or gaps in preventive services. Ongoing activities include:

- Monitoring, tracking, and researching the problem. State and local agencies work together to gather data that enable policy and community leaders to make informed decisions about violence prevention programs and strategies. Other CDC research focuses on the relationship between different forms of violent behavior and suicide among adolescent and school-associated violent deaths.

- Supporting and enhancing prevention programs that are university- and school-based as well as multistate and national prevention and education initiatives that promote awareness of suicide as a preventable public health problem.

- Providing prevention resources, such as a toll-free hotline, a website, or a fax-on-demand service that supplies prevention information and print publications.

- Encouraging research and development on violence, injury, and suicide prevention in specific populations such as adolescents making the transition to early adulthood, urban youth, and youth identified as at risk for suicidal behavior by screening programs.

ACTIVE MILITARY AND VETERANS ARE AT RISK FOR SUICIDE

According to Robin B. McFee, in "Gulf War Servicemen and Servicewomen: The Long Road Home and the Role of Health Care Professionals to Enhance the Troops' Health and Healing" (*Disease-a-Month*, vol. 54, no. 5, May 2008), returning from war presents a wide range of physical and psychological risks, injuries, and therapeutic challenges. Troops must reenter society after experiencing the horrors of war, the loss of friends, injuries, and deprivation not encountered in the United States. Unlike earlier wars, such as World War II (1939–1945) or the Korean War (1950–1953), most U.S. citizens are not involved with the war in Afghanistan (nor were they with the war in Iraq) on a daily basis, and as a result many communities lack support for returning veterans.

In "Rising Military Suicides" (November 25, 2009, http://www.congress.org/news/2009/11/25/rising_military_suicides), John Donnelly observes that "more U.S. military personnel have taken their own lives so far in 2009 than have been killed in either the Afghanistan or Iraq wars." Between January and November 2009, 334 members of the U.S. military had committed suicide, compared with 297 killed in Afghanistan and 144 killed in Iraq. Of the 334 military personnel who committed suicide, 211 were in the U.S. Army, 47 were in the U.S. Navy, 42 were in the U.S. Marine Corps (active duty only), and 34 were in the U.S. Air Force. These numbers are alarming because members of the U.S. military have generally had much lower rates of suicide than the U.S. population, which according to the CDC is about 20 per 100,000 among men aged 20 to 29 years. For example, the army reported just 9 suicides per 100,000 active duty troops in 2001, and the Marine Corps reported 12.5 per 100,000 in 2002. By 2008 the army rate had risen to 20.2 per 100,000 and the Marine Corps rate was 19.5 per 100,000. Even though it may not be the sole contributing factor to the rising number, Donnelly observes that "the rising number of suicides has coincided with U.S. military forces redeploying frequently to Iraq and Afghanistan."

Amanda Edwards-Stewart et al. report in "Military and Civilian Media Coverage of Suicide" (*Archives of Suicide Research*, vol. 15, no. 4, October 2011) that "military suicide has increased over the past decade."

The researchers caution that media attention to military suicides can potentially increase the risk for both military and civilian suicide. Edwards-Stewart et al. looked at 240 media reports of suicide to determine how well they complied with the guidelines from the Suicide Prevention Resource Center and found that nearly all the accounts strayed from the guidelines. Accounts of military suicides tended to reference failed psychological treatment, whereas those of civilians were more likely to romanticize the victim. Edwards-Stewart et al. call for further research to better characterize media bias in reporting suicide and the impact of bias on the occurrence of suicide.

Identifying Troops and Veterans Who Are at Risk for Suicide

The U.S. Department of Veterans Affairs (VA) identifies in "How to Recognize When to Ask for Help" (August 30, 2011, http://www.mentalhealth.va.gov/suicide_prevention/whentoaskforhelp.asp) veteran-specific risks for suicide, including:

- Frequent deployments

- Deployments to hostile environments

- Exposure to extreme stress

- Physical/sexual assault while in the service (not limited to women)

- Length of deployments

- Service-related injury

The VA also instructs health professionals about how to identify and respond to risk for suicide. Table 2.7 enumerates the warning signs for suicide risk.

Jitender Sareen and Shay-Lee Belik note in "The Need for Outreach in Preventing Suicide among Young Veterans" (*PLoS Medicine*, vol. 6, no. 3, March 3, 2009) that suicide is the second-most common cause of death in the U.S. military and that most service members with mental health problems do not seek or receive treatment. One study finds that just one out of five veterans who committed suicide had any contact with a mental health professional. Sareen and Belik describe five major areas of suicide prevention:

- Education and awareness programs for the general public and professionals

- Screening methods for high-risk people

- Treatment of psychiatric disorders

- Restricting access to lethal means

- Safe media reporting of suicide to minimize the risk of so-called copycat suicides, especially in youth

In "Military Veteran Mortality Following a Survived Suicide Attempt" (*BMC Public Health*, May 23, 2011),

TABLE 2.7

Warning signs for suicide risk

Look for the warning signs

- Threatening to hurt or kill self
- Looking for ways to kill self
- Seeking access to pills, weapons or other means
- Talking or writing about death, dying or suicide

Presence of any of the above warning signs requires immediate attention and referral. Consider hospitalization for safety until complete assessment may be made.

Additional warning signs

- Hopelessness
- Rage, anger, seeking revenge
- Acting reckless or engaging in risky activities, seemingly without thinking
- Feeling trapped—like there is no way out
- Increasing alcohol or drug abuse
- Withdrawing from friends, family and society
- Anxiety, agitation, unable to sleep or sleeping all the time
- Dramatic changes in mood
- No reason for living, no sense of purpose in life

For any of the above refer for mental health treatment or assure that follow-up appointment is made.

SOURCE: "Look for the Warning Signs," in *Suicide Risk Assessment Guide*, U.S. Department of Veterans Affairs, December 11, 2009, http://www.mentalhealth.va.gov/docs/Suicide-Risk-Assessment-Guide.pdf (accessed December 19, 2011)

Janet Weiner et al. analyze the deaths of U.S. military veterans after they were hospitalized for a suicide attempt. The researchers find that the veterans who attempted suicide had a greater risk of death from all causes—the risk of mortality among veterans was about three times higher than expected among their age peers. Much of the excess mortality was attributable to heart disease, suicide, unintentional injury, and cancer.

The VA Suicide Prevention Program Expands

The VA describes its Veterans Crisis Line in "How to Recognize When to Ask for Help." The crisis line is available 24 hours per day, seven days per week, and is staffed by trained mental health counselors. In "About the Veterans Crisis Line" (2012, http://www.veteranscrisisline.net/About/AboutVeteransCrisisLine.aspx), the VA states that since 1997 the line "has answered more than 500,000 calls and made more than 18,000 life-saving rescues."

In July 2009 the VA launched an online chat service that provides a forum where veterans, their families, and friends can chat anonymously with a trained VA counselor. Should the counselor identify the person's problem as a crisis or emergency, he or she can provide immediate assistance by connecting the person online to the Veterans Crisis Line for counseling and crisis intervention services. The online service is an outreach program that is intended to communicate with and inform all veterans—not only those enrolled in the VA health care system—and offer them immediate online access to peer support and trained counselors who can provide anonymous suicide prevention services. According to the VA, the online chat service has helped over 28,000 people.

The U.S. Air Force Suicide Prevention Program

The suicide prevention program initiated by the U.S. Air Force is comprehensive and acts to increase knowledge and change attitudes within a community, dispel barriers to treatment, and improve access to support and intervention. According to Kerry L. Knox et al., in "The US Air Force Suicide Prevention Program: Implications for Public Health Policy" (*American Journal of Public Health*, vol. 100, no. 12, December 2010), the program is effective. Since its launching in 1997 the program has helped decreased suicides from an average of 3 per 100,000 people per quarter to 2 per 100,000 people per quarter.

The Air Force Suicide Prevention Program is a population-based, community approach to suicide risk prevention and behavioral health promotion. It integrates human, medical, and mental health services by uniting a coalition of community agencies from within and outside the health care delivery system to significantly reduce suicide among air force personnel, which had risen to an all-time high during the mid-1990s.

The program attempts to reduce risk factors, such as problems with finances, intimate relationships, mental health, job performance, substance abuse, social isolation, and poor coping skills. It simultaneously seeks to strengthen protective factors such as effective coping skills, a sense of social connectedness, and policies and norms that encourage effective help-seeking behaviors. To stimulate help-seeking behaviors, the program stresses the urgent need for air force leaders, supervisors, and frontline workers to support one another during times of heightened life stress. It exhorts members of the air force to seek help from mental health clinics and observes that seeking help early is likely to enhance careers rather than hinder them. The program instructs commanders and supervisors to support and protect those who seek mental health care and eliminates policies that previously served as barriers to seeking and obtaining mental health care.

To improve surveillance, a web-based database is used to capture demographic, risk factor, and protective factor information about individuals who attempted or completed suicide. This extremely secure tool protects privacy and permits timely detection of changes in patterns in suicidal behavior that can be used to strengthen policies and enhance practices throughout the air force community. To improve crisis management, critical incident stress management teams are assembled and sent to installations that are hit hard by potentially traumatizing events such as combat deployments, serious aircraft accidents, natural disasters, and suicides within the units.

The air force experience is not necessarily applicable to the general population, because the air force is a tightly controlled and relatively homogenous community with identifiable leaders readily able to influence community norms and priorities. Regardless, it can still serve as a model for comparable hierarchical organizations and offer insight into prevention program planning. The program's overarching principles, such as engaging community leaders to change cultural norms, improving coordination of diverse human and health services, and providing educational programs to community members, can inform national efforts and may be replicable in other populations.

PREVENTION RESEARCH AND GOALS

In 1986 Congress funded the first Prevention Research Centers. In "Prevention Research Centers—Building the Public Health Research Base with Community Partners: At a Glance 2011" (May 4, 2011, http://www.cdc.gov/chronicdisease/resources/publications/AAG/prc.htm), the CDC indicates that as of 2011, 37 such centers were affiliated with medical schools or schools of public health. The centers explore and research a wide range of public health problems and test strategies to address these problems. In 2011 hundreds of funded projects were examining programs that addressed myriad prevention efforts such as childhood obesity, reducing smoking, promoting healthy aging, and workplace safety.

Primary prevention research and programming in the past aimed to prevent illness by more effectively encouraging people to avoid behaviors (such as smoking, abusing drugs, engaging in unsafe sexual practices, or overeating) that were linked to health risk. By 2012 prevention research and education also emphasized preventing falls among older adults, helping teens to delay sexual behavior, and reducing environmental exposures (such as sun, water pollution, radon, ozone, pesticides, and hazardous chemicals) that increase health risk.

SATISFYING WORK, SOCIAL ACTIVITIES, AND PERSONAL RELATIONSHIPS ARE KEY TO HEALTH AND WELLNESS

Family, friends, active interests, and community involvement may do more than simply help people enjoy their lives. Social activities and relationships may actually enable people to live longer by preventing or delaying the development of many diseases, including dementia. During the past two decades research has demonstrated that social experiences, activities, relationships, and work stress are related to health, well-being, and longevity. The kind of work stress that causes the greatest harm to physical and mental health is effort-reward imbalance—when great effort is made and the effort is neither recognized nor rewarded. Even though women appear more vulnerable to work stress, men's health seems more dependent on the availability of social relationships and emotional support.

Several studies, such as the landmark RAND Corporation's "Health, Marriage, and Longer Life for Men" (1998, http://www.rand.org/pubs/research_briefs/RB5018/index1.html), show that marriage or living with a partner has greater health benefits for men than for women, because traditionally women are caregivers. More recent findings, such as a comparison of blood pressure and mental health among people who are happily married, unhappily married, and single, question whether the nurturing qualities of women are solely responsible for married men's improved health. Julianne Holt-Lunstad, Wendy Birmingham, and Brandon Q. Jones find in "Is There Something Unique about Marriage? The Relative Impact of Marital Status, Relationship Quality, and Network Social Support on Ambulatory Blood Pressure and Mental Health" (*Annals of Behavioral Medicine*, vol. 35, no. 2, April 2008) that both marital status and marital quality influence health status. Married people reported greater satisfaction with life and lower blood pressure than single individuals. Among married people, those who deemed their marital quality "higher" had lower blood pressure, lower stress, less depression, and reported higher levels of overall satisfaction with life. Holt-Lunstad, Birmingham, and Jones also observe that men and women living alone had better health than those with unsatisfactory relationships with their partner.

Cheryl A. Frye of the University at Albany, State University of New York, finds in "Neurosteroids' Effects and Mechanisms for Social, Cognitive, Emotional, and Physical Functions" (*Psychoneuroendocrinology*, vol. 34, suppl. 1, December 2009) that social supports—their presence or absence—may influence the course of age-related changes in physical, mental, and emotional health and well-being. The loss of close relationships, especially among older adults, is one of the greatest risk factors for mental and physical decline. Emerging research suggests that these changes may be hormonally mediated, and Frye indicates that "further understanding of these neurobiological and/or behavioral factors may lead to findings that ultimately can promote health and prevent disease."

Along with personal relationships, social activities also seem to protect against disease and increase longevity, even when the activities do not involve physical exercise. In "The Quality of Dyadic Relationships, Leisure Activities and Health among Older Women" (*Health Care for Women International*, vol. 30, no. 12, December 2009), Tanya R. Fitzpatrick of McGill University examines the influence of social relationships and leisure activities on the health of older women and finds that the quality of interpersonal relationships "has a strong influence on mental health measured by spirit,

happiness, and an interesting life." Furthermore, Fitzpatrick observes that leisure activities not only predict but also improve physical health as measured by self-report and the number of chronic health conditions. There is also evidence that close relationships can substitute for other close relationships. This is a key concern because the death of a spouse or a close friend may increase the survivor's risk for social isolation. The observation that strong connections with children, relatives, and friends can substitute for relationships with spouses or partners is especially significant for widowed, divorced, or never-married older adults.

There is mounting evidence of the health benefits of socialization. The National Social Life, Health, and Aging Project (NSHAP) considers indicators of social connectedness, social participation, social support, and loneliness among older adults. Erin York Cornwell and Linda J. Waite analyze in "Measuring Social Isolation among Older Adults Using Multiple Indicators from the NSHAP Study" (*Journals of Gerontology Series B: Psychological Sciences and Social Sciences*, vol. 64, supp. 1, November 2009) two aspects of social isolation: social disconnectedness (defined as physical separation from others) and perceived isolation. The researchers find that, in general, social disconnectedness does not vary across age groups, but that the oldest older adults (aged 75 years and older) do feel more isolated than younger older adults (aged 65 to 75 years). Furthermore, Cornwell and Waite reconfirm the association between social supports and health outcomes reported in earlier studies, in that social disconnectedness and perceived isolation are greater among those who have worse health.

In "Trajectories of Social Engagement and Limitations in Late Life" (*Journal of Health and Social Behavior*, vol. 52, no. 4, December 2011), Patricia A. Thomas of the University of Texas, Austin, confirms the observation that maintaining high levels of social interaction and engagement exerts a protective effect on the health of older adults. Thomas looked at how changing frequency and intensity of social interaction influenced the physical health and cognitive abilities of older adults. Survey participants were asked how often they attended religious services, visited with friends and family, and participated in volunteer activities, organizations, or special-interest clubs. Thomas posits that social interaction and engagement may act to prevent cognitive and physical decline by giving older adults a sense of purpose in their lives and motivating them to engage in healthy behaviors.

Pets Are More Than Best Friends; They Can Help Keep People Healthy

Research conducted during the late 1990s found that pet ownership was associated with better health. At first it was believed that the effects were simply increased well-being—the obvious delight of hospital and nursing home patients petting puppies, watching kittens play, or viewing fish in an aquarium clearly demonstrated pets' abilities to enhance mood and stimulate social interactions.

However, in March 1999 Parminder Raina et al. reported in "Influence of Companion Animals on the Physical and Psychological Health of Older People: An Analysis of a One-Year Longitudinal Study" (*Journal of the American Geriatrics Society*, vol. 47, no. 3) that attachment to a companion animal was linked to maintaining or slightly improving the physical and psychological well-being of older adults. The researchers followed 1,054 older adults for one year and found that pet owners were better able to perform the activities of daily living and were more satisfied with their physical health, mental health, family relationships, living arrangements, finances, and friends. These findings were confirmed by Karen Allen, Jim Blascovich, and Wendy B. Mendes in "Cardiovascular Reactivity and the Presence of Pets, Friends, and Spouses: The Truth about Cats and Dogs" (*Psychosomatic Medicine*, vol. 64, no. 5, September 1, 2002).

Other research reveals the specific health benefits of human interaction with animals. Erika Friedmann et al. examine in "Relation between Pet Ownership and Heart Rate Variability in Patients with Healed Myocardial Infarcts" (*American Journal of Cardiology*, vol. 91, no. 6, March 2003) the differences in survival between pet owners and nonowners who suffered heart attacks over a two-year period. The researchers find that subjects without pets had reduced heart rate variability, which was associated with an increased risk of cardiac disease and mortality. Several researchers observe that petting dogs and cats actually lowers blood pressure. The physiologic mechanisms responsible for these health benefits are as yet unidentified; however, some researchers think that pets connect people to the natural world, enabling them to focus on others, rather than simply on themselves. Other researchers observe that dog owners walk more than people without dogs and credit pet owners' improved health to exercise. Nearly all agree that the nonjudgmental affection pets offer boosts health and wellness.

Erika Friedmann and Heesook Son assert in "The Human-Companion Animal Bond: How Humans Benefit" (*Veterinary Clinics of North America Small Animal Practice*, vol. 39, no. 2, March 2009) that pet ownership, or just the presence of a companion animal, is associated with health benefits, including improvements in mental, social, and physiologic health status. In "The Benefits of Human-Companion Animal Interaction: A Review" (*Journal of Veterinary Medical Education*, vol. 35, no.

4, Winter 2008), a review of research published since 1980 about the benefits of human-companion animal bonds, Sandra B. Barker and Aaron R. Wolen conclude that many studies support the health benefits of interacting with companion animals. The researchers call for more rigorous research to increase the understanding of the dynamics of these interactions and how they exert benefits on human health.

In "Friends with Benefits: On the Positive Consequences of Pet Ownership" (*Journal of Personality and Social Psychology*, vol. 101, no. 6, December 2011), Allen R. McConnell et al. assert that the emotional benefits of pet ownership rival those of human friendship. The researchers observe that "pet owners had greater self-esteem, were more physically fit, tended to be less lonely, were more conscientious, were more extraverted, tended to be less fearful and tended to be less preoccupied than non-owners" and find "considerable evidence that pets benefit the lives of their owners, both psychologically and physically, by serving as an important source of social support."

Healthy People 2020

Since 1979 the U.S. Department of Health and Human Services has been compiling scientific insights and advances in medicine from each decade to develop 10-year national objectives for promoting health and preventing disease. In *Healthy People 2020 Framework* (December 19, 2011, http://healthypeople.gov/2020/consortium/HP2020Framework.pdf), the Department of Health and Human Services explains that Healthy People 2020 builds on previous public health objectives and aims to "expand its focus to emphasize health-enhancing social and physical environments. Integrating prevention into the continuum of education—from the earliest ages on—is an integral part of this ecological and determinants approach." Its overarching goals are to:

- Attain high-quality, longer lives free of preventable disease, disability, injury, and premature death.

- Achieve health equity, eliminate disparities, and improve the health of all groups.

- Create social and physical environments that promote good health for all.

- Promote quality of life, healthy development, and healthy behaviors across all life stages.

Nearly all the Healthy People 2020 goals and objectives involve one or more of the three levels of prevention that were discussed in this chapter. Figure 2.6 displays a graphic framework of the determinants of health and the overarching goals of Healthy People 2020.

FIGURE 2.6

Healthy People 2020 goals

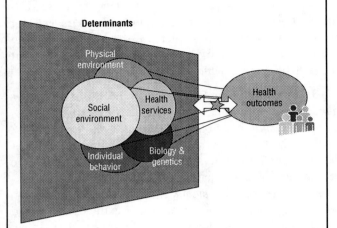

Determinants

Overarching goals:
- Attain high quality, longer lives free of preventable disease, disability, injury, and premature death.
- Achieve health equity, eliminate disparities, and improve the health of all groups
- Create social and physical environments that promote good health for all.
- Promote quality of life, healthy development and healthy behaviors across all life stages.

SOURCE: "Healthy People 2020," in *Healthy People 2020 Framework*, U.S. Department of Health and Human Services, December 19, 2011, http://healthypeople.gov/2020/consortium/HP2020Framework.pdf (accessed December 19, 2011)

CHAPTER 3
DIAGNOSING DISEASE: THE PROCESS OF DETECTING AND IDENTIFYING ILLNESS

"Diagnosis" means finding the cause of a disorder, not just giving it a name.

—Sydney Walker III, *A Dose of Sanity: Mind, Medicine, and Misdiagnosis* (1996)

The practice of medicine is often considered to be both science and art because identifying the underlying causes of disease and establishing a diagnosis require that health care practitioners (physicians, nurses, and allied health professionals) use a combination of scientific method, intuition, and interpersonal (communication and human relations) skills. Diagnosis relies on the powers of observation; listening and communication skills; analytical ability; knowledge of human anatomy (structure and parts of the human body) and physiology (the functions and life processes of body systems); and an understanding of the natural course of illness.

The editors of the 17th edition of *Harrison's Principles of Internal Medicine* (2008) explain that diagnosis requires a logical approach to problem solving that involves analysis and synthesis. In other words, health care practitioners must systematically break down the information they obtain from a patient's medical history, physical examination, and laboratory test results and then reassemble it into a pattern that fits a well-defined syndrome (a group of symptoms that collectively describe a disease).

MEDICAL HISTORIES

Obtaining a complete and accurate medical history is the first step in the diagnostic process. In fact, many health care practitioners believe that the patient's medical history is the key to diagnosis and that the physical examination and results of any diagnostic testing (laboratory analyses of blood or urine, x-rays, or other imaging studies) simply serve to confirm the diagnosis that is made on the basis of the medical history.

A medical history is developed using data that are collected during the health care practitioner's interview with the patient. The medical history may also include data from a health history form or health questionnaire that is completed by the patient before the visit with the practitioner. The objectives of taking a medical history are to:

- Obtain, develop, and document (in writing) a clear, accurate, and chronological account of the individual's medical history (including a family history, employment history, social history, and other relevant information) and current medical problems

- List, describe, and assign priority to each symptom, complaint, and problem presented

- Observe the patient's emotional state as reflected in voice, posture, and demeanor

- Establish and enhance communication, trust, understanding, and comfort in the physician-patient (or nurse-patient) relationship

Besides eliciting a history of all the patient's previous medical problems and illnesses, the health care practitioner asks questions to learn about the history of the present illness or complaint—how and when it began, the nature of symptoms, aggravating and relieving factors, its effect on function, and any self-care measures the patient has taken.

The medical history also includes a review of physiological systems—such as the cardiovascular (related to heart and circulation), gastrointestinal (GI; digestive disorders), psychiatric (mental and emotional health), and neurologic (brain and nerve disorders) systems—through which the patient may experience symptoms of disease. The review of physiological systems frequently helps the practitioner obtain information to help assess the severity of the present problem and confirm the diagnosis.

Because it relies on the patient's assessment of the severity, duration, and other characteristics of symptoms, as well as the patient's memories and interpretation of past illnesses, the medical history provides the practitioner with subjective information. With the objective findings of the physical examination and other diagnostic tests, it helps the practitioner to identify disease correctly.

PHYSICAL EXAMINATION

The National Institutes of Health's U.S. National Library of Medicine notes in "Physical Examination" (February 17, 2012, http://www.nlm.nih.gov/medlineplus/ency/article/002274.htm) that during a physical examination "a health care provider studies a patient's body to determine the presence or absence of physical problems." It includes inspection (looking), palpation (feeling), auscultation (listening), and percussion (tapping to produce sounds).

Vital Signs

In a clinic or office-based medical practice, the physical examination may begin with a nurse or medical assistant measuring the patient's vital signs: temperature, respiration, pulse, and blood pressure. Temperature is measured using a thermometer. Normal oral temperature (measured by mouth) is 98.6 degrees Fahrenheit (37 degrees Celsius). Temperature may also be measured rectally, under the arm (axillary), or aurally with an electronic thermometer placed in the ear.

Respiration is measured by observing the patient's rate of breathing. Besides determining the rate of respiration (the average adult takes 12 to 20 breaths per minute), the practitioner also notes any difficulties in breathing.

Pulse rate and rhythm are assessed by compressing the resting patient's radial artery at the wrist. The normal resting pulse rate is between 60 and 100 beats per minute, and the rhythm should be regular, with even spaces between beats. Pulse rates higher than 100 beats per minute are called tachycardia, and rates lower than 60 beats per minute are called bradycardia. Some variations in pulse rates are considered normal and do not signify disease. Athletes who engage in high levels of physical conditioning often have pulse rates of less than 60 beats per minute at rest. Similarly, pulse rates increase naturally in response to exercise or emotional stress.

Blood pressure is measured using an inflatable blood pressure cuff, also known as a sphygmomanometer. Blood pressure is measured in millimeters of mercury (mm Hg). Two readings are recorded: systolic pressure and diastolic pressure. Systolic pressure is the top number of a blood pressure reading and represents the pressure at which beats are first heard in the artery; diastolic pressure is the bottom number and is the pressure at which the beat can no longer be heard. As with pulse rates, blood pressure varies in response to exercise and emotional stress. Normally, the systolic blood pressure of an adult is less than 140 mm Hg and diastolic blood pressure is less than 90 mm

Hg. Repeated blood pressure readings higher than 140/90 mm Hg lead to a diagnosis of hypertension (high blood pressure).

Head and Neck

Physical examination of the head and neck involves inspection of the head (including the skin and hair), ears, nose, throat, and neck. An instrument called an otoscope is used to examine the ear canal and tympanic membrane for swelling, redness, lesions, drainage, discharge, or deformity. When examining the throat, the practitioner looks for abnormalities and, by depressing the tongue, can inspect the mouth, oropharynx, and tonsils.

The practitioner notes any scars, asymmetry, or masses (lumps or thickenings) in the neck and systematically palpates (presses) to examine the chains of lymph nodes (also called lymph glands, which are clusters of cells that filter fluid known as lymph) that run in front and behind the ear, near the jaw, and at the base of the neck. The practitioner also inspects and palpates the thyroid gland (the largest gland in the endocrine system, located where the larynx and trachea meet).

Eye Examination

An eye examination consists of a vision test and visual inspection of the eye and surrounding areas for abnormalities, deformities, and signs of infection. Two numbers describe visual acuity (vision). The first number is the distance (in feet) that the patient is standing from the test chart, and the second number is the distance that the eye can read a line of letters from the test chart. Because 20/20 is considered normal vision, a person with 20/60 vision can read a line of letters from 20 feet (6.1 m) away that a person with normal vision can read from a distance of 60 feet (18.3 m) away from the test chart. Using an ophthalmoscope, the practitioner examines the inner structures of the eye by looking through the pupil.

Chest and Lungs

The examination of the chest and lungs focuses on identifying disorders of breathing, which consists of inspiration and expiration (inhaling and exhaling). Changes in the length of either action could be a sign of disease. For example, prolonged expiration may be the result of an obstruction in the airway due to asthma.

Percussion is a tapping technique used to produce sounds on the chest wall that may be distinguished as normal, dull, or hyperresonant. Dull sounds may indicate the presence of pneumonia (infection of the lungs), whereas hyperresonant sounds may be signs of pneumothorax (collapsed lung) or emphysema (a disease in which the alveoli [microscopic air sacs] of the lung are destroyed).

The practitioner listens to breath sounds with a stethoscope. Listening with the stethoscope is called auscultation.

Decreased breath sounds may be signs of emphysema or pneumothorax, whereas high-pitched wheezes are associated with asthma. Another device that is used to monitor the breathing of patients with asthma is a peak flow meter. After taking a deep breath, the patient exhales into the peak flow meter, which measures the velocity of exhaled breath.

Back and Extremities

The examination of the back and extremities (arms and legs) focuses on the anatomy of the musculoskeletal system. Major muscle groups and all joints are examined, and pulses on the arms, legs, and feet (radial, posterior tibial, and dorsalis pedis, respectively) are checked to be certain that blood flow to the extremities is adequate. Monitoring capillary refill time is another way to assess the adequacy of blood flow. To do this, the practitioner presses the patient's fingernail or toenail until it pales and then observes how long it takes to regain color once the pressure is released. Longer capillary refill time may be a sign of peripheral vascular disease or blocked arteries.

Cardiovascular System

The examination of the cardiovascular system focuses on the rate and rhythm of the radial and carotid artery pulses (located at the wrist and neck), blood pressure, and the sounds that are associated with blood flow through the carotid arteries and the heart. After measuring and recording the rate and rhythm of the radial and carotid pulses, the practitioner may listen with a stethoscope for abnormal sounds in the carotid arteries. Rushing sounds, called bruits, may indicate a narrowing of the arteries and an increased risk for stroke.

Examination also entails assessment of jugular vein pressure and listening with a stethoscope to heart sounds. Heart murmurs, clicks, and extra sounds are abnormal heart sounds that are associated with the functioning of heart valves. Some murmurs are considered innocent (normal variations), whereas others are indicators of serious malfunctioning of heart valves.

Abdominal Examination

Inspection of the abdomen focuses on the shape of the abdomen and the presence of scars, lesions, rashes, and hernias (protrusion of an organ through a wall that usually encloses it). Using a stethoscope, the practitioner listens to the arteries that supply blood to the kidneys, listens to the aorta (the main artery that supplies blood to all the organs except the lungs), and listens for bowel sounds.

Percussion of the abdomen that produces a dull sound may indicate an abnormality, such as an abdominal mass. Percussion is also used to determine the size of the liver (the largest gland in the body, which produces bile to aid in the digestion of fats) that measures 2.5 to 5 inches (6 to 12.7 cm) in a healthy adult. An expanse of dullness

around the liver or spleen (an organ on the left side of the body, below the diaphragm, that filters and stores blood) may indicate that these organs are enlarged.

Breast and Pelvic Examination

Visual inspection of the breast focuses on symmetry, dimpling, swelling, or discoloration of the skin and position of the nipple. Manual breast examination is performed by slowly and methodically palpating breast tissue in overlapping vertical strips using small circular movements from the midline to the axilla (armpit). The practitioner presses the nipple to observe whether there is any discharge (fluid) and palpates the axilla for the presence of lymph nodes.

A pelvic examination may be performed after the breast examination, during a woman's physical examination. At this time, a sample of tissue may be obtained for a Papanicolaou (Pap) test, which is examined microscopically by the cytology laboratory for cervical cancer cells.

Neurologic and Mental Status Examinations

Neurologic examination considers mental status, cranial nerves (the 12 cranial nerves are abducens, accessory, acoustic, facial, glossopharyngeal, hypoglossal, oculomotor, olfactory, optic, trigeminal, trochlear, and vagus), muscle strength, coordination and gait, reflexes, and the senses. Figure 3.1 shows the nervous system and describes each of the four types of nerves. The cranial nerves connect the brain to the eyes, mouth, ears, and other parts of the head. The central nerves are in the brain and spinal cord. The peripheral nerves go from the spinal cord to the arms, hands, legs, and feet. The autonomic nerves go from the spinal cord to internal organs—lungs, heart, stomach, intestines, bladder, and sex organs.

Generally, the cranial nerves are assessed by observation as the health care practitioner asks the patient to demonstrate their use. For example, the facial nerve may be tested by watching patients open their mouth and clench their teeth. The practitioner also tests sensation to the parts of the face that are supplied by branches of the trigeminal nerve by applying sharp and dull objects to these areas and asking the patient to distinguish between them. Finally, the practitioner touches the patient's cornea lightly to observe whether the corneal reflex is functioning properly; if it is, the patient will blink.

Evaluating the motor system involves the assessment of muscle symmetry, tone, strength, gait, and coordination. Patients are observed performing different skills and walking. Reflexes are tested and graded as normal, hypoactive, or hyperactive. An example of reflex testing is when the practitioner strikes the patellar tendon just below the kneecap to observe contraction of the quadriceps muscle in the thigh and extension of the knee.

The sensory system test determines whether there is a loss of sensation in any body part. The practitioner may use

FIGURE 3.1

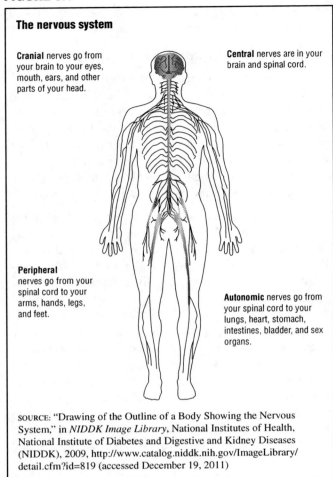

The nervous system

Cranial nerves go from your brain to your eyes, mouth, ears, and other parts of your head.

Central nerves are in your brain and spinal cord.

Peripheral nerves go from your spinal cord to your arms, hands, legs, and feet.

Autonomic nerves go from your spinal cord to your lungs, heart, stomach, intestines, bladder, and sex organs.

SOURCE: "Drawing of the Outline of a Body Showing the Nervous System," in *NIDDK Image Library*, National Institutes of Health, National Institute of Diabetes and Digestive and Kidney Diseases (NIDDK), 2009, http://www.catalog.niddk.nih.gov/ImageLibrary/detail.cfm?id=819 (accessed December 19, 2011)

the vibrations from a tuning fork or hot, cold, or sharp objects to evaluate the patient's ability to perceive sensation accurately. The practitioner may also test discrimination (the ability to accurately interpret touch and position) by tracing a number on the patient's palm and asking the patient to name the number.

A preliminary evaluation of mental status aims to determine the patient's orientation, immediate and short-term memory, and ability to follow simple verbal and written commands. Patients are considered "oriented" if they can identify time, place, and person accurately. Immediate and short-term memories are tested when the practitioner poses simple questions for the patient to answer, and the ability to follow commands is assessed by observing the patient perform tasks in response to verbal or written instructions.

Weighing the Value of Annual Physicals

In recent years the American Medical Association and other medical professional societies have down-played the importance of traditional "head-to-toe" annual physical examinations. Instead, they favor a periodic health examination—an individualized screening and examination that is based on the patient's age, health status, lifestyle, and risk factors.

In "Preventive Health Examinations and Preventive Gynecological Examinations in the United States" (*Archives of Internal Medicine*, vol. 167, no. 17, September 24, 2007), Ateev Mehrotra, Alan M. Zaslavsky, and John Z. Ayanian report the results of their research, which analyzed 8,413 physician visits for preventive medical examinations that were conducted between 2002 and 2004. The researchers find that about 21% of Americans had preventive physical examinations each year and about 18% of adult women obtained an annual preventive gynecological examination. The number of adults varied geographically—people living in the Northeast had a 60% greater chance of having a physical examination than those living on the West Coast.

Mehrotra, Zaslavsky, and Ayanian also find that Americans received most of their preventive medical care when they visited physicians for reasons other than an annual physical examination, so the relatively low percentage of annual physical examinations did not mean that preventive care was not obtained. The researchers opine that the value of annual physical examinations has not been confirmed by research and observe that critical preventive care is often received during other visits.

Bonnie Darves asserts in "Rethinking the Value of the Annual Exam" (*ACP Internist*, January 2010) that even though there is no strong evidence of the benefit of the annual physical examination, many consumers expect it and many physicians are unwilling to forgo it. Darves opines that focused examinations that concentrate on detecting conditions where intervention is likely to have a significant impact (e.g., screening for certain kinds of cancer) or tailored examinations that address specific issues (e.g., obesity, smoking, and physical activity) may be a better use of time and resources.

DIAGNOSTIC TESTING

Once the history and physical examination have been completed, the health care practitioner is often relatively certain about the cause of illness and the diagnosis. However, occasions occur when the history and physical examination point to more than one possible diagnosis. In such instances, the practitioner develops a differential diagnosis (a list of several likely diagnoses). The practitioner may then order specific diagnostic tests to narrow the list of possibilities. The results of these tests are evaluated in the context of the patient's history and physical examination.

There are scores of diagnostic tests—including blood tests, x-rays, computed tomography (CT) scans, ultra-sounds, and magnetic resonance imaging (MRI) scans—to help the health care practitioner identify the cause of disease. It is important for practitioners to choose tests that not only improve their understanding of the disease but also affect treatment decisions. The decision to order a specific diagnostic test takes into account the test's reliability, validity, sensitivity, and specificity besides its risks to the patient and costs in terms of time and dollars.

The Reliability and Validity of Diagnostic Tests

The reliability of diagnostic testing refers to the test's ability to be repeated and to produce equivalent results in comparable circumstances. A reliable test is consistent and measures the same way each time it is used with the same patients in the same circumstances. For example, a well-calibrated balance scale is a reliable instrument for measuring body weight.

Validity is the accuracy of the diagnostic test. It is the degree to which the diagnostic test measures the disease, blood level, or other quality or characteristic it is intended to detect. A valid diagnostic test is one that can distinguish between those who have the disease from those who do not. There are two components of validity: sensitivity and specificity.

THE SENSITIVITY AND SPECIFICITY OF DIAGNOSTIC TESTS. Sensitivity refers to a test's ability to identify people who have the disease. By contrast, specificity refers to a test's ability to identify people who do not have the disease. Ideally, diagnostic tests should be highly sensitive and highly specific, thereby accurately classifying all people tested as either positive or negative. In practice, however, sensitivity and specificity are frequently inversely related—most tests with high levels of sensitivity have low specificity, and the reverse is also true.

The likelihood that a test result will be incorrect can be gauged based on the sensitivity and specificity of the test. For example, if a test's sensitivity is 95%, then when 100 patients with the disease are tested, 95 will test positive and five will test "false negative"—they have the disease but the test has failed to detect it. If a test is 90% specific, when 100 healthy, disease-free people are tested, 90 will receive negative test results and 10 will be given "false-positive" results—they do not have the disease but the test has inaccurately classified them as positive.

The advantages of highly sensitive tests are that they produce few false-negative results, and people who test negative are almost certain to be truly negative. Highly sensitive tests may be useful as preliminary screening measures for diseases where early detection is vitally important, such as the enzyme-linked immunosorbent assay (ELISA) screening test for the human immunodeficiency virus (HIV), the virus that produces the acquired immunodeficiency syndrome (AIDS).

In contrast, highly specific tests produce few false-positive results and those who test positive are nearly certain to be positive. Highly specific tests are useful when

confirming a diagnosis and in cases where the risks of treatment are high, such as the Western blot test to confirm the presence of HIV after it has been detected by the highly sensitive, but less specific, ELISA test.

Laboratory Tests

The editors of *Harrison's Principles of Internal Medicine* observe that the growing number and availability of laboratory tests has encouraged physicians and other health care practitioners to become increasingly reliant on them as diagnostic tools. Laboratory tests are easy and convenient screening measures because multiple tests may be performed on a single sample of blood, urine, or other tissue and abnormal test results can provide valuable clues for diagnosis.

For screening purposes (to detect disease at its earliest stage, before it produces symptoms), the health care practitioner may order a complete blood count (a measurement of the size, number, and maturity of the different blood cells in a specific volume of blood), as well as a variety of other blood tests, including:

- Fasting blood glucose—this is a screening and diagnostic test for diabetes; values consistently greater than 126 milligrams per deciliter (mg/dl) indicate diabetes. Fasting blood glucose levels between 100 mg/dl and 125 mg/dl are considered impaired and are called prediabetes.

- Calcium—blood levels of calcium can be elevated as a result of hyperactive parathyroid glands.

- Lipids—elevated cholesterol, triglycerides, and low-density lipoproteins are associated with an increased risk of heart disease.

- Thyroid stimulating hormone (TSH)—high levels of TSH indicate hypothyroidism (underactivity of the thyroid gland), and abnormally low levels indicate hyperthyroidism (overly active thyroid gland).

- Venereal Disease Research Laboratory or rapid plasma reagin—these tests screen for syphilis, a sexually transmitted disease.

- HIV—it is important to screen for the presence of this virus.

- Prostate specific antigen—this blood test is used to screen for prostate cancer and to monitor treatment of the disease.

- Stool occult blood (also called fecal occult blood test)—this tests for the presence of blood in the stool, which could be an indicator of colon cancer.

Diagnostic Imaging Techniques

Imaging studies are another form of diagnostic testing. In the past all diagnostic imaging studies were obtained using ionizing radiation (x-rays) and recorded on transparent film. Modern imaging studies such as ultrasound and

MRI use nonionizing radiation and can be recorded digitally, viewed on computer monitors, sent via e-mail, and stored on compact discs, digital tape, or transparent film. Most imaging studies are painless and pose little risk to patients apart from minimal exposure to radiation.

X-RAYS AND ULTRASOUND. The images produced by x-rays are the result of varying radiation absorption rates of different body tissues—the calcium in bone has the highest x-ray absorption, soft tissue such as fat absorbs less, and air absorbs the least. Chest x-rays, which offer images of the lungs, ribs, heart, and diaphragm, are among the most frequently ordered imaging studies.

To view tissues that are normally invisible on x-ray, contrast agents, such as barium and iodine, may be introduced into the body. For example, contrast agents are often used for imaging studies of the GI tract to diagnose digestive disorders.

Another common use of diagnostic x-rays is the measurement of bone density. Bone mass measurement (also called bone mineral density) is performed to evaluate the risk of bone fractures. Bone density is usually measured in the spine, hip, and/or wrist because these are the most common sites of fractures resulting from osteoporosis, a disease in which bones become weak, thin, fragile, and more likely to break.

Mammography also relies on x-ray technology to detect and pinpoint changes or abnormalities in the breast tissue that are too small to be felt by hand. Another imaging technique for breast examination is ultrasound, which can accurately distinguish solid tumors (lumps or masses) from fluid-filled cysts.

Ultrasound images are produced using the heat that is reflected from body tissues in response to high-frequency sound waves. Whereas x-ray is ideal for examining bone, ultrasound is used to examine soft tissue, such as the ovaries, uterus, breast, and prostate. It is not suitable for looking at bones, because calcium-containing tissues such as bone absorb, rather than reflect, sound waves.

COMPUTED TOMOGRAPHY, MAGNETIC RESONANCE IMAGING, AND POSITRON EMISSION TOMOGRAPHY. For conventional flat x-rays, the patient, x-ray source, and camera remain fixed and immobile. CT scans use a mobile x-ray source and generate a series of cross-section pictures, or slices, that are assembled by computer into images. Because CT distinguishes differences in soft tissue more effectively and with higher resolution than conventional x-rays, it is often used to examine internal organs in the abdomen, such as the liver, pancreas, spleen, kidneys, and adrenal gland, and the aorta and vena cava (large blood vessels that pass through the abdomen).

MRI scans generate images that are based on the interaction between a large magnet, radio waves, and hydrogen atoms in the body. Stimulated by ordinary radio waves within the powerful magnetic field, these atoms give off weak signals that a computer builds into images. MRI is frequently used to create images of the brain, spinal cord, heart, abdomen, bone marrow, and knee.

A variety of specialized MRI techniques are also available, including:

- Diffusion MRI—this technique, which is principally used to image the brain, reveals the movement of water molecules in tissue and the microstructure of the tissue. It also detects swelling in tissues.

- Dynamic contrast enhanced MRI—this technique, which is often used to assess blood flow to a tumor, creates a series of images before, during, and after injection of a contrast agent.

- Fluid attenuated inversion recovery—this technique removes the effect of fluid from MRI images, enabling differentiation of brain and spine lesions. It is used to assess stroke (when blood flow to the brain is reduced below the threshold for irreversible cell death) and degenerative neurological diseases such as multiple sclerosis.

- Functional MRI—this technique measures changes in blood flow in the brain and produces high-resolution images that help assess the activity of different parts of the brain.

- Magnetic resonance angiography—this technique enables examination of blood vessels and is frequently used to look at the arteries in or near the heart, brain, abdomen, or legs. The use of a contrast agent helps produce a clear image of the blood vessels.

- Magnetic resonance spectroscopy (MRS)—this technique detects chemical activity in cells. Because tumors contain high levels of specific chemicals, MRS may be used to identify and characterize a tumor.

- Perfusion MRI—this technique, which is generally used to assess problems in the brain such as tumors or stroke, detects capillary blood flow—both the amount and transit time of blood flow in the smallest blood vessels in the body. The use of a contrast agent helps identify blood flow in the capillaries and enables the identification of regions of brain tissue with diminished blood flow.

CT and MRI scans generate images of the body's structure (anatomy), whereas positron emission tomography (PET) scans offer insight into body function or processes (physiology). To create PET images, positron-emitting atoms are injected into the body, where they travel and strike other electrons, producing gamma rays. The gamma rays are then interpreted into images by a computer. Unlike CT and MRI scans, PET scans are rarely used for screening or diagnostic purposes. Instead, they are used to track the progress and treatment of patients with diagnosed diseases such as cancer.

Diagnostic Procedures

Other diagnostic tests that are commonly performed to screen for the presence of disease include:

- Throat culture—this test is used to determine whether streptococcus pyrogenes (commonly called strep) bacteria are the cause of a sore throat. To obtain a sample of the mucus in the throat, the health care practitioner swabs the back of the throat and places the swab in a tube. The swab is transferred into a culture in the laboratory, where it is examined for bacterial growth. The results of this test are available in two to three days. A rapid strep test that produces results in minutes is also available.

- Urinalysis and urine culture—chemical and microscopic examination of urine allow the identification of infection, diabetes, and the presence of blood in the urine.

- Colonoscopy—using a long tube that is fitted with a lens, the health care practitioner is able to look at the entire colon; identify and remove polyps; detect cancer; and diagnose other causes of blood in the stool, abdominal pain, and digestive disorders. To prepare for a colonoscopy, patients must empty their intestines completely before the examination.

- Flexible sigmoidoscopy—this test is similar to the colonoscopy, in that it uses a tube that is fitted with a camera to examine the colon. However, because the instrument is shorter than a colonoscope, it does not enable views of the entire colon. Through the flexible sigmoidoscope, the practitioner can examine only the sigmoid (lower portion) of the colon to detect polyps and cancers.

- Electrocardiogram—this test assesses the electrical function of the heart, detects abnormal heart rhythms, and aids in the diagnosis of myocardial infarction (heart attack) and other heart diseases.

Prenatal Diagnostic Testing

Ultrasound is routinely used to monitor the progress of pregnancy; evaluate the size, health, and position of the fetus; and detect some birth defects. Fetal ultrasound assists in the prediction of multiple births (more than one baby) and sometimes provides information about the gender of the unborn child. Table 3.1 describes how and why ultrasound and other common prenatal tests are performed.

Chorionic villus sampling (CVS) enables obstetricians and perinatologists (physicians specializing in the evaluation and care of high-risk expectant mothers and babies) to assess the progress of pregnancy during the first trimester (the first three months). A physician passes a small, flexible tube called a catheter through the cervix to extract chorionic villi tissue—cells that will become the placenta and are genetically identical to the baby's cells. The cells are examined in the laboratory for indications of genetic disorders such as cystic fibrosis (an inherited disease that is characterized by chronic respiratory and digestive problems), Down syndrome (a genetic condition that is caused by having an extra copy of chromosome 21), Tay-Sachs disease (a fatal disease that generally affects children of east European Jewish ancestry), and thalassemia (an inherited disorder of hemoglobin in red blood cells). The results of the testing are available within seven to 14 days. CVS provides the same diagnostic information as amniocentesis; however, the risks (miscarriage, infection, vaginal bleeding, and birth defects) that are associated with CVS are slightly higher.

Amniocentesis involves analyzing a sample of the amniotic fluid that surrounds the fetus in the uterus. The fluid is obtained when a physician inserts a hollow needle through the abdominal wall and the uterine wall. Like CVS, amniocentesis samples and analyzes cells that are derived from the baby to enable parents to learn of chromosomal abnormalities and the gender of the unborn child. Results are usually available about two weeks after the test is performed.

Blood tests are also available to help diagnose fetal abnormalities. The enhanced alpha-fetoprotein test (also called a triple screen) measures the levels of protein and hormones that are produced by the fetus and can identify some birth defects, such as Down syndrome and neural tube defects. Two of the most common neural tube defects are anencephaly (absence of the majority of the brain) and spina bifida (incomplete development of the back and spine). Test results are available within two to three days. Women with abnormal results are often advised to undergo additional diagnostic testing, such as CVS or amniocentesis.

DIAGNOSING MENTAL ILLNESS

Unlike physical health problems and medical conditions, there are no laboratory tests such as blood and urine analyses or x-rays to assist practitioners to definitively diagnose mental illnesses. Instead, practitioners generally rely on listening carefully to patients' complaints and observing their behavior to assess their moods, motivations, and thinking. Sometimes mental health disorders may accompany physical complaints or medical conditions. The presence of more than one disease or disorder is called comorbidity.

Even though there are varying opinions about the personality traits and characteristics that taken together constitute optimal mental health, historically it has been somewhat easier to define and identify mental illness—deviations from, or the absence of, mental health. Within the broad diagnosis of mental illness, there is more consensus about the origins, nature, and symptoms of mental disorders—serious and often long-term conditions in which changes in cognition (thought processes), behavior, or mood impair functioning—than exists about mental health problems—shorter term, less intense conditions that often resolve spontaneously and without treatment.

TABLE 3.1

Common prenatal tests

Test	What it is	How it is done
Amniocentesis (AM-nee-oh-sen-TEE-suhss)	This test can diagnosis certain birth defects, including: • Down syndrome • Cystic fibrosis • Spina bifida It is performed at 14 to 20 weeks. It may be suggested for couples at higher risk for genetic disorders. It also provides DNA for paternity testing.	A thin needle is used to draw out a small amount of amniotic fluid and cells from the sac surrounding the fetus. The sample is sent to a lab for testing.
Biophysical profile (BPP)	This test is used in the third trimester to monitor the overall health of the baby and to help decide if the baby should be delivered early.	BPP involves an ultrasound exam along with a nonstress test. The BPP looks at the baby's breathing, movement, muscle tone, heart rate, and the amount of amniotic fluid.
Chorionic villus (KOR-ee-ON-ihk VIL-uhss) sampling (CVS)	A test done at 10 to 13 weeks to diagnose certain birth defects, including: • Chromosomal disorders, including Down syndrome • Genetic disorders, such as cystic fibrosis CVS may be suggested for couples at higher risk for genetic disorders. It also provides DNA for paternity testing.	A needle removes a small sample of cells from the placenta to be tested.
First trimester screen	A screening test done at 11 to 14 weeks to detect higher risk of: • Chromosomal disorders, including Down syndrome and trisomy 18 • Other problems, such as heart defects It also can reveal multiple births. Based on test results, your doctor may suggest other tests to diagnose a disorder.	This test involves both a blood test and an ultrasound exam called nuchal translucency (NOO-kuhl trans-LOO-sent-see) screening. The blood test measures the levels of certain substances in the mother's blood. The ultrasound exam measures the thickness at the back of the baby's neck. This information, combined with the mother's age, help doctors determine risk to the fetus.
Glucose challenge screening	A screening test done at 26 to 28 weeks to determine the mother's risk of gestational diabetes. Based on test results, your doctor may suggest a glucose tolerance test.	First, you consume a special sugary drink from your doctor. A blood sample is taken one hour later to look for high blood sugar levels.
Glucose tolerance test	This test is done at 26 to 28 weeks to diagnose gestational diabetes.	Your doctor will tell you what to eat a few days before the test. Then, you cannot eat or drink anything but sips of water for 14 hours before the test. Your blood is drawn to test your "fasting blood glucose level." Then, you will consume a sugary drink. Your blood will be tested every hour for three hours to see how well your body processes sugar.
Group B streptococcus (STREP-tuh-KOK-uhss) infection	This test is done at 36 to 37 weeks to look for bacteria that can cause pneumonia or serious infection in newborn.	A swab is used to take cells from your vagina and rectum to be tested.
Maternal serum screen (alsocalled quad screen, triple test,triple screen, multiple markerscreen, or AFP)	A screening test done at 15 to 20 weeks to detect higher risk of: • Chromosomal disorders, including Down syndrome and trisomy 18 • Neural tube defects, such as spina bifida Based on test results, your doctor may suggest other tests to diagnose a disorder.	Blood is drawn to measure the levels of certain substances in the mother's blood.
Nonstress test (NST)	This test is performed after 28 weeks to monitor your baby's health. It can show signs of fetal distress, such as your baby not getting enough oxygen.	A belt is placed around the mother's belly to measure the baby's heart rate in response to its own movements.
Ultrasound exam	An ultrasound exam can be performed at any point during the pregnancy. Ultrasound exams are not routine. But it is not uncommon for women to have a standard ultrasound exam between 18 and 20 weeks to look for signs of problems with the baby's organs and body systems and confirm the age of the fetus and proper growth. It also might be able to tell the sex of your baby. Ultrasound exam is also used as part of the first trimester screen and biophysical profile (BPP). Based on exam results, your doctor may suggest other tests or other types of ultrasound to help detect a problem.	Ultrasound uses sound waves to create a "picture" of your baby on a monitor. With a standard ultrasound, a gel is spread on your abdomen. A special tool is moved over your abdomen, which allows your doctor and you to view the baby on a monitor.

TABLE 3.1

Common prenatal tests [CONTINUED]

Test	What it is	How it is done
Urine test	A urine sample can look for signs of health problems, such as: • Urinary tract infection • Diabetes • Preeclampsia If your doctor suspects a problem, the sample might be sent to a lab for more in-depth testing.	You will collect a small sample of clean, midstream urine in a sterile plastic cup. Testing strips that look for certain substances in your urine are dipped in the sample. The sample also can be looked at under a microscope.

SOURCE: "Common Prenatal Tests," in *Prenatal Care and Tests*, U.S. Department of Health and Human Services, Office on Women's Health in the Office of the Assistant Secretary for Health, September 27, 2010, http://www.womenshealth.gov/pregnancy/you-are-pregnant/prenatal-care-tests.cfm (accessed December 19, 2011)

Because many mental health disorders are identified by primary-care physicians (general practitioners, family practitioners, internists, and pediatricians), the World Health Organization (WHO) developed educational materials and guidelines to assist practitioners in general medical settings—as opposed to psychiatric or other mental health settings—to assess and treat the mental health problems and disorders of patients in their care. The guidelines call for an assessment interview, during which a series of screening questions are asked. If a patient provides predominantly positive answers, the patient has an "identified mental disorder." If a patient responds positively to many questions but not enough to fulfill the diagnostic criteria for a disorder, the patient has a "subthreshold disorder." These disorders are defined by the WHO's 10th revision of the *International Classification of Diseases: Classification of Mental and Behavioural Disorders* (*ICD-10*), the European guide for the diagnosis of mental disorders. In North America the fourth edition of the *Diagnostic and Statistical Manual of Mental Disorders* (*DSM-IV*) by the American Psychiatric Association (APA) is used for the same purpose as the *ICD-10*. *DSM-IV* is the authoritative encyclopedia of diagnostic criteria for mental disorders. This definitive guide, which expands on the *ICD-10*, is the most widely used psychiatric reference in the world and catalogs more than 300 mental disorders. A new version of the *DSM*, *DSM-V*, is slated for release in mid-2013. Practitioners are encouraged to ask open-ended questions that enable patients to freely express their emotions, to ensure confidentiality, to acknowledge patients' responses, and to closely observe their body language and tone of voice.

Changing Criteria for Mental Illness

There are many controversies in mental health diagnosis, beginning with the definitions and classification of mental illnesses. Which criteria distinguish conditions as mental illness rather than as normal variations in thinking and behavior? Should conditions such as attention deficit/hyperactivity disorder (ADHD) be classified as a learning problem or a mental disorder? Should practitioners distinguish between neurological conditions that cause brain dysfunction and cognitive impairment such as Alzheimer's disease (a type of dementia that causes confusion, memory failure, speech disturbances, and an inability to function) and mental illness involving brain dysfunction such as depression that may result from an imbalance of chemicals in the brain?

An examination of past versions of the *DSM* reveals that the definitions of mental illnesses have changed dramatically from one edition to another. People diagnosed with a specific mental disorder based on diagnostic criteria in one edition might no longer be considered mentally ill according to the next edition. Critics of the *DSM*, which has expanded more than 10-fold since its inception in 1952, claim that diseases are added arbitrarily by the APA and that even though some entries represent changing ideas about mental health and illness, others are politically motivated. For example, homosexuality was once considered a mental illness, but in the 21st century, largely in response to changing societal attitudes, it is no longer considered an illness.

Skeptics also question the sharp increase in the number of diagnoses and the number of Americans receiving these diagnoses. Does the increasing number of diagnoses reflect rapid advances in mental health diagnostic techniques? Have mental health professionals (psychiatrists, psychologists, clinical social workers, marriage and family therapists, and other mental health practitioners) simply improved their diagnostic skills? Are the stresses of 21st-century life precipitating an epidemic of mental illness in the United States? Or are mental health professionals simply labeling more behaviors and aspects of everyday life as pathological (diseased)?

Furthermore, there is dissent even within the mental health field about diagnosis that is rooted in the ongoing debate about the origins of mental illness. After taking into account all the relevant medical research, the Office of the Surgeon General concludes in the landmark report *Mental Health: A Report of the Surgeon General* (1999, http://www.surgeongeneral.gov/library/mentalhealth/home.html) that for most mental illnesses there is no demonstrable physiological cause. This means there is no laboratory test, imaging study (x-ray, MRI, or PET), or abnormality in brain tissue that has been definitively identified as causing mental illness. As of February 2012, there were no published studies refuting this contention. As such, the majority of people suffering from mental illness apparently have normal brains, and those with abnormal brain structure or function are diagnosed with neurological disorders rather than with mental illnesses.

Debut of *DSM-V*

The fifth edition of the *DSM*, *DSM-V*, is scheduled to debut in May 2013. According to the APA, in the press release "DSM-5 Development Process Includes Emphasis on Gender and Cultural Sensitivity" (February 10, 2011, http://www.dsm5.org/Newsroom/Documents/Race-Gender-Ethnicity%20Release%20FINAL%202.05.pdf), the proposed diagnostic criteria for the fifth edition emphasize gender and cultural sensitivity and how gender, race, and ethnicity may influence the diagnosis of mental illness. Furthermore, the APA explains in the press release "DSM-5 Proposed Revisions Include New Category of Autism Spectrum Disorders" (February 10, 2011, http://www.dsm5.org/Newsroom/Documents/Autism%20Release%20FINAL%202.05.pdf) that the fifth edition may include new categories for learning disorders and a single diagnostic category, autism spectrum disorders, that encompasses a variety of diagnoses currently in use such as Asperger's disorder (which affects the ability to socialize and communicate with others), childhood disintegrative disorder (a serious loss or absence of social, communication, and other skills), and pervasive developmental disorder (a group of disorders that are characterized by delays in the development of socialization and communication skills).

Other proposed changes include revision of eating disorder diagnoses and a new category, behavioral addictions, that will contain a single disorder: gambling. In the press release "DSM-5 Revisions for Personality Disorders Reflect Major Change" (July 7, 2011, http://www.dsm5.org/Newsroom/Documents/DSM-5-Revisions-for-Personality-Disorders-Reflect-Major-Change-.pdf), the APA indicates that the fifth edition may offer "a significant reformulation in how personality disorders are identified and assessed." The term *dimensional assessments* may be added to diagnostic evaluations of mental disorders to enable practitioners to assess the severity of symptoms and to consider symptoms such as insomnia and anxiety that occur in many different diagnoses.

Changing Views of Mental Illness

Finally, there are those who view mental illness as a social condition rather than as one requiring medical diagnosis. They observe that even the surgeon general's report, which favors biological explanations of the origin, diagnosis, and treatment of mental illness, concedes that mental health is poorly understood and defined differently across cultures. If mental health and illness are rooted in cultural mores and values, then they are likely socioeconomic and political in origin. The proponents of societal causes of mental illness contend that mental illness is in part defined as a functional impairment and that during the course of their lives an estimated 28.5% of Americans will be impaired (according to the National Institute of Mental Health [NIMH], which measures the burden of disease in units called disability-adjusted life years [DALYs]). (See Figure 3.2.) In "Leading Categories of Diseases/Disorders" (2011, http://www.nimh.nih.gov/statistics/2LEAD_CAT .shtml), the NIMH observes that neuropsychiatric disorders are the lead contributor to DALYs. Given the prevalence of impairment, perhaps it is not the individual who is ailing, but the society.

Despite the challenges of diagnosing mental illnesses, the NIMH finds that only 58.7% of adults in the United States with a serious mental illness received treatment for a mental health problem in 2008. (See Figure 3.3.) There are public health implications for those who do not receive treatment or who experience delays in treatment. Untreated psychiatric disorders can lead to more frequent and more severe episodes and are more likely to become resistant to treatment.

FIGURE 3.2

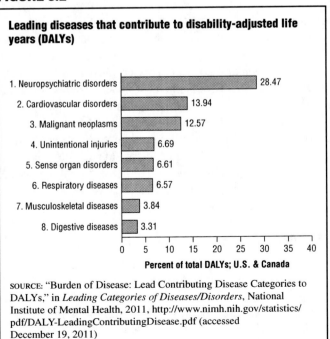

Leading diseases that contribute to disability-adjusted life years (DALYs)

1. Neuropsychiatric disorders	28.47
2. Cardiovascular disorders	13.94
3. Malignant neoplasms	12.57
4. Unintentional injuries	6.69
5. Sense organ disorders	6.61
6. Respiratory diseases	6.57
7. Musculoskeletal diseases	3.84
8. Digestive diseases	3.31

Percent of total DALYs; U.S. & Canada

SOURCE: "Burden of Disease: Lead Contributing Disease Categories to DALYs," in *Leading Categories of Diseases/Disorders*, National Institute of Mental Health, 2011, http://www.nimh.nih.gov/statistics/pdf/DALY-LeadingContributingDisease.pdf (accessed December 19, 2011)

FIGURE 3.3

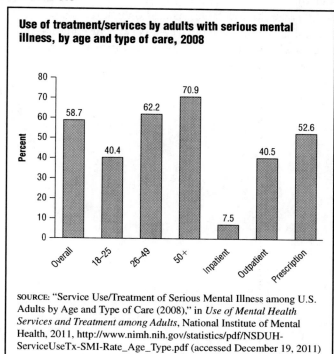

Use of treatment/services by adults with serious mental illness, by age and type of care, 2008

SOURCE: "Service Use/Treatment of Serious Mental Illness among U.S. Adults by Age and Type of Care (2008)," in *Use of Mental Health Services and Treatment among Adults*, National Institute of Mental Health, 2011, http://www.nimh.nih.gov/statistics/pdf/NSDUH-ServiceUseTx-SMI-Rate_Age_Type.pdf (accessed December 19, 2011)

In addition, early onset mental disorders that are left untreated are associated with school failure, teenage childbearing, unstable employment, early marriage, and marital instability and violence.

ONLY HALF OF CHILDREN AND TEENS WITH MENTAL HEALTH DISORDERS SEEK TREATMENT. Kathleen Ries Merikangas et al. find in "Service Utilization for Lifetime Mental Disorders in U.S. Adolescents: Results of the National Comorbidity Survey-Adolescent Supplement (NCS-A)" (*Journal of the American Academy of Child and Adolescent Psychiatry*, vol. 50, no. 1, January 2011) that between 2002 and 2004 an estimated 36% of American children and young teens with any mental health disorder received treatment. Of greater concern is the finding that only half of the children and teens who were severely impaired by their mental disorder received professional mental health treatment. The majority (68%) of the children who did receive services had fewer than six visits with a provider of mental health care. Merikangas et al. report that children with ADHD were the most likely to receive services (60%), followed by children and teens with behavior disorders (45%). Just 38% of youth with depression and 18% with anxiety received services. Fewer received services for a substance use disorder (15%) or eating disorder (13%).

Boys were more likely than girls to receive services for ADHD, and girls were more likely to receive services for anxiety disorders. Noting that African-Americans and Mexican-Americans were much less likely to receive treatment than whites, Merikangas et al. call for increased efforts "to increase awareness of mood and anxiety disorders among ethnic minority communities, improve access to services, and improve the assessment skills of clinicians and pediatricians who are often the 'front line' treatment providers of youth with mental disorders."

Technological Advances Offer New Diagnostic Tools

In "Integration of Diagnostic and Communication Technologies" (*Journal of Telemedicine and Telecare*, vol. 15, no. 7, 2009), Nafees N. Malik of the University of Cambridge describes key areas of diagnostics that have benefited from advances in communication and computer technologies, including point-of-care testing (analysis of clinical specimens such as blood at the site where care is delivered such as the patient's bedside), microelectromechanical systems (technology that combines computers with tiny mechanical devices such as sensors that are embedded in semiconductor chips), and the discovery of additional biomarkers (biological molecules found in blood or other body fluids that indicate or predict normal or abnormal processes or that detect a condition or disease). Malik observes that a growing number of people are able to send data (such as blood glucose readings, changes in body weight and diet, and medication logs) from their home to their physicians using their telephones and the Internet. The widespread availability of broadband enables patients to interact in real-time videoconferences with physicians and other health professionals and also allows physicians immediate access to specialists around the world.

Malik notes that many patients are already monitoring their heart rates and blood pressure at home and sending the results using communication technologies to their physicians, who can promptly review the information to diagnose problems. As diagnostic and communication technologies converge, it will be possible for patients to transmit increasingly complex health care data to their physicians, who will then be able to promptly identify problems and institute timely treatment to prevent complications of patients' medical conditions. These advances promise to improve patient care in a wide range of health care settings, from improving the proportion of the population that makes use of preventive measures such as screenings to management of acute medical conditions and chronic diseases.

In 2011 technological advances produced a variety of handheld diagnostic devices that offer rapid results. For example, in "A Hematoma Detector: A Practical Application of Instrumental Motion as Signal in Near Infra-red Imaging" (*Biomedical Optics Express*, vol. 3, no. 1, December 2011), Jason D. Riley et al. of the National Institutes of Health explain their design of a handheld device that uses motion as a signal for detecting changes in blood volume in the membrane that encloses the brain and spinal cord. The device can rapidly detect brain injuries such as hematomas, which occur when blood vessels are damaged and blood enters the surrounding tissues where it can cause dangerous swelling. One of the primary applications for the device will be the rapid screening of traumatic brain injury patients in settings where CT and MRI imaging facilities are not available, such as on battlefields or at the scene of accidents. The device can also be used to monitor patients who are diagnosed with hematomas in the hospital or in an outpatient clinic.

CHAPTER 4

GENETICS AND HEALTH

Even at birth the whole individual is destined to die, and perhaps his organic disposition may already contain the indication of what he is to die from.

—Sigmund Freud, "The Dissolution of the Oedipus Complex" (1924)

Genetics, which is the branch of biology that studies heredity, concerns the biochemical instructions that convey information from generation to generation. To appreciate the role of genetics in health and illness, it is important to understand the interaction of genes, chromosomes, and genomes and to learn how deoxyribonucleic acid (DNA) functions as the information molecule of living organisms.

Genes are units of hereditary information that are made of DNA and located on chromosomes, which are separate strands of DNA wrapped in a double helix (two intertwined three-dimensional spirals) around a core of proteins contained in the nuclei of cells. Genes contain the instructions for the production of proteins, which make up the structure of cells and direct their activities. They exist in corresponding pairs, and a genome is a complete set of paired genes for an organism. The Human Genome Project explains in "The Science behind the Human Genome Project" (March 26, 2008, http://www.ornl.gov/sci/techresources/Human_Genome/project/info.shtml) that humans have 46 chromosomes arranged in 23 pairs and that the human genome contains between 20,000 and 25,000 genes and 600,000 base pairs of DNA. Changes in the number, size, shape, or structure of chromosomes can result in a variety of physical and mental abnormalities and diseases.

GENETIC INHERITANCE

The inheritance of simple genetic traits involves two inherited copies of the gene that determines the phenotype (the observable characteristic) for that trait. When genes for a particular trait, such as eye color or hair color, exist in two or more different forms that may differ between individuals and populations, they are called alleles. For every gene, the offspring receives two alleles, one from each parent. The specific combination of inherited alleles is known as the genotype of the organism, and its expression, which can be observed, is its phenotype.

For many traits the phenotype results from an interaction between the genotype and environmental influences. For example, many readily apparent traits in humans, such as height, weight, and skin color, result from interactions between genetic and environmental factors. Height and weight are strongly influenced by nutrition as well as by genetic predisposition, and skin color may be influenced by exposure to ultraviolet radiation from sunlight. Along with these easily observed traits, there are other complex phenotypes that involve multiple gene-encoded proteins and the alleles of these particular genes that are influenced by a subtle and intricate interplay of genetic and environmental factors. So even though the presence of specific genes indicates a susceptibility or a likelihood to develop a certain trait, it does not guarantee expression of the trait.

For a specific trait, some alleles may be dominant whereas others are recessive. The phenotype of a dominant allele is always expressed, but the phenotype of a recessive allele is expressed only when both alleles are recessive. Recessive genes are passed from one generation to the next, and they can only be expressed in individuals who do not inherit a copy of the dominant gene for the specific trait.

In some instances, known as incomplete dominance, one allele does not completely dominate over the other, and the resulting phenotype is a blend of both traits. For example, skin color is a trait often governed by incomplete dominance, with offspring appearing to be a blend of the skin tones of each parent. Furthermore, some traits are multigenic or polygenic, which means that they are determined by a combination of several genes, and the resulting phenotype is determined by the final combination of alleles of all the genes that govern the particular trait.

Some multigenic traits are governed by many genes, and each contributes equally to the expression of the trait. In cases such as these, a defect in a single gene pair may have little impact on the expression of the trait. Other multigenic traits are predominantly directed by one major gene pair and only mildly influenced by the effects of other gene pairs. For these traits, the impact of a defective gene pair depends on whether it is the major pair governing expression of the trait or one of the minor pairs influencing its expression.

Genetic inheritance can be quite complex, and a broad array of other factors enters into whether a trait will appear and the extent to which it is expressed. For example, different individuals may express a trait with different levels of intensity or severity. When this occurs, it is known as variable expressivity.

The Influence of Heredity on Health

It has long been understood that heredity exerts a profound influence on health. Genetic inheritance explains how and why certain traits such as the propensity to obesity, eye color, and blood types run in families. Genomics (the study of more than single genes) considers the functions and interactions of all the genes in the genome. Genomics is a relatively recent discipline, because it has only been about two decades since the human genome was fully elaborated, but it already has important applications in advancing an understanding of health and disease.

Genomics relies on knowledge of and access to the entire genome and has already been applied to understanding the causes of many serious and increasingly prevalent diseases such as breast and colorectal cancer, Parkinson's disease (a disease affecting the part of the brain that is associated with movement), and Alzheimer's disease (a type of dementia that causes confusion, memory failure, speech disturbances, and an inability to function). Furthermore, genomics has also played a key role in understanding susceptibility to, and treatment of, infectious diseases, which were, until recently, thought to be caused exclusively by environmental factors. Examples of infectious diseases in which multiple genes and environmental exposures influence the risk of developing the disease include infection with the human immunodeficiency virus (HIV; the virus that produces the acquired immunodeficiency syndrome [AIDS]) and tuberculosis. Genetic variations may confer protection against disease or may have a causative role in the expression of disease.

Even though most conditions involve an interplay in which genetics and environmental factors make important, though not necessarily equal, contributions, it is nonetheless conventional to classify diseases as primarily genetic in origin or largely attributable to environmental causes. As understanding of genomics advances and scientists identify genes involved in more diseases, the distinction between

these two classes of disorders is blurring. This chapter considers genetic testing, some of the disorders that are believed to be predominantly genetic in origin, and some that are the result of genes acted on by environmental factors.

GENETIC DISORDERS

There are two types of genes: dominant and recessive. When a dominant gene is passed on to offspring, the feature or trait it determines will appear independent of the characteristics of the corresponding gene on the chromosome that is inherited from the other parent. If the gene is recessive, the feature it determines cannot appear in the offspring unless both of the parents' chromosomes contain the recessive gene for that characteristic. Similarly, among diseases and conditions that are primarily attributable to a single gene or multiple genes, there are autosomal (a non-sex-related chromosome) dominant disorders and autosomal recessive disorders. Figure 4.1 shows an example of how X-linked recessive inheritance of Duchenne/Becker muscular dystrophy (this is similar to Duchenne muscular dystrophy but is a milder form of the disease with later onset and slower progression) occurs.

Another way to characterize genetic disorders is by their pattern of inheritance, as single gene, multifactorial, chromosomal, or mitochondrial. Single-gene disorders (also called Mendelian or monogenic) are caused by mutations in the DNA sequence of one gene. According to the U.S. National Library of Medicine, in "Genetics" (February 7, 2012, http://www.nlm.nih.gov/medlineplus/ency/article/002048.htm), there are approximately 18,000 known single-gene disorders. Examples are cystic fibrosis (an inherited disease that is characterized by chronic respiratory and digestive problems), sickle-cell anemia (an inherited disease that produces abnormal hemoglobin in the blood), Huntington disease (an inherited disease that affects the functioning of both the body and brain), and hereditary hemochromatosis. Hemochromatosis is a disorder in which the body absorbs too much iron from food. Instead of excreting the excess iron, the body stores it throughout the body, and this buildup of iron eventually damages the pancreas, liver, skin, and other tissues. Single-gene disorders are the result of either autosomal dominant, autosomal recessive, or X-linked inheritance (involving a gene on the X chromosome that is passed down through the family).

Multifactorial disorders (also called polygenic disorders) involve a complex interaction of environmental factors and mutations in multiple genes. For example, different genes that influence breast cancer susceptibility have been found on different chromosomes, rendering it more difficult to analyze than single-gene or chromosomal disorders. Until 2009, it was thought that breast cancer risk was associated with genes on seven chromosomes. However, in May 2009 Shahana Ahmed et al. identified in "Newly

FIGURE 4.1

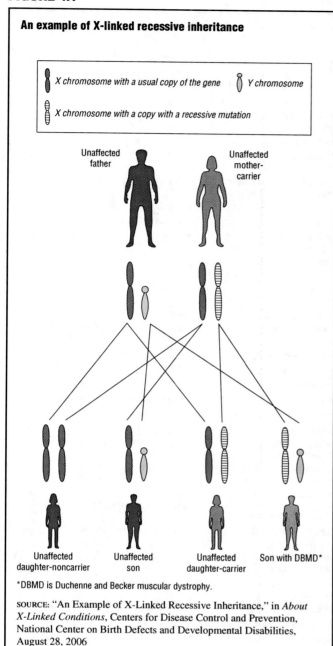

An example of X-linked recessive inheritance

| | X chromosome with a usual copy of the gene | | Y chromosome |
| | X chromosome with a copy with a recessive mutation | |

Unaffected father

Unaffected mother-carrier

Unaffected daughter-noncarrier

Unaffected son

Unaffected daughter-carrier

Son with DBMD*

*DBMD is Duchenne and Becker muscular dystrophy.

SOURCE: "An Example of X-Linked Recessive Inheritance," in *About X-Linked Conditions*, Centers for Disease Control and Prevention, National Center on Birth Defects and Developmental Disabilities, August 28, 2006

Discovered Breast Cancer Susceptibility Loci on 3p24 and 17q23.2" (*Nature Genetics*, vol. 41, no. 5) new genetic variations in two regions of DNA—on chromosomes 1 and 14—that may be associated with the risk of developing breast cancer. Many common chronic diseases such as heart disease, Alzheimer's disease, arthritis, diabetes, and cancer are multifactorial in origin.

Chromosomal disorders result from abnormalities in chromosome structure, missing or extra copies of chromosomes, or errors such as the movement of a chromosome section from one chromosome to another, which is called translocation. Down syndrome is a chromosomal disorder that results when an individual has an extra copy, or a total of three copies, of chromosome 21. Mitochondrial disorders, which occur infrequently compared with other inherited disorders, result from mutations in the nonchromosomal DNA of mitochondria, which are organelles involved in cellular respiration.

The possibility of preventing and changing genetic legacies appears to be within the reach of modern medical science in the 21st century. Genomic medicine has the capacity to predict the risk of disease—from disorders that are highly probable as in the case of some of the well-established single-gene disorders to those in which increased susceptibility may be triggered by environmental factors. The promise of genomic medicine is to make preventive medicine more powerful and to individualize and customize treatment for each individual. Such treatment takes into account an individual's genetic susceptibilities and the characteristics of the specific disease or disorder.

GENETIC TESTING

A genetic test analyzes DNA, ribonucleic acid (RNA), chromosomes, and proteins to detect heritable diseases for the purposes of diagnosis, treatment, and other clinical decision making. A simple blood sample, which allows the extraction of the DNA from white blood cells, enables most genetic tests to be performed, but other body fluids and tissues may also be used for genetic testing. Genetic tests are used to screen for and diagnose genetic disease in newborns, children, and adults; to identify future health risks; to predict drug responses; and to assess the risk of disease in future generations.

Genetic tests that are performed to establish a diagnosis are different from those that are used to screen for a disease. Diagnostic tests are intended to definitively determine whether a patient has a particular problem. Such tests are generally quite complex and often require sophisticated analysis and interpretation. Because they are complex, require highly trained personnel to interpret them, and may be expensive, they are usually performed only on people who are believed to be at risk, such as patients who already have symptoms of a specific disease.

By contrast, screening is performed on healthy people with no symptoms of disease and may often be applied to the entire population or to people who are considered to be at risk of developing a specific disorder. By definition, a good screening test is relatively inexpensive, easy to use and interpret, and assists to identify which individuals in the population are at higher risk for a specific disease. Screening tests identify people who require further testing or people who should take special preventive measures or precautions. For example, people who are deemed especially susceptible to genetic conditions with specific environmental triggers, such as people with life-threatening allergic sensitivities, are advised to avoid specific environmental triggers.

Commonly used genetic tests include screening people of Ashkenazi Jewish heritage (the east European Jewish population primarily from Germany, Poland, and Russia, as opposed to the Sephardic Jewish population, which is primarily from Spain, parts of France, Italy, and North Africa) for Tay-Sachs disease; screening African-Americans for sickle-cell disease; and screening expectant mothers over the age of 35 years whose fetuses are at an increased risk for Down syndrome. Table 4.1 lists some of the more than 1,000 DNA-based genetic tests that are currently available.

The most common form of genetic testing is the screening of newborn infants for genetic abnormalities. This screening is accomplished by testing blood that is obtained from a prick of the newborn's heel within the first few days of being born. Newborn infants are screened for specific genetic disorders such as phenylketonuria, an inherited error of metabolism resulting from a deficiency of an enzyme called phenylalanine hydroxylase. If left undiagnosed and untreated, the deficiency of this enzyme can cause mental retardation, organ damage, and postural problems.

Genetic screening aims to identify disorders that require early detection and benefit from timely treatment to prevent serious illness, disability, or death. The determination of which disorders to include in screening programs is made by each state; as such, the tests that are conducted vary from state to state. To determine which disorders to screen for, states generally consider criteria such as how often the disorder occurs in the population, whether screening is effective, and whether the disease or disorder is treatable. Figure 4.2 shows a method developed by the Health Resources and Services Administration's (HRSA) Maternal and Child Health Bureau that may be used to score and evaluate conditions to determine whether they should be included in routine newborn screening. The American College of Medical Genetics (ACMG) explains in *Newborn Screening: Toward a Uniform Screening Panel and System* (March 2005, ftp://ftp.hrsa.gov/mchb/genetics/screeningdraftforcomment.pdf) that it used this method to conduct, at the behest of the HRSA, an analysis of the scientific literature on the effectiveness of newborn screening and consider expert opinion to develop recommendations about the conditions to include in newborn screening. The ACMG was also asked to develop a uniform condition panel to help standardize screening.

In April 2008 the Newborn Screening Saves Lives Act was signed into law. Thereafter, the HRSA and the Centers for Disease Control and Prevention (CDC) began developing programs to help support state newborn screening programs and provide technical assistance for laboratories that are responsible for evaluating newborn screening tests. In "Newborn Screening: The Tandem Mass Spectrometry Revolution" (*Clinical Laboratory News*, June 2011), Suzanne T. Kotkin-Jaszi and John E. Sherwin state that "all 50 states

TABLE 4.1

Currently available DNA-based gene tests

Alpha-1-antitrypsin deficiency (AAT; emphysema and liver disease)

Amyotrophic lateral sclerosis (ALS; Lou Gehrig's Disease; progressive motor function loss leading to paralysis and death)

Alzheimer's disease* (APOE; late-onset variety of senile dementia)

Ataxia telangiectasia (AT; progressive brain disorder resulting in loss of muscle control and cancers)

Gaucher disease (GD; enlarged liver and spleen, bone degeneration)

Inherited breast and ovarian cancer* (BRCA 1 and 2; early-onset tumors of breasts and ovaries)

Hereditary nonpolyposis colon cancer* (CA; early-onset tumors of colon and sometimes other organs)

Central core disease (CCD; mild to severe muscle weakness)

Charcot-Marie-Tooth (CMT; loss of feeling in ends of limbs)

Congenital adrenal hyperplasia (CAH; hormone deficiency; ambiguous genitalia and male pseudohermaphroditism)

Cystic fibrosis (CF; disease of lung and pancreas resulting in thick mucous accumulations and chronic infections)

Duchenne muscular dystrophy/Becker muscular dystrophy (DMD; severe to mild muscle wasting, deterioration, weakness)

Dystonia (DYT; muscle rigidity, repetitive twisting movements)

Emanuel syndrome (severe mental retardation, abnormal development of the head, heart and kidney problems)

Fanconi anemia, group C (FA; anemia, leukemia, skeletal deformities)

Factor V-Leiden (FVL; blood-clotting disorder)

Fragile X syndrome (FRAX; leading cause of inherited mental retardation)

Galactosemia (GALT; metabolic disorder affects ability to metabolize galactose)

Hemophilia A and B (HEMA and HEMB; bleeding disorders)

Hereditary demochromatosis (HFE; excess iron storage disorder)

Huntington's disease (HD; usually midlife onset; progressive, lethal, degenerative neurological disease)

Marfan syndrome (FBN1; connective tissue disorder; tissues of ligaments, blood vessel walls, cartilage, heart valves and other structures abnormally weak)

Mucopolysaccharidosis (MPS; deficiency of enzymes needed to break down long chain sugars called glycosaminoglycans; corneal clouding, joint stiffness, heart disease, mental retardation)

Myotonic dystrophy (MD; progressive muscle weakness; most common form of adult muscular dystrophy)

Neurofibromatosis type 1 (NF1; multiple benign nervous system tumors that can be disfiguring; cancers)

Phenylketonuria (PKU; progressive mental retardation due to missing enzyme; correctable by diet)

Polycystic kidney disease (PKD1, PKD2; cysts in the kidneys and other organs)

Adult polycystic kidney disease (APKD; kidney failure and liver disease)

Prader Willi/Angelman syndromes (PW/A; decreased motor skills, cognitive impairment, early death)

Sickle cell disease (SS; blood cell disorder; chronic pain and infections)

Spinocerebellar ataxia, type 1 (SCA1; involuntary muscle movements, reflex disorders, explosive speech)

Spinal muscular atrophy (SMA; severe, usually lethal progressive muscle-wasting disorder in children)

Tay-Sachs Disease (TS; fatal neurological disease of early childhood; seizures, paralysis)

Thalassemias (THAL; anemias—reduced red blood cell levels)

Timothy syndrome (CACNA1C; characterized by severe cardiac arrhythmia, webbing of the fingers and toes called syndactyly, autism)

SOURCE: "Some Currently Available DNA-Based Gene Tests," in *Gene Testing*, U.S. Department of Energy Office of Science, Office of Biological and Environmental Research, Human Genome Program, September 17, 2010, http://www.ornl.gov/sci/techresources/Human_Genome/medicine/genetest.shtml (accessed December 22, 2011)

FIGURE 4.2

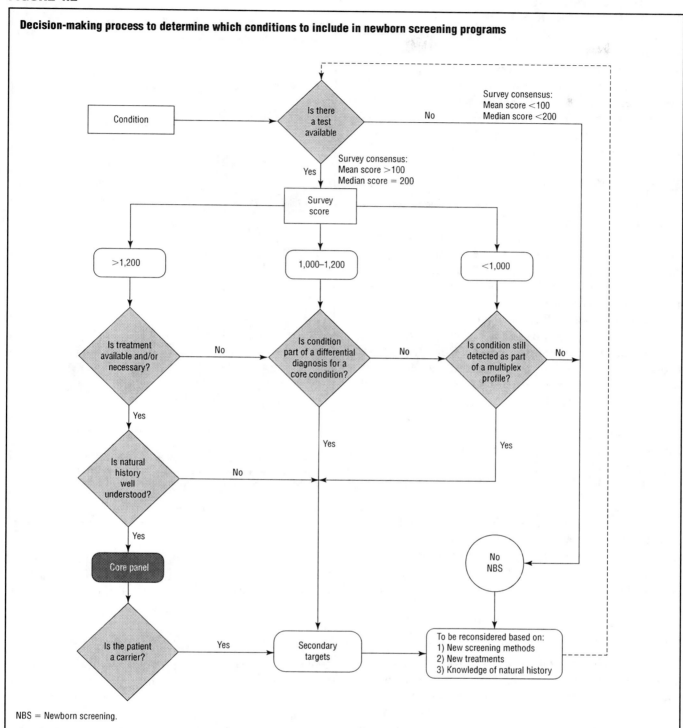

Decision-making process to determine which conditions to include in newborn screening programs

NBS = Newborn screening.

SOURCE: "Figure 9. Survey Scores Sorted by Testing Platforms," In *Newborn Screening: Toward a Uniform Screening Panel and System*, Health Resources and Services Administration, Maternal and Child Health Bureau, September 23, 2011, http://www.hrsa.gov/advisorycommittees/mchbadvisory/heritabledisorders/uniformscreening.pdf (accessed December 22, 2011)

offer newborn screening services and virtually all (>99%) of the more than 4 million babies born in the U.S. each year are screened for conditions such as phenylketonuria (PKU), congenital hypothyroidism, galactosemia, and hemoglobinpathies." (Congenital hypothyroidism is a condition in which the thyroid gland is underactive. Galactosemia is a condition in which the body is unable to metabolize galactose, a simple sugar. Hemoglobinpathies are disorders of hemoglobin, the oxygen-carrying protein of the red blood cells.)

GENETIC TESTING AND HUMAN REPRODUCTION

By February 2012 thousands of genetic diseases, both frequently occurring disorders and extremely rare ones, had been identified that may be conveyed from one generation to the next. As genetic research advances, many more genetic diseases will be uncovered and additional tests will be developed to screen parents who are at risk of passing on genetic disease to their children and to identify embryos, fetuses, and newborns that suffer from genetic diseases.

Carrier Identification

Carrier identification is used to determine whether a healthy individual has a gene that may cause disease if passed on to his or her offspring. It is nearly always performed on populations that are deemed to be at a higher-than-average risk, such as those of Ashkenazi Jewish descent. Carrier testing is important because many people have just one copy of a gene for an autosomal recessive trait and because they are unaffected by the trait or disorder and are unaware that they may pass it on to their children. Only an individual with two copies of the gene will actually have the disorder. So even though it is generally assumed that everyone is an unaffected carrier of at least one autosomal recessive gene, it only becomes a problem in terms of genetic inheritance when both parents are carriers—meaning that the mother and the father both have the same recessive disorder gene. When both parents are carriers, the offspring each have a one in four chance of receiving a defective copy of the gene from each parent and developing the disorder. (See Figure 4.3.)

Another example of carrier identification is the test for a deletion in the dystrophin gene, which results in Duchenne muscular dystrophy (DMD; the most common form of muscular dystrophy in children). Carriers may avoid having an affected child by preventing pregnancy or by undergoing prenatal testing for DMD, with the option of ending the pregnancy if the fetus is found to be affected.

Using genetic testing to detect carriers poses some challenges. Typically, a carrier has inherited a mutant gene from one parent and a normal gene from another parent. If, however, the carrier harbors a mutation that is only found in germ cells (the sperm or eggs), and only in some of these germ cells, then conventional genetic testing, which is performed on white blood cells, will miss the mutation.

Preimplantation Genetic Diagnosis

Preimplantation genetic diagnosis (PGD) permits prospective parents using in vitro fertilization (fertilization that takes place outside the body) to screen an embryo for specific genetic mutations before it is implanted in the uterus—when it is no larger than six or eight cells. One

FIGURE 4.3

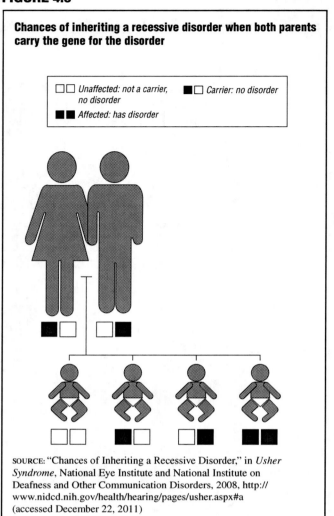

Chances of inheriting a recessive disorder when both parents carry the gene for the disorder

□□ *Unaffected: not a carrier, no disorder* ■□ *Carrier: no disorder*
■■ *Affected: has disorder*

SOURCE: "Chances of Inheriting a Recessive Disorder," in *Usher Syndrome*, National Eye Institute and National Institute on Deafness and Other Communication Disorders, 2008, http://www.nidcd.nih.gov/health/hearing/pages/usher.aspx#a (accessed December 22, 2011)

advantage of PGD is that it can screen any congenital disorder for which the causative gene is known and may be used by couples who wish to avoid traditional prenatal diagnosis and the possibility of termination of pregnancy.

Prenatal Genetic Testing

Most prenatal genetic tests examine blood or other tissue from the mother to detect abnormalities in the fetus. The most common prenatal genetic blood test is the triple-marker screen, which measures the levels of three substances in the blood—alpha fetoprotein, human chorionic gonadotropin, and unconjugated estriol—and can identify selected birth defects such as Down syndrome and neural tube defects. (Two common neural tube defects are anencephaly—absence of the majority of the brain—and spina bifida—incomplete development of the back and spine.) The results of triple-marker screens are available within several days, and women with abnormal results are often advised to undergo further diagnostic testing such as chorionic villus sampling (CVS), amniocentesis, or percutaneous umbilical blood sampling. Table 4.2 describes five

TABLE 4.2

Prenatal tests

Amniocentesis	This test takes a small sample of the amniotic fluid surrounding the baby.	This test can be given after 14 weeks or during the third trimester. The former checks for genetic defects like Down Syndrome; the latter checks for abnormal lung development.
Chorionic Villus Sampling (CVS)	This test withdraws a small sample of tissue from just outside the amniotic sac in which the baby grows.	Taken between 10 and 12 weeks, this test checks for the possibility of such genetic diseases as Huntington's Disease and Duchenne muscular dystrophy.
Quad-screen test	This is a blood test taken from the mother that checks several different components.	This test is usually performed in the second trimester (15–20 weeks). The screening looks for several things, particularly the risk of Down Syndrome.
Rh incompatibility	This test determines whether the mother and baby have incompatible blood types.	This test can be done before pregnancy or at the first prenatal visit. If there is Rh incompatibility, treatments can help prevent later complications.
Ultrasound	This test uses high frequency sound waves to show internal organs and the growing baby within the womb.	Ultrasound can be used during the first, second, and third trimesters to show the gender, status, position, health, and growth of the baby.

SOURCE: "Understanding Prenatal Tests," in "What Makes a Healthy Pregnancy?" *Medline Plus*, vol. 3, no.1, Winter 2008, http://www.nlm.nih.gov/medlineplus/magazine/issues/winter08/articles/winter08pg22.html (accessed December 22, 2011)

prenatal diagnostic procedures and when they are performed in terms of the weeks or trimesters of pregnancy.

CVS permits physicians who specialize in the evaluation and care of high-risk expectant mothers and infants to monitor the progress of pregnancy during the first trimester (the first three months). Laboratory examination of cells obtained via CVS can detect chromosomal abnormalities that produce genetic disorders such as Down syndrome, Tay-Sachs disease, cystic fibrosis, and thalassemia (an inherited disorder of the hemoglobin in red blood cells). Some test results are available within a few days and others take one to two weeks, depending on the complexity of the laboratory analysis. CVS provides comparable diagnostic information as amniocentesis; however, the risks (miscarriage, infection, vaginal bleeding, and birth defects) that are associated with CVS are slightly higher. CVS may also be performed earlier in pregnancy, at 10 to 12 weeks, than amniocentesis, which is generally performed at 15 to 20 weeks. Approximately one out of 100 pregnancies is miscarried as a result of CVS.

Amniocentesis involves taking a sample of the fluid that surrounds the fetus in the uterus for chromosome analysis. Like CVS, amniocentesis samples and analyzes cells that are derived from the baby to enable parents to learn of chromosomal abnormalities and the gender of the unborn child. The results are available in about two weeks after the test is performed. The risk of miscarriage (about one out of 200 pregnancies) resulting from amniocentesis is lower than the risk that is associated with CVS.

Down syndrome is the genetic disease most often identified by amniocentesis or CVS. Down syndrome is rarely inherited; most cases arise from an error in the formation of the egg or sperm, which results in the addition of an extra chromosome 21 at conception. Like most prenatal diagnoses for inherited genetic diseases, this use of genetic testing is intended to help prospective parents make informed decisions about the viability of a pregnancy. The CDC reports in "Down Syndrome Cases at Birth Increased" (July 2011,

TABLE 4.3

Prevalence of Down Syndrome, 1979–2003

[per 10,000 live births]

Interval	Prevalence
1979–1983	9.5
1984–1988	10.3
1989–1993	10.8
1994–1998	11.0
1999–2003	11.8

SOURCE: "Down Syndrome at Birth per 10,000 Live Births, 1979–2003," in *Down Syndrome Cases at Birth Increased*, Centers for Disease Control and Prevention, National Center on Birth Defects and Developmental Disabilities, Division of Birth Defects, July 2011, http://www.cdc.gov/Features/dsDownSyndrome/ (accessed December 27, 2011)

http://www.cdc.gov/Features/dsDownSyndrome/) that the prevalence of Down syndrome has increased since 1979. Between the interval 1979–83 and the interval 1999–2003 the prevalence of Down syndrome increased by 24.2%, from 9.5 per 10,000 live births to 11.8 per 10,000 live births. (See Table 4.3.) The number of infants born with Down syndrome was nearly five times higher among older mothers (38.6 per 10,000 live births) than among births to younger mothers (7.8 per 10,000 live births). In 2010 Samantha E. Parker et al. published new prevalence estimates for Down syndrome based on data that were collected between 2004 and 2006. In "Updated National Birth Prevalence Estimates for Selected Birth Defects in the United States, 2004–2006" (*Birth Defects Research Part A: Clinical and Molecular Teratology*, vol. 88, no. 12, December 2010), the researchers indicate that there are approximately 6,000 diagnoses of Down syndrome each year in the United States—one out of every 691 babies is born with Down syndrome.

Periumbilical blood sampling (PUBS) is the most invasive prenatal genetic test. Using a high-resolution ultrasound, a physician inserts a needle through the expectant mother's abdominal wall to extract a sample of fetal blood from the umbilical cord. PUBS may be performed from approximately 16 weeks' gestation to term. PUBS poses a high risk to the fetus—one out of 50 procedures results in miscarriage. Because it is an invasive, relatively high-risk procedure, it is primarily used when a diagnosis must be made quickly. For example, if an expectant mother is exposed to an infectious agent with the potential to produce birth defects, PUBS may be used to detect an infection in the blood of the fetus.

GENETIC TESTING IN CHILDREN AND ADULTS

Genetic testing may also be performed to find out which children and adults are at an increased risk for developing specific diseases. Predictive genetic testing can identify which individuals are at risk for many heritable diseases including cystic fibrosis, Tay-Sachs disease, Huntington disease, and amyotrophic lateral sclerosis (a degenerative neurologic condition commonly known as Lou Gehrig's disease), as well as some cancers (including some cases of breast, colon, and ovarian cancer).

The presence of a defective or altered gene is considered a "positive" result from predictive genetic testing. However, a positive result does not guarantee that the person will develop the disease; it simply identifies the individual as being genetically susceptible and at an increased risk for developing the disease. Also, like other types of diagnostic medical testing, genetic tests are not 100% predictive—the results rely on the quality of laboratory procedures and the accuracy of interpretations—and there is always the chance of obtaining false-positive and false-negative test results.

Health professionals and researchers are optimistic that positive test results will motivate people at higher-than-average risk of developing a disease to be particularly attentive to disease prevention activities and to seek regular and periodic screening to detect the disease early, when it is most successfully treated. There is an expectation that genetic information will increasingly be used in routine population screening to determine individual susceptibility to common disorders such as heart disease, diabetes, and cancer. This type of screening will identify groups at risk so that primary prevention efforts such as diet and exercise or secondary prevention efforts such as early detection can be directed to them.

Symptomatic Genetic Testing

Even though the majority of genetic testing is performed on people who are healthy and symptom-free to determine if they are carriers or to assess their risk of developing a specific disease or disorder, some testing is performed on people with symptoms of a disease to clarify or to establish the diagnosis and calculate the risk of developing the disease for other family members. This type of testing is known as symptomatic genetic testing

(it is also called diagnostic genetic testing or predictive genetic testing).

Symptomatic genetic testing is used to predict the likelihood that a healthy person with a family history of a disorder will develop the disease. Testing positive for a specific genetic mutation indicates an increased susceptibility to the disorder but does not confirm the diagnosis. For example, a woman may opt to undergo testing to learn whether she has a genetic mutation (BRCA1 or BRCA2, respectively) that would indicate the likelihood of developing hereditary breast or ovarian cancer. If she tests positive for the genetic mutation, she may then choose to undergo some form of preventive treatment. Preventive measures may include increased surveillance, such as more frequent mammography and breast ultrasound examinations; chemoprevention (prescription drug therapy that is intended to reduce risk); or surgical prophylaxis, such as mastectomy (surgical removal of one or both breasts) and/or oophorectomy (surgical removal of one or both ovaries).

Interestingly, researchers have discovered that these preventive measures are not as widely used as might be expected. For example, chemoprevention for breast cancer can cause serious side effects such as increased risk of developing endometrial cancer (cancer of the lining of the uterus) and increased risk of developing cataracts. In "Women's Decisions Regarding Tamoxifen for Breast Cancer Prevention: Responses to a Tailored Decision Aid" (*Breast Cancer Research and Treatment*, vol. 119, no. 3, February 2010), Angela Fagerlin et al. note that women considered to be at high risk for developing the disease were apprised of the risks and benefits of chemoprevention. Just 29% of the study subjects said they intended to seek more information or talk to their physician about chemoprevention, and only 6% thought they would use it. Many of the subjects said the benefits of chemoprevention did not outweigh the risks.

Symptomatic genetic testing may also assist in directing the treatment for symptomatic patients in whom a mutation in a single gene (or in a gene pair) accounts for a disorder. Cystic fibrosis and myotonic dystrophy (the most common adult form of muscular dystrophy) are examples of disorders that may be confirmed or ruled out by symptomatic genetic testing and other methods (the sweat test for cystic fibrosis and a neurologic evaluation for myotonic dystrophy).

One issue involved in symptomatic genetic testing is the appropriate frequency of testing in view of rapidly expanding genetic knowledge and identification of genes that are linked to disease. Physicians frequently see symptomatic patients for whom there is neither a definitive diagnosis nor a genetic test. The as yet unanswered question is: Should such people be recalled for genetic testing each time a new test becomes available? Even though clinics that perform genetic testing counsel patients to maintain regular contact so they may learn about the availability of new tests, there is no uniform guideline or recommendation about the frequency of testing.

Testing Children for Adult-Onset Disorders

In 2000 the American Academy of Pediatrics Committee on Genetics recommended genetic testing for people under the age of 18 years only when testing offers immediate medical benefits or when there is a benefit to another family member and there is no anticipated harm to the person being tested. Rebekah Hamilton of the University of Illinois, Chicago, observes in "Genetics: Breast Cancer as an Exemplar" (*Nursing Clinics of North America*, vol. 44, no. 3, September 2009) that genetic counseling before and after testing for adult-onset diseases is an essential component of the process.

The American Academy of Pediatrics Committee on Bioethics and Newborn Screening Task Force recommends that genetic tests included in the newborn-screening battery should be based on scientific evidence. The committee also advocates informed consent for newborn screening. (As of February 2012, most states did not require informed consent.) The committee does not endorse carrier screening in people under the age of 18 years, except in the case of a pregnant teenager. It also recommends against predictive testing for adult-onset disorders in people under the age of 18 years.

The American College of Medical Genetics, the American Society of Human Genetics, and the World Health Organization (WHO) have also weighed in about genetic testing of asymptomatic (exhibiting no symptoms of illness or disease) children, asserting that decision making should emphasize the children's well-being. One issue involves the value of testing asymptomatic children for genetic mutations that are associated with adult-onset conditions such as Huntington disease. Because treatment can only begin with the onset of the disease and because there is no treatment to alter the course of the disease, it may be ill advised to test for it. Another concern is testing for the carrier status of autosomal-recessive or X-linked conditions such as cystic fibrosis or DMD. Experts caution that children might confuse carrier status with actually having the condition, which in turn might provoke needless anxiety.

There are, however, circumstances in which genetic testing of children may be appropriate and useful. Examples are children with symptoms of suspected hereditary disorders or those who are at risk for cancers in which inheritance plays a primary role. In "Developmental Defects and Childhood Cancer" (*Current Opinions in Pediatrics*, vol. 21, no. 6, December 2009), Thomas P. Slavin and Georgia L. Wiesner observe that genetic testing is available for many disorders and that guidelines for screening are evolving rapidly. The researchers assert that

genetic testing can help improve diagnostic accuracy and "allow for targeted surveillance in appropriate individuals; for example, presymptomatic genetic testing in a family with a known cancer-predisposing mutation." However, they caution that in children with no known family mutation, gene testing may not be fully predictive because some children with certain cancer syndromes may not have identifiable genetic defects.

Regardless, Michael Parker of the University of Oxford notes in "Genetic Testing in Children and Young People" (*Familial Cancer*, vol. 9, no. 1, March 2010) that nearly all recommendations for genetic testing of children concur "that where there are no 'urgent medical reasons,' presymptomatic and predictive testing for adult-onset disorders and carrier testing should be postponed until a child is able to give his or her own consent." Parker explains that there are "situations in which this requirement can be in tension with genetics professionals' and others' judgement of what is in the child's best interests."

ETHICAL CONSIDERATIONS AND GENETIC TESTING

Since the 1990s, rapid advances in genetic research have challenged scientists, health care professionals, ethicists, government regulators, legislators, and consumers to stay abreast of new developments. Understanding the scientific advances and their implications is critical for everyone involved in making informed decisions about the ways in which genetic research and information will affect the lives of current and future generations. As of February 2012, consideration of these ethical issues had not produced simple or universally applicable answers to the many questions that are posed by the increasing availability of genetic information. Ongoing public discussion and debate are intended to inform, educate, and assist people in every walk of life to make personal decisions about their health and participate in decisions that concern others.

In "Ethical and Policy Issues in Newborn Screening: Historical, Current, and Future Developments" (*NeoReviews*, vol. 10, no. 2, February 1, 2009), Lainie Friedman Ross of the University of Chicago reviews the controversies and as yet unresolved questions and ethical considerations of newborn screening. Some of the issues she addresses are obtaining informed consent from parents, whether to disclose incidental discoveries such as carrier status, whether an effective treatment must exist as a rationale for screening, when to screen, and determining whether specific tests should be universal or target selected populations.

As researchers learn more about the genes that are responsible for a variety of illnesses, they can design more tests with ever-increasing accuracy and reliability to predict whether an individual is at risk of developing specific diseases. However, the ethical issues involved in genetic testing have turned out to be far more complicated than originally anticipated. Physicians and researchers initially believed that at-risk families would welcome a test to determine in advance who would develop or escape a disease. They would be able to plan more realistically about having children, choosing jobs, obtaining insurance, and living their lives. Nevertheless, many people with family histories of a genetic disease have decided that not knowing is better than anticipating a grim future and an agonizing, slow death. They prefer to live with the hope that they will not develop the disease rather than having the certain knowledge that they will.

The discovery of genetic links and the development of tests that predict the likelihood or certainty of developing a disease raise ethical questions for people who carry a defective gene. Should women who are carriers of Huntington disease or cystic fibrosis have children? Should a fetus with a defective gene be carried to term or aborted? There is already some evidence that prenatal screening has influenced parents' decisions about continuing pregnancies when as yet unborn children will be born with specific genetic diseases. For example, Marilynn Marchione reports in "Genetic Disease Testing Leads Some Adults Not to Have Kids" (Associated Press, February 17, 2010) that "Kaiser Permanente, a large health maintenance organization, offered prenatal screening. From 2006 through 2008, 87 couples with cystic fibrosis mutations agreed to have fetuses tested, and 23 were found to have the disease. Sixteen of the 17 fetuses projected to have the severest type of disease were aborted, as were four of the six fetuses projected to have less severe disease."

Concerns persist about privacy and the confidentiality of medical records, as well as the possibility that the results of genetic testing can lead to stigmatization despite legislation passed in 2008 that prevents such discrimination. Some people remain reluctant to be tested because they still fear they may lose their health, life, and disability insurance, or even their jobs, if they are found to have an increased risk of developing a chronic disease that is costly to treat or that may produce significant disability.

Historically, the fear of stigmatization and discrimination by insurance companies and employers when they learn the results of genetic testing was often justified. An insurance carrier might deny coverage or charge an individual a higher rate on the basis of test results, and an employer might choose not to hire or to deny an affected employee a promotion. Most medical professional associations agreed that people should not be forced to forgo taking a genetic test that could provide lifesaving information to retain their health insurance coverage or to save their job.

Until May 2008, when the Genetic Information Nondiscrimination Act (GINA) became law, Americans' dissemination of genetic information was protected by an uneven array of federal and state regulations. Considered to be the first major civil rights bill of the 21st century, GINA prevents health insurers from denying coverage, adjusting premiums on the basis of genetic test results, or requesting that an individual undergo genetic testing. The law prohibits employers from using genetic information to make hiring, firing, or promotion decisions. It also sharply restricts an employer's right to request, require, or purchase workers' genetic information.

Current Controversies about Predictive and Personalized DNA Testing

Direct-to-consumer genomic testing to assess disease risk is now available, and offers information about a person's genetic risk of 20 to 40 common polygenic diseases. The tests are sold via the Internet and cost between $400 and $2,000. Consumers may purchase the tests and receive their results without any contact with a health care professional. Advocates of direct-to-consumer genomic testing contend that providing this type of information may motivate consumers to obtain timely health screening and pursue healthful lifestyle choices. Detractors allege that this type of testing may cause undue harm, including anxiety about the results and their interpretation, and increase the use of unnecessary and expensive screening and medical procedures. In "Effect of Direct-to-Consumer Genomewide Profiling to Assess Disease Risk" (*New England Journal of Medicine*, vol. 364, no. 6, February 10, 2011), Cinnamon S. Bloss, Nicholas J. Schork, and Eric J. Topol report that because "the clinical validity and utility of these tests have not been demonstrated, and given their cost, many observers argue that their sale raises consumer-protection issues."

Bloss, Schork, and Topol analyze data from the Scripps Genomic Health Initiative, a study that measured the effects of direct-to-consumer genome-wide scans. Subjects purchased a commercially available genome-wide risk scan and underwent web-based standardized assessments before testing and three months after to measure changes in their anxiety level, diet, exercise, and test-related distress. The researchers found "no significant differences in the level of anxiety, dietary fat intake, or exercise behavior between baseline and follow-up" and no significant test-related distress. Bloss, Schork, and Topol conclude that the results of their study support the hypothesis that "provision of the results of a direct-to-consumer genomic risk test does not affect health-related behavior."

COMMON GENETICALLY INHERITED DISEASES

Even though many diseases, disorders, and conditions are called genetic, classifying a disease as genetic simply means that there is an identified genetic component to either its origin or expression. Many medical geneticists contend that most diseases cannot be classified as strictly genetic or environmental. Environmental factors can greatly influence the way disease-causing genes express themselves. They can even prevent the genes from being expressed at all. Similarly, environmental (infectious) diseases may not be expressed because of some genetic predisposition to immunity. Each disease, in each individual, exists along a continuum between a genetic disease and an environmental disease.

A multitude of diseases are believed to have strong genetic contributions, including:

- Heart disease—coronary atherosclerosis (a disease in which cholesterol and other deposits build up on the inner walls of the arteries and limit the flow of blood), hypertension (high blood pressure), and hyperlipidemia (elevated blood levels of cholesterol and other lipids)

- Diabetes

- Cancer—retinoblastomas (cancer of the eye), colon, stomach, ovarian, uterine, lung, bladder, breast, skin (melanoma), pancreatic, and prostate

- Neurological disorders—Alzheimer's disease, amyotrophic lateral sclerosis, Gaucher's disease (a disease of fat processing that is linked to the lack of an enzyme), Huntington disease, multiple sclerosis, narcolepsy (a neurological disorder that is marked by a sudden recurrent uncontrollable compulsion to sleep), neurofibromatosis (a hereditary disorder that is characterized by widespread abnormalities in the nervous system, skin, and bones), Parkinson's disease, Tay-Sachs disease, and Tourette syndrome (a neurological disorder that is characterized by repeated, involuntary movements and uncontrollable vocal sounds)

- Mental illnesses, mental retardation, and behavioral conditions—alcoholism, anxiety disorders, attention deficit/hyperactivity disorder, eating disorders, Lesch-Nyhan's syndrome (a rare disorder that disrupts the ability to build and break down purines and can produce self-destructive behavior), manic depression, and schizophrenia

- Other disorders—cleft lip and cleft palate, clubfoot, cystic fibrosis, DMD, hemophilia (a genetic blood disorder in which blood does not clot properly), Hurler's syndrome (a rare disorder in which the enzyme that breaks down long chains of sugar molecules is absent), Marfan's syndrome (a disease that is characterized by elongated bones, especially in limbs and digits, and by abnormalities of the eyes and circulatory system), phenylketonuria, sickle-cell disease, and thalassemia

- Medical and physical conditions with genetic links—alpha-1-antitrypsin deficiency (the lack of this liver protein may result in emphysema and liver and skin disease), arthritis, asthma, baldness, congenital adrenal hyperplasia (lack of an enzyme that is necessary to make the hormones cortisol and aldosterone), migraine headaches, obesity, periodontal disease, porphyria (a genetic abnormality of metabolism that causes abdominal pains and mental confusion), and selected speech disorders

Cystic Fibrosis

Cystic fibrosis (CF) is the most common inherited fatal disease of children and young adults in the United States. The National Library of Medicine's Genetics Home Reference reports in "Genetic Conditions: Cystic Fibrosis" (February 20, 2012, http://ghr.nlm.nih.gov/condition/cystic-fibrosis) that CF occurs in about one out of 2,500 to 3,500 whites, one out of 17,000 African-Americans, and one out of 31,000 Asian-Americans. In "Learning about Cystic Fibrosis" (September 27, 2011, http://www.genome.gov/10001213), the National Institutes of Health's National Human Genome Research Institute (NHGRI) observes that one out of 31 Americans—over 10 million people—are symptom-free carriers of the CF gene. Because it is a recessive genetic disorder, a child must receive the CF gene from both parents to inherit CF.

The CF gene was identified in 1989 and was cloned and sequenced in 1991. The gene was originally called cystic fibrosis transmembrane conductance regulator because it encodes a cell membrane protein that controls the movement of chloride ions across the plasma membrane of cells. Chloride transport is crucial because chloride is a component of salt, which is involved in fluid absorption and volume regulation. Mutations of this gene prevent the chloride ions from operating properly, which can cause disease that affects organs and tissues throughout the body, provoking abnormal, thick secretions from glands and epithelial cells. Over time, a thick, viscous mucus fills the lungs and pancreas, which produces difficulty in breathing and interference with digestion. Eventually, affected children die of respiratory failure.

CF is usually diagnosed by the time an affected child is three years old. Often, the only signs are a persistent cough, a large appetite but poor weight gain, an extremely salty taste to the skin, and large, foul-smelling bowel movements. A simple sweat test is the standard diagnostic test for CF. The test measures the amount of salt in the sweat; abnormally high levels are the hallmark of CF.

The U.S. Food and Drug Administration (FDA) reports in *Aztreonam for Inhalation Solution (NDA 50-814) for Improvement of Respiratory Symptoms in Cystic Fibrosis Patients* (December 10, 2009, http://www.fda.gov/downloads/AdvisoryCommittees/CommitteesMeetingMaterials/Drugs/Anti-InfectiveDrugsAdvisoryCommittee/UCM193023.pdf) that aztreonam, an inhaled drug used to treat life-threatening lung infections in CF patients in Europe and Canada, is safe and effective and recommends that it be approved for sale in the United States. The drug combats lung infections that are caused by pseudomonas aeruginosa bacteria, for which there are few inhaled antibiotics available.

Huntington Disease

Huntington disease (HD) is one of the more common hereditary diseases. It is an inherited, progressive brain disorder that causes the degeneration of cells in a pair of nerve clusters deep in the brain that affect both the body and the mind. HD is caused by a single dominant gene and affects men and women of all races and ethnic groups.

According to Genetics Home Reference, in "Genetic Conditions: Huntington Disease" (February 20, 2012, http://ghr.nlm.nih.gov/condition/huntington-disease), HD affects 3 to 7 per 100,000 people of European ancestry. It seems to be less common in other populations, including people of Japanese, Chinese, and African descent. In "Learning about Huntington's Disease" (November 17, 2011, http://www.genome.gov/10001215), the NHGRI reports that 30,000 people in the United States have HD, an additional 35,000 display some symptoms, and 75,000 carry the gene mutation that will cause them to develop the disease.

The gene mutation responsible for HD was mapped to chromosome 4 in 1983 and was cloned in 1993. The mutation occurs in the DNA that codes for the protein called huntingtin. The number of repeated triplets of nucleotides—cytosine (C), adenine (A), and guanine (G), known as CAG (nucleotides are nitrogen-containing molecules that link together to form strands of DNA and RNA)—is inversely related to the age when the individual first experiences symptoms: the more repeated triplets, the younger the age at which the disease first appears.

HD generally begins during the third and fourth decades of life; however, there is a form of the disease that can affect children and adolescents. It is easy to overlook early symptoms, such as forgetfulness, a lack of muscle coordination, or a loss of balance, and as a result the diagnosis is often delayed. The disease progresses gradually, usually over a 10- to 25-year period.

As HD progresses, patients develop involuntary movement (chorea) of the body, limbs, and facial muscles; speech becomes slurred; and swallowing becomes increasingly difficult. HD patients' cognitive abilities decline and there are distinct personality changes—depression and withdrawal, sometimes countered with euphoria. By the late stages of the illness, nearly all patients must be institutionalized, and they usually die as a result of choking or infections.

PREDICTION TEST. In 1983 researchers identified a DNA marker that made it possible to offer a test to determine, before symptoms appear, whether an individual has inherited the HD gene. It is even possible to make a prenatal diagnosis by testing DNA from fetal cells that are removed via CVS or amniocentesis. However, some people prefer not to know whether or not they carry the defective gene.

PROMISING RESEARCH FINDINGS. According to the National Institute of Neurological Disorders and Stroke,

in "NINDS Huntington's Disease Information Page" (August 13, 2010, http://www.ninds.nih.gov/disorders/huntington/huntington.htm), in August 2008 the FDA approved tetrabenazine to treat the involuntary writhing movements that are characteristic of HD; the drug is the first approved for use in the United States to treat the disease. In "Tetrabenazine as Anti-chorea Therapy in Huntington Disease: An Open-Label Continuation Study" (*BMC Neurology*, vol. 9, December 18, 2009), Samuel Frank and the Huntington Study Group/TETRA-HD Investigators report the results of research concerning the long-term safety and efficacy of the new drug. The study followed 45 patients for 80 weeks and concluded that the drug effectively suppressed HD-related involuntary movements and was generally well tolerated but did produce some undesirable side effects such as sleep disturbances, depression, and anxiety.

Muscular Dystrophy

Muscular dystrophy (MD) is a term that describes a group of hereditary muscle-destroying disorders. The CDC estimates in "Prevalence of Duchenne/Becker Muscular Dystrophy among Males Aged 5–24 Years—Four States, 2007" (*Morbidity and Mortality Weekly Report*, vol. 58, no. 40, October 16, 2009) that DMD is diagnosed in one out of 3,500 (2.9 per 10,000) male births and Becker MD is diagnosed in one out of 18,518 (0.5 per 10,000) male births. All forms of the disease are caused by defects in genes that play key roles in the growth and development of muscles. The gene is passed from the mother to her children. Females who inherit the defective gene generally do not display symptoms—instead they become carriers, and their children have a 50% chance of inheriting the disease.

Because the proteins that are produced by the defective genes are abnormal, the muscles begin to atrophy (waste away). As the muscle cells die, they are replaced by fat and connective tissue. The symptoms of MD often progress slowly, so they may not be noticed until as much as 50% of the muscle tissue has been affected.

Even though all the various forms of MD cause progressive weakening and wasting of muscle tissues, they vary in terms of the usual age when symptoms appear, the rate of progression, and the initial group of muscles affected. The most common childhood type, DMD, affects young boys, who exhibit symptoms in early childhood and generally die from respiratory weakness or damage to the heart before adulthood. Other forms of MD develop later in life and are usually not fatal.

In 1992 scientists discovered the defect in the gene that causes myotonic dystrophy, the most common adult form of MD. In people with this disorder, a segment of the gene is enlarged and unstable. This finding helps physicians to diagnose myotonic dystrophy. Researchers have since identified genes that are linked to other types of MD, including DMD, Becker MD, limb-girdle MD, and Emery-Dreifuss MD.

TREATMENT AND HOPE. Even though there is no cure for MD, treatment modalities such as physical therapy, exercise programs, and orthopedic devices (special shoes, braces, or powered wheelchairs) can help patients maintain mobility and independence as long as possible.

Many researchers believe that genetic research holds the key to development of effective treatments, and even cures, for these diseases. Because defective or absent proteins cause MD, researchers hope that experimental treatments to transplant normal muscle cells into wasting muscles will replace the diseased cells. Muscle cells, unlike other cells in the body, fuse together to become giant cells. It is hoped that by introducing cells with healthy genes the muscle cells will start to produce the deficient or entirely absent proteins.

The challenge is to get the body to accept the new muscle cells without mounting an immune attack against them. Researchers are experimenting with new delivery methods called vectors to help the healthy genes gain access to the body. One such vector implants a healthy gene into a virus that has been stripped of all its harmful properties. The modified virus containing the gene is then injected into a patient. Researchers hope this will sharply reduce the patient's immune system response, which will enable the healthy gene to restore the missing muscle protein.

In "The Contribution of Human Synovial Stem Cells to Skeletal Muscle Regeneration" (*Neuromuscular Disorders*, vol. 20, no. 1, January 2010), Jinhong Meng et al. assert that because human stem cells have some ability to regenerate muscle fibers, stem cell therapy, in which undifferentiated cells are used to repair and renew tissues, holds promise for treating muscle diseases such as MD. Stem cell therapy may also be able to repair damaged muscle cells and revive their ability to make the correct form of dystrophin, the protein that is defective in DMD.

Sickle-Cell Disease

Sickle-cell disease (SCD) is a group of inherited blood disorders (including sickle-cell anemia, sickle-hemoglobin C disease, sickle beta-plus thalassemia, and sickle beta-zero thalassemia) that affects red blood cells. In SCD the red blood cells contain an abnormal type of hemoglobin, called hemoglobin S, that is responsible for hemolysis (the premature destruction of red blood cells). It also causes the red blood cells to stiffen and change shape; they become sickle, or crescent shaped, particularly in parts of the body where the amount of oxygen is relatively low. These abnormally shaped cells have shorter life spans than normal red blood cells and they have difficulty passing through the smaller blood vessels and capillaries. Unlike normal red blood cells, they tend to clog the vessels, which prevents blood and oxygen from reaching vital tissues. The lack of oxygen damages the tissue, which in turn causes more sickling and more damage. Figure 4.4 shows how a mutation in an amino

FIGURE 4.4

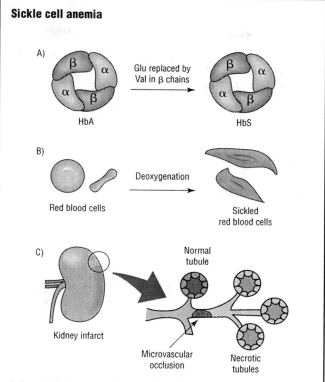

Sickle cell anemia

A) Hemoglobin is made up of 4 chains: 2 α and 2 β. In sickle cell anemia, a point mutation causes the amino acid glutamic acid (Glu) to be replaced by valine (Val) in the β chains of HbA, resulting in the abnormal HbS.
B) Under certain conditions, such as low oxygen levels, red blood cells with HbS distort into sickled shapes.
C) These sickled cells can block small vessels producing microvascular occlusions which may cause necrosis (death) of the tissue.

SOURCE: "Anemia, Sickle Cell," in *Genes and Disease*, National Institutes of Health, National Center for Biotechnology Information, 2007, http://www.ncbi.nlm.nih.gov/books/bv.fcgi?call=bv.View..Show Section&rid=gnd.section.98 (accessed December 23, 2011)

acid produces the abnormal hemoglobin, which in turn can produce the sickled cells that cause illness.

SYMPTOMS OF SCD. SCD produces symptoms that are comparable to those of anemia, including fatigue, weakness, fainting, and palpitations or an increased awareness of the heartbeat. The palpitations result from the heart's attempts to compensate for the anemia by pumping blood faster than normal.

Sickle-cell patients experience periodic sickle-cell crises—attacks of pain in the bones and stomach. Blood clots may also develop in the lungs, kidneys, brain, and other organs. A severe crisis or several acute crises can damage the organs of the body by impeding blood flow. The frequency of these crises varies from patient to patient. However, sickle-cell crises are more likely to occur during times of stress, such as when the body is combating an infection or after an accident or injury. Cumulative damage can lead to death from heart failure, kidney failure, or stroke.

WHO CONTRACTS SCD? SCD occurs most frequently in people of African, Native American, and Hispanic descent. However, it also occurs in Portuguese, Spanish, French-Corsicans, Sardinians, Sicilians, mainland Italians, Greeks, Turks, and Cypriots. There are also occurrences of SCD in the Middle East and Asia. According to the WHO, in "Genes and Human Disease: Monogenic Diseases" (2012, http://www.who.int/genomics/public/geneticdiseases/en/index2.html), SCD is the most com- mon inherited blood disorder in the United States, affecting an estimated 72,000 Americans, most of whom have African ancestry. SCD occurs in approximately one out of 500 African-American births and in one out of 1,000 to 1,400 Hispanic-American births.

When one parent has the sickle-cell gene, the offspring will carry the trait, but only when both the mother and the father have the trait can they produce a child with SCD. Figure 4.5 shows the inheritance pattern for the

FIGURE 4.5

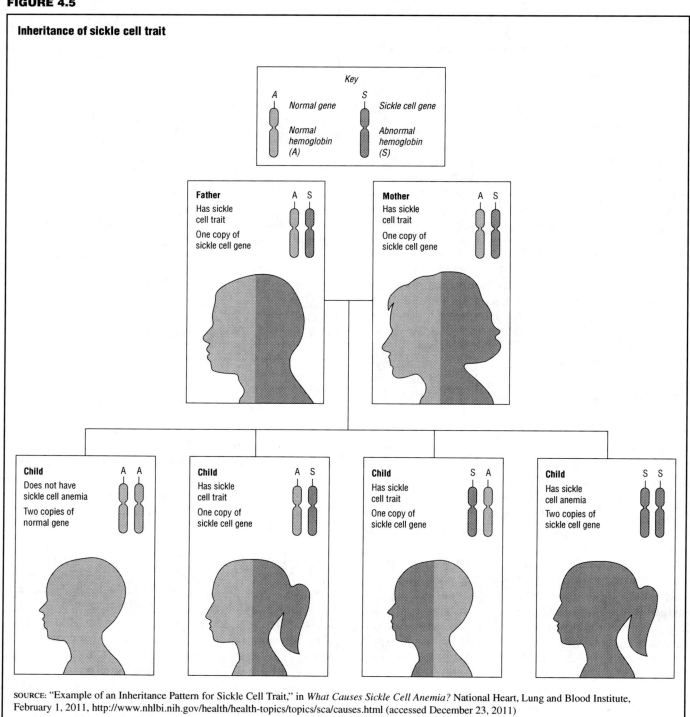

Inheritance of sickle cell trait

SOURCE: "Example of an Inheritance Pattern for Sickle Cell Trait," in *What Causes Sickle Cell Anemia?* National Heart, Lung and Blood Institute, February 1, 2011, http://www.nhlbi.nih.gov/health/health-topics/topics/sca/causes.html (accessed December 23, 2011)

sickle-cell trait. The sickle-cell trait is present in one out of 12 African-Americans, or about 2 million people.

Examining amniotic fluid or tissue that is taken from the placenta as early as the first trimester of pregnancy enables detection of the likelihood the unborn child will have the sickle-cell trait or SCD. A genetic counselor evaluates the results and can inform the expectant parents of the chances that their child will have the sickle-cell trait or SCD.

BENEFITS OF UNIVERSAL SCREENING. The National Heart Lung and Blood Institute notes in "What Is Sickle Cell Anemia?" (February 1, 2011, http://www.nhlbi.nih .gov/health/dci/Diseases/Sca/SCA_WhatIs.html) that SCD screening of all newborns is important because early diagnosis and treatment significantly improves future health. Early diagnosis and timely treatments such as penicillin reduce the number of deaths that are attributable to SCD and enable most children who are born with SCD to live well into adulthood.

THE CURE FOR SCD. According to the CDC, in "Facts about Sickle Cell Disease" (September 16, 2011, http:// www.cdc.gov/ncbddd/sicklecell/facts.html), bone marrow transplant and stem cell treatment can cure SCD. Bone marrow is the spongy tissue in the cavities of bones that creates and contains blood cells. A bone marrow/ stem cell transplant procedure extracts blood stem cells (the cells that form blood) from a healthy donor and places them into a person whose bone marrow is not functioning properly. Bone marrow/stem cell transplants carry significant risks, which even include death of the recipient. To be optimally effective, the bone marrow must be a close match and the ideal donor is most often a sibling. Because of the associated risks, bone marrow/ stem cell transplants are reserved for children with severe cases of SCD.

Tay-Sachs Disease

Tay-Sachs disease (TSD) is a fatal genetic disorder in children that causes the progressive destruction of the central nervous system. It is named for Warren Tay (1843–1927), a British ophthalmologist, and Bernard Sachs (1858–1944), an American neurologist, the physicians who first identified and described the disease. It is caused by insufficient activity of, or the complete absence of, an important enzyme called hexosaminidase A (hex-A). Without hex-A, a fatty substance called ganglioside GM2 builds up abnormally in the cells, particularly the brain's nerve cells. Ultimately, this buildup causes these cells to degenerate and die. This destructive process begins well before birth, but the disease is usually not diagnosed until the baby is several months old.

SYMPTOMS OF TSD. A baby with TSD appears healthy at birth and usually develops normally during the first months of life, but then development slows. The child begins to regress and loses skills one by one—the ability to crawl, to sit, to reach out, and to turn over. The victim gradually becomes blind, deaf, and unable to swallow. Muscles atrophy, and paralysis sets in. Mental retardation occurs, and the child is unable to interact with the outside world. There is no cure for this disease. Even with optimal medical care and treatment, death from infection usually occurs by age four.

HOW IS TSD INHERITED? TSD is transmitted from parent to child the same way eye or hair color is inherited. It is an autosomal recessive genetic disorder caused by mutations in both alleles of the HEXA gene on chromosome 15. Both parents must be carriers of the TSD gene to give birth to a child with the disease.

People who carry the TSD gene have no signs of the disease and are generally unaware that they have the potential to pass this disease on to their offspring. When just one parent is a carrier, the offspring will not have TSD, but there is a 50% chance of having a child who is a carrier. When both parents carry the recessive TSD gene, there is a 25% chance of having a child with the disease and a 50% chance of bearing a child who is a carrier. Prenatal diagnosis early in pregnancy, using CVS or amniocentesis, can accurately predict if the fetus is affected by TSD.

WHO IS AT RISK? Like SCD, TSD occurs most frequently in specific populations. People of east European (Ashkenazi) Jewish descent have the highest risk of being carriers of TSD. According to the National Tay-Sachs and Allied Diseases Association of Delaware Valley, in "Tay-Sachs Disease" (2012, http://www.tay-sachs.org/ taysachs_disease.php), approximately one out of 27 Jews in the United States is a carrier of the TSD gene. French-Canadians and Cajuns also have the same carrier rate as Ashkenazi Jews, and one out of 50 Irish-Americans is a carrier. The Pennsylvania Dutch population as well as people of British Isle and Italian descent also have a higher carrier rate than that observed in the general population, where the carrier rate is one out of 250.

CHAPTER 5
CHRONIC DISEASES: CAUSES, TREATMENT, AND PREVENTION

The Centers for Disease Control and Prevention (CDC) defines chronic diseases as prolonged illnesses that do not resolve spontaneously and are rarely cured completely. According to the CDC, in "Chronic Diseases and Health Promotion" (July 7, 2010, http://www.cdc.gov/nccdphp/overview.htm), chronic illnesses such as cardiovascular disease, cancer, respiratory disease, cerebrovascular disease, and diabetes account for 70% of all deaths in the United States and are among the most common and potentially preventable of all health problems in the United States.

CARDIOVASCULAR DISEASES

Cardiovascular disease, which includes coronary heart diseases, arrhythmias, diseases of the arteries, congestive heart failure, rheumatic heart disease, cerebrovascular disease (stroke), and congenital heart defects, was the leading cause of death in the United States in 2007. (See Figure 5.1.) In *NHLBI Fact Book, Fiscal Year 2010* (January 2011, http://www.nhlbi.nih.gov/about/factbook/FactBook_2010.pdf), the National Heart Lung and Blood Institute reports that in 2007 cardiovascular disease accounted for 814,000 deaths—34% of all deaths—and cerebrovascular disease, the third-leading cause of death after cancer, accounted for 136,000 deaths. In terms of death rate and years of potential life lost, heart disease was second only to all cancers combined.

Véronique L. Roger et al. indicate in "Heart Disease and Stroke Statistics—2012 Update" (*Circulation*, vol. 125, no. 1, December 15, 2011) that based on 2008 data more than 2,200 Americans die from cardiovascular disease each day—about one death every 39 seconds. Coronary heart disease claimed 405,309 lives in the United States in 2008, or about one out of every six deaths. Each year about 785,000 Americans will have a new coronary attack, and 470,000 will have a recurrent (second or third) attack. An additional 195,000 silent first myocardial infarctions

(heart attacks that produce no symptoms or such mild symptoms that they go unnoticed) occur each year. Roger et al. estimate that "every 25 seconds, an American will have a coronary event, and approximately every minute, someone will die of one."

According to Donald Lloyd-Jones et al., in "Heart Disease and Stroke Statistics—2010 Update" (*Circulation*, vol. 127, no. 7, December 17, 2009), if all forms of major cardiovascular disease were eliminated, life expectancy in the United States would rise by almost seven years. If all forms of cancer were eliminated, the estimated gain would be three years.

Heart Attack and Angina Pectoris

A heart attack, or myocardial infarction, occurs when the blood supply from a coronary artery to the heart muscle (the myocardium) is cut off abruptly. This happens when one of the coronary arteries that supply blood to the heart is obstructed (blocked). When the blood supply is eliminated, the heart's muscle cells are deprived of oxygen and die. Disability or death can result, depending on how much of the heart muscle has been damaged.

Angina pectoris is not a disease; it is a symptom and the name for chest pain or pressure that occurs when poor blood flow through a partially occluded (blocked) artery to the heart quickly and temporarily reduces its supply of oxygen. When the blood flow is restored, the pain subsides. A common condition, angina is often a warning sign of the risk of heart attack. Its dull, constricting pain typically occurs when an individual is physically active or excited but subsides when activity ceases. In men, angina usually occurs after the age of 50 years, whereas women tend to develop angina later in life. Roger et al. note in that in 2008 an estimated 9 million people in the United States suffered from angina.

WARNING SIGNALS OF A HEART ATTACK. In "Warning Signs of Heart Attack, Stroke and Cardiac Arrest" (2012, http://www.heart.org/HEARTORG/Conditions/

FIGURE 5.1

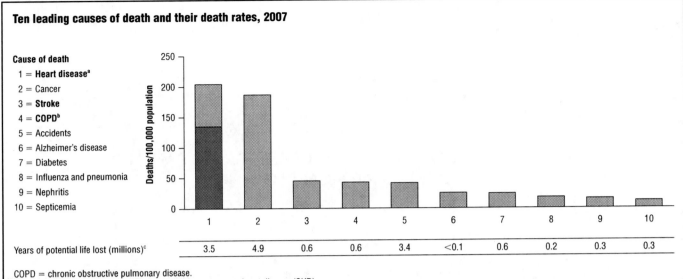

Ten leading causes of death and their death rates, 2007

Cause of death

1 = **Heart disease**[a]
2 = Cancer
3 = **Stroke**
4 = **COPD**[b]
5 = Accidents
6 = Alzheimer's disease
7 = Diabetes
8 = Influenza and pneumonia
9 = Nephritis
10 = Septicemia

	1	2	3	4	5	6	7	8	9	10
Years of potential life lost (millions)[c]	3.5	4.9	0.6	0.6	3.4	<0.1	0.6	0.2	0.3	0.3

COPD = chronic obstructive pulmonary disease.
[a]Includes 134.7 deaths per 100,000 population from coronary heart disease (CHD).
[b]COPD and allied conditions (including asthma); the term in the International Classification of Diseases/10 is "chronic lower respiratory diseases."
[c]Based on the average remaining years of life up to age 77 years.
Note: Diseases shown in bold are those addressed in National Institutes of Health, National Heart, Lung, and Blood Institute programs.

SOURCE: "Ten Leading Causes of Death: Death Rates, U.S., 2007," in *NHLBI Factbook, Fiscal Year 2010*, National Institutes of Health, National Heart, Lung, and Blood Institute, April 2011, http://www.nhlbi.nih.gov/about/factbook/FactBook_2010.pdf (accessed December 23, 2011)

Conditions_UCM_305346_SubHomePage.jsp), the American Heart Association (AHA) describes several warning signs of a heart attack:

- An uncomfortable pressure, squeezing, fullness, or pain in the center of the chest behind the breastbone

- Pain that spreads to the shoulders, neck, arms, back, jaw, or stomach

- Chest discomfort that is accompanied by sweating, nausea, shortness of breath, or a feeling of weakness

IMMEDIATE CARE IS CRUCIAL. Immediate medical care dramatically improves the odds of surviving a heart attack. Treatments are most effective if given within an hour of when the attack begins. According to the AHA, intensive emergency care during the first 12 hours after a heart attack improves the patient's chance of survival and recovery. Researchers believe that patients who suffer heart attacks benefit from early intensive treatment—such as improved monitoring of their conditions and aggressive use of pharmacologic (drug) therapy, including appropriate reperfusion therapies and "clot-busting" medications—that is initiated with as little delay as possible. There are a variety of drugs that dissolve clots, but tissue plasminogen activator, which was approved by the U.S. Food and Drug Administration (FDA) in 1996, is currently used most often.

Treatments for Heart Disease

Drug treatment for heart disease focuses on improving blood flow to the heart, controlling abnormal heart rhythms, reducing the heart's workload, and preventing blood clots. Frequently prescribed heart disease medications include:

- Angiotensin converting enzyme (ACE) inhibitors, which widen blood vessels to ease the heart's workload and reduce blood pressure

- Angiotensin II receptor blockers, which exert the same effects as ACE inhibitors but act using a different mechanism

- Antiarrhythmia drugs, which help regulate abnormal heart rhythms that are caused by erratic electrical activity of the heart

- Antiplatelet drugs, which help prevent blood clots from forming

- Aspirin, which reduces inflammation and pain and inhibits blood clots

- Beta-blockers, which ease the heart's workload by slowing the heart rate and improving the heart's ability to pump blood through the body

- Digoxin, which slows the heart rate, strengthens contractions, and boosts blood circulation

- Diuretics, which remove excess water and salt from the body to reduce the heart's workload and help lower blood pressure

- Nitrates, which widen and relax the coronary arteries, thereby easing blood flow to the heart

- Warfarin, which prevents blood clots from forming

Once it is clear that a person is having a heart attack, immediate treatment usually includes administering drugs to help open the blocked artery, which restores blood flow to the heart and prevents clots from forming again. If the patient gets to an emergency department quickly, reperfusion (the action of restoring the flow of blood to the heart) might be done. Drugs may be administered to decrease the workload of the heart, relieve chest pain, reduce blood pressure, and thin the blood to prevent clot formation in the arteries and promote reperfusion. Patients with heart disease may also undergo other procedures, including:

- Balloon angioplasty or percutaneous transluminal coronary angioplasty to widen narrowed arteries with an inflated balloon

- Placement of wire mesh tubes, called stents, into arteries after angioplasty to prevent later collapse or restenosis (renarrowing)

- Coronary artery bypass graft (CABG) surgery to improve blood supply to parts of the heart muscle that have decreased blood flow

Once emergency care and immediate treatment is completed, most communities have cardiac rehabilitation programs that help people recover from a heart attack and reduce the chances of having another one.

Bypass Surgery

CABG, commonly known as bypass surgery, can improve blood flow to the heart, relieve chest pains, and help the heart pump more efficiently. Generally, a segment of a large healthy vein, usually taken from the patient's leg, is spliced between the aorta (the main vessel carrying blood from the left side of the heart to all the arteries of the body and limbs) and the blocked coronary arteries. The coronary bypass operation thus supplies blood to the area of the heart that has a deficient blood supply. During the operation the patient is placed on a heart-lung machine that takes over the function of the heart and lungs while the surgery is proceeding. Usually, patients recovering from CABG surgery spend two or three days in the intensive care unit and several days to one week in the hospital following the surgery. Roger et al. report that in 2008 CABG surgeries were performed on 242,000 patients in the United States.

Lloyd-Jones et al. note that between 1996 and 2006 the total number of cardiovascular operations and procedures increased by 33%, from 5.4 million to 7.2 million per year. During this period CABG surgery volume declined, and the numbers of selected procedures such as cardiac catheterizations also decreased slightly. In contrast, the numbers of other kinds of catheter-based interventions increased as did the use of newer techniques such as minimally invasive direct coronary bypass surgery. In this procedure, the surgeon makes one or more small incisions (about 3 inches [7.6 cm] long) in the chest wall and works directly on the clogged artery while the heart is beating. Some surgeons use fiber-optic techniques similar to those that are used in gallbladder and other procedures. Anesthesiologists slow the heartbeat with drugs such as calcium channel blockers and beta-blockers to allow surgeons more control. Another technique actually stops the heartbeat and uses a modified heart-lung machine that is connected to a large artery in the groin while the surgeon operates through small incisions using a video camera and long-handled instruments.

Research studies, such as Alexander Iribarne et al.'s "Eight-Year Experience with Minimally Invasive Cardiothoracic Surgery" (*World Journal of Surgery*, vol. 34, no. 4, April 2010), find that minimally invasive procedures have delivered the anticipated benefits, including shorter recovery times, less time spent in the hospital, and the possibility of combining the new procedure with angioplasty or other procedures. After following more than 900 patients for an average of eight years, Iribarne et al. conclude that "minimally invasive approaches are effective and reproducible for a variety of cardiac operations, with acceptable operating time durations, morbidity, and mortality."

Catheter-Based Interventions

A growing number of patients are candidates for much simpler procedures called catheter-based interventions because the procedures are performed via a thin tube that is inserted into an artery, rather than operating on the coronary artery by cutting through the chest wall. One such catheter-based intervention, performed under a local anesthetic, is percutaneous coronary intervention (PCI; this procedure is also called percutaneous transluminal coronary angioplasty). A physician punctures an artery in the patient's groin and threads a balloon-tipped catheter into the artery. The tip of the catheter is slowly advanced up through the arterial system and positioned in the coronary artery at the point of the blockage or stenosis (narrowing). The small, sausage-shaped balloon on the end of the catheter is then inflated, flattening the fatty plaque and widening the artery. The balloon is sometimes inflated and deflated several times to clear the artery.

PCI has several obvious advantages over bypass surgery. First, it is performed under a local rather than a general anesthetic and does not involve opening the chest or using a heart-lung machine. It is less expensive, and the patient is usually out of the hospital and recovering in a few days. Still, PCI is not always completely effective, and nearly one-third of patients who have had PCI eventually require bypass surgery or another PCI because the initial procedure is unsuccessful or the blockage recurs.

According to Lloyd-Jones et al., 1.3 million PCI procedures were performed in the United States in 2006. Of these procedures, 65% were performed on men.

As technology advances, catheter-based interventions using devices such as fiber optics and laser methods may replace angioplasty as the treatments of choice. Some physicians are also using a tiny cutting blade that is attached to the end of a fiber-optic tube to remove accumulated plaque, although this method has not yet been proven to be more effective than balloon angioplasty.

Physicians are also placing stents into arteries after angioplasty or PCI to prevent later collapse or restenosis. However, even with stents, arteries renarrow in about a quarter of patients.

In "Effects of Percutaneous Coronary Interventions in Silent Ischemia after Myocardial Infarction" (*Journal of the American Medical Association*, vol. 297, no. 18, May 9, 2007), Paul Erne et al. report the results of a study following patients who had PCI after having a heart attack. The researchers find that PCI and drug therapy reduced the subjects' risk of suffering another major cardiac event. By 2009 PCI was considered to be the "treatment of choice" for the majority of patients who experience heart attack, as noted by Nevio Taglieri and Carlo Di Mario of the Royal Brompton Hospital and Imperial College, in London, England, in "Percutaneous Coronary Intervention following Thrombolysis: For Whom and When?" (*Acute Cardiac Care*, vol. 11, no. 4, 2009).

In "Trends in Coronary Revascularization in the United States from 2001 to 2009: Recent Declines in Percutaneous Coronary Intervention Volumes" (*Circulation: Cardiovascular Quality and Outcomes*, vol. 4, no. 2, March 2011), Robert F. Riley et al. look at utilization trends for PCI, coronary angiography, and CABG surgery procedures in Medicare patients (people aged 65 years and older) between 2001 and 2009. The researchers find that all forms of coronary revascularization have been declining since 2004 and that PCI has declined slightly in recent years. The overall number of diagnostic catheterizations per 1,000 Medicare beneficiaries decreased by 2.7% per year between 2004 and 2009. Even though the average annual increase in PCI (stenting and angioplasty alone) per 1,000 beneficiaries was 1.3% over this nine-year period, the increase occurred between 2001 and 2004; by contrast, an annual rate of decline of 2.5% was seen between 2004 and 2009. CABG procedures declined consistently between 2001 and 2008 by about 4% to 7% per year followed by a slight increase in 2009.

Riley et al. attribute these declines to improved risk-factor modifications and cardiovascular therapies such as the use of statins (drugs that reduce cholesterol) and beta-blockers (drugs that decrease the force and rate of the heart's contractions, which lowers blood pressure and reduces the heart's demand for oxygen) for people with diagnosed coronary artery disease. For example, the prevalence of smoking among adults decreased by 3.5% between 1998 and 2008. During this period an increasing percentage of the U.S. population achieved target blood pressure and cholesterol goals. Riley et al. also posit that more patients with stable angina are medically managed—meaning that they are given drug treatment or evaluated with noninvasive imaging before diagnostic catheterization or coronary revascularization procedures.

HEART TRANSPLANTS. In December 1967 Christiaan Barnard (1922–2001) of South Africa performed the first successful heart transplant. This feat was repeated one month later in the United States by Norman Shumway (1923–2006) at Stanford University Hospital in California. According to the Health Resources and Services Administration's (HRSA) Organ Procurement and Transplantation Network (December 26, 2009, http://optn.transplant.hrsa .gov/latestData/rptData.asp), in 2010, 2,333 heart transplants were performed in the United States, and in 2011, 2,151 heart transplants were performed. As of February 2012, 3,136 patients were awaiting heart transplants in the United States.

Risk Factors for Heart Disease

Various risk factors exist for heart disease. Even though some cannot be changed, others can be modified.

UNCHANGEABLE RISK FACTORS. Four risk factors for heart disease that cannot be altered are heredity, race, gender, and increasing age. People whose parents had or have cardiovascular diseases are more likely to develop them. Race is also a significant factor. For example, Lloyd-Jones et al. indicate that African-American adults have the highest rates of high blood pressure in the world (greater than 43%), which increases the risk for heart disease. Men have a greater risk of heart attack than do women. Heart attacks are the leading cause of death among men older than the age of 40 years, but heart disease is not a major cause of death among women until they reach the age of 60 years. Heart attacks are also more likely to occur as a person ages. More than half of the Americans who experience heart attacks are aged 65 years or older. Of those who die from their attacks, the vast majority are older than the age of 65 years.

CHANGEABLE RISK FACTORS. Cigarette smoking doubles the risk of heart attack. A smoker who suffers a heart attack is more likely to die from it and more likely to die suddenly than a nonsmoker. Once people stop smoking, however, regardless of the length of time or the amount they smoked, the risk of heart disease decreases significantly. Between 1999 and 2009 the prevalence of cigarette smoking among male and female high school students in grades nine to 12 declined from 35% to 20% and 19%, respectively, and among male and female adults aged 18 to 44 years there was a similar decrease. (See Figure 5.2.) In contrast, among male and female adults aged 45 to 64 years and 65 years and older the percentage of smokers remained relatively constant.

FIGURE 5.2

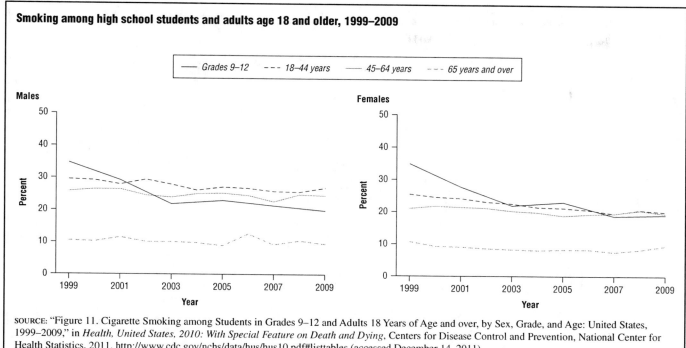

Smoking among high school students and adults age 18 and older, 1999–2009

— Grades 9–12   - - - 18–44 years   — 45–64 years   - - - 65 years and over

Males

Females

SOURCE: "Figure 11. Cigarette Smoking among Students in Grades 9–12 and Adults 18 Years of Age and over, by Sex, Grade, and Age: United States, 1999–2009," in *Health, United States, 2010: With Special Feature on Death and Dying*, Centers for Disease Control and Prevention, National Center for Health Statistics, 2011, http://www.cdc.gov/nchs/data/hus/hus10.pdf#listtables (accessed December 14, 2011)

High blood pressure, which usually has no symptoms or warning signs, is called the "silent killer." High blood pressure means that it is more difficult for blood to pump through the arteries, which increases the heart's workload, causing it to weaken and enlarge over time. Generally, blood pressure increases with age. Men have a higher incidence of high blood pressure than women until 45 to 54 years of age, when the risks become equal for both sexes. The prevalence of high blood pressure for men and women of all age groups increased between 1988–94 and 2005–08. (See Figure 5.3.) The largest increase during this period was for men and women aged 65 to 74 years, who experienced a rise of 10% and 12%, respectively. In *Health, United States, 2010* (2011, http://www.cdc.gov/nchs/data/hus/hus10.pdf), the National Center for Health Statistics (NCHS) defines hypertension as having elevated blood pressure and/or taking antihypertensive medication. Those with elevated blood pressure may also be taking prescribed medication for high blood pressure. Those taking antihypertensive medication may not have measured elevated blood pressure but are still classified as having hypertension. In most cases, high blood pressure can be controlled through diet, exercise, and medication.

High serum cholesterol levels increase the risk of coronary heart disease. High serum cholesterol is defined as greater than or equal to 240 milligrams per deciliter (mg/dL). Borderline high serum cholesterol is defined as greater than or equal to 200 mg/dL and less than 240 mg/dL. According to the NCHS, 14.9% of adults aged 20 years and

older had high cholesterol levels in 2005–08, down from 20.8% in 1988–1994. This decline is likely the result of heightened awareness of the importance of reducing cholesterol levels and increased use of cholesterol-lowering drugs. Figure 5.4 shows increasing use of statin drugs (the most commonly prescribed class of cholesterol-lowering drugs) for both men and women between 1988–1994 and 2005–2008. A reduction of dietary fat, especially artery-clogging saturated fat, can reduce blood cholesterol levels, as can exercise. Maintaining a healthy weight, eating a proper diet, and exercising can also enhance the effectiveness of cholesterol-lowering drugs.

A lack of physical exercise is also a risk factor for heart disease. According to the NCHS, between 1999 and 2009 the percentage of men aged 18 years and older who met the 2008 federal aerobic activity and muscle-strengthening guidelines increased from 18.5% to 22.1%. However, in 2009 the percentage of Americans who were engaged in regular leisure-time physical activity declined with increasing age, from 27.7% of men and 19% of women aged 18 to 44 years to just 11.8% of men and 8.6% of women aged 65 years and older. (See Figure 5.5.)

For adults aged 18 to 64 years, the U.S. Department of Health and Human Services recommends in "Physical Activity Guidelines for Americans" (September 16, 2011, http://www.health.gov/paguidelines/) 2 hours and 30 minutes per week of moderate-intensity, or 1 hour and 15 minutes (75 minutes) per week of vigorous-intensity aerobic physical activity, or an equivalent combination of moderate- and vigorous-intensity aerobic physical

FIGURE 5.3

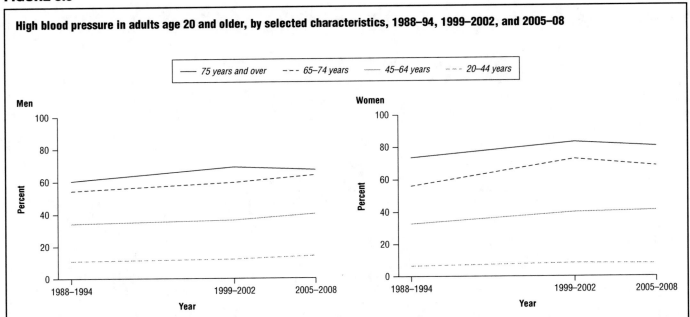

High blood pressure in adults age 20 and older, by selected characteristics, 1988–94, 1999–2002, and 2005–08

Legend: —— 75 years and over   – – – 65–74 years   ········ 45–64 years   - - - 20–44 years

SOURCE: "Figure 15. Hypertension among Adults 20 Years of Age and over, by Sex and Age: United States, 1988–94, 1999–2002, and 2005–08," in *Health, United States, 2010: With Special Feature on Death and Dying*, Centers for Disease Control and Prevention, National Center for Health Statistics, 2011, http://www.cdc.gov/nchs/data/hus/hus10.pdf#listtables (accessed December 14, 2011)

FIGURE 5.4

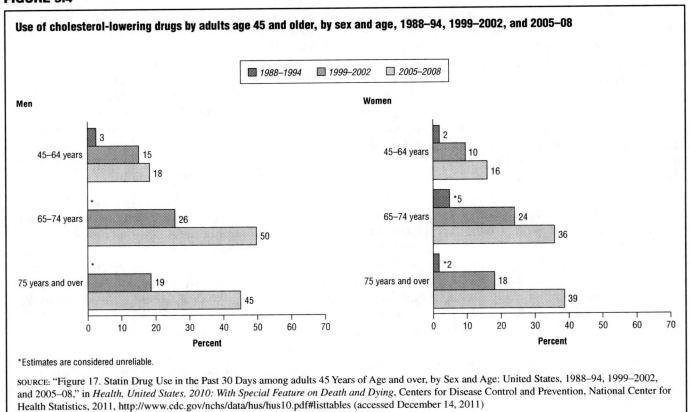

Use of cholesterol-lowering drugs by adults age 45 and older, by sex and age, 1988–94, 1999–2002, and 2005–08

Legend: ■ 1988–1994   ■ 1999–2002   □ 2005–2008

*Estimates are considered unreliable.

SOURCE: "Figure 17. Statin Drug Use in the Past 30 Days among adults 45 Years of Age and over, by Sex and Age: United States, 1988–94, 1999–2002, and 2005–08," in *Health, United States, 2010: With Special Feature on Death and Dying*, Centers for Disease Control and Prevention, National Center for Health Statistics, 2011, http://www.cdc.gov/nchs/data/hus/hus10.pdf#listtables (accessed December 14, 2011)

activity. Aerobic activity should be performed in episodes of at least 10 minutes, preferably spread throughout the week. Adults should also engage in muscle-strengthening activities that involve all the major muscle groups on two or more days per week. The Department of Health and Human Services asserts that additional health benefits are

FIGURE 5.5

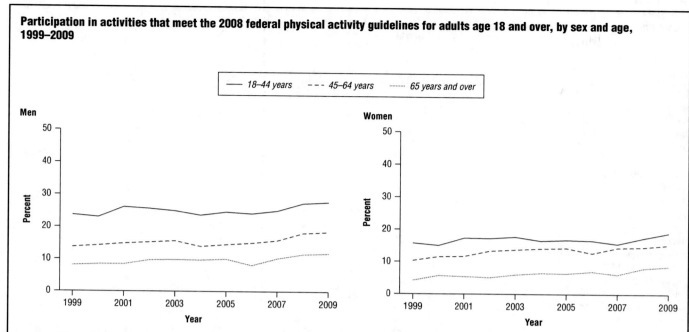

Participation in activities that meet the 2008 federal physical activity guidelines for adults age 18 and over, by sex and age, 1999–2009

SOURCE: "Figure 12. Participation in Leisure-Time Aerobic and Muscle-Strengthening Activities That Meet the 2008 Federal Physical Activity Guidelines for Adults 18 Years of Age and over, by Sex and Age: United States, 1999–2009," in *Health, United States, 2010: With Special Feature on Death and Dying*, Centers for Disease Control and Prevention, National Center for Health Statistics, 2011, http://www.cdc.gov/nchs/data/hus/hus10.pdf#listtables (accessed December 14, 2011)

provided by increasing to 5 hours (300 minutes) per week of moderate-intensity aerobic physical activity, or 2 hours and 30 minutes per week of vigorous-intensity physical activity, or an equivalent combination of both.

CONTRIBUTING FACTORS. Diabetes, or elevated blood glucose, affects cholesterol and triglyceride levels. The disease can sharply increase the risk of heart attack, especially when blood glucose is uncontrolled or poorly controlled. According to the National Institute of Diabetes and Digestive and Kidney Diseases, in "National Diabetes Statistics, 2011" (February 2011, http://diabetes.niddk .nih.gov/dm/pubs/statistics/index.htm), in 2004 approximately 68% of deaths among people aged 65 years and older who had diabetes resulted from heart disease and stroke. Adults with diabetes have heart disease death rates that are two to four times higher than adults without diabetes. Table 5.1 shows that 11.9% of adults over the age of 20 years had diabetes in 2007–08.

Obesity is also a factor that contributes to heart disease. Research shows that the location of body fat may affect the risk of suffering a heart attack significantly. Men with a waist measurement that exceeds their hip measurement and women whose waistline measurement is more than 80% of their hip measurement are at greater risk. Even though obesity is directly associated with an increased risk for cardiovascular disease, being overweight to any degree strains the heart.

The prevalence of obesity among adults aged 20 years and older in the United States has increased from 19.4% in 1997 to 29.4% in 2011. (See Figure 5.6.) The NCHS notes in *Early Release of Selected Estimates Based on Data from the January–June 2011 National Health Interview Survey* (December 2011, http://www.cdc.gov/ nchs/data/nhis/earlyrelease/201112_06.pdf) that even though the prevalence of overweight and obesity increased in both males and females in all racial and ethnic groups between 1997 and 2011, non-Hispanic white women were less likely to be obese than Hispanic and non-Hispanic African-American women. Obesity was highest among non-Hispanic African-American women (45.8%). (See Figure 5.7.)

Women and Heart Disease

Until the early 1990s almost all research on heart disease was carried out on middle-aged men. However, heart disease affects women, too. When a woman enters menopause, she begins to lose the protection provided by the hormones that appear to reduce the risk of heart disease. As a result, the rates of coronary heart disease are two to three times higher among postmenopausal women than among premenopausal women. According to Roger et al., 43% of deaths among women are attributable to cardiovascular disease. The researchers also note that more than one out of three women suffers from some form of cardiovascular disease. In fact,

TABLE 5.1

Selected health conditions and risk factors, 1988–94 through 2007–08

[Data are based on interviews and physical examinations of a sample of the civilian noninstitutionalized population]

Health condition	1988–1994	1999–2000	2001–2002	2003–2004	2005–2006	2007–2008
Diabetes[a]			Percent of persons 20 years of age and over			
Total, age-adjusted[b]	9.1	9.0	10.5	10.8	10.4	11.5
Total, crude	8.4	8.5	10.1	10.8	10.7	11.9
High cholesterol[c]						
Total, age-adjusted[d]	22.8	25.0	24.4	27.5	27.0	27.2
Total, crude	21.5	24.0	23.9	27.5	27.6	28.3
High serum total cholesterol[e]						
Total, age-adjusted[d]	20.8	18.3	16.5	16.9	15.6	14.2
Total, crude	19.6	17.7	16.4	17.0	15.9	14.6
Hypertension[f]						
Total, age-adjusted[d]	25.5	30.0	29.7	32.1	30.5	31.2
Total, crude	24.1	28.9	28.9	32.5	31.7	32.6
Uncontrolled high blood pressure among persons with hypertension[g]						
Total, age-adjusted[d]	77.2	71.9	68.3	63.8	63.0	56.2
Total, crude	73.9	69.1	65.4	60.8	56.6	51.8
Overweight (includes obesity)[h]						
Total, age-adjusted[d]	56.0	64.0	65.3	66.0	66.6	67.9
Total, crude	54.9	63.6	65.2	66.2	67.0	68.1
Obesity[i]						
Total, age-adjusted[d]	22.9	30.1	29.9	32.0	33.9	33.5
Total, crude	22.3	29.9	30.0	32.0	34.2	33.7
Untreated dental caries[j]						
Total, age-adjusted[d]	27.7	24.3	21.3	30.0	23.6	21.2
Total, crude	28.2	25.0	21.6	30.3	23.7	21.2
Obesity[k]			Percent of persons under 20 years of age			
2–5 years	7.2	10.3	10.6	14.0	11.0	10.4
6–11 years	11.3	15.1	16.3	18.8	15.1	19.6
12–19 years	10.5	14.8	16.7	17.4	17.8	18.1
Untreated dental caries[j, l]						
6–19 years	23.6	22.7	20.6	25.2	—	16.1

—Data not available.

[a]Includes physician-diagnosed and undiagnosed diabetes. Physician-diagnosed diabetes was obtained by self-report and excludes women who reported having diabetes only during pregnancy. Undiagnosed diabetes is defined as a fasting blood glucose (FBG) of at least 126 mg/dl or a hemoglobin A1c of at least 6.5% and no reported physician diagnosis. Respondents had fasted for at least 8 hours and less than 24 hours. Estimates in some prior editions of *Health, United States* included data from respondents who had fasted for at least 9 hours and less than 24 hours. In 2005–2006 and 2007–2008, testing was performed at a different laboratory and using different instruments than testing in earlier years. National Health and Nutrition Examination Survey (NHANES) conducted a crossover study to evaluate the impact of these changes on FBG and A1c measurements. As a result of that study, NHANES recommended that 2005–2008 data on FBG and A1c measurements be adjusted to be compatible with earlier years. Undiagnosed diabetes estimates in *Health, United States* were produced after adjusting the 2005–2008 lab data as recommended. The definition of undiagnosed diabetes in previous editions of *Health, United States* did not consider hemoglobin A1c. The revised definition of undiagnosed diabetes was based on recommendations from the American Diabetes Association.
[b]Age-adjusted to the 2000 standard population using three age groups: 20–44 years, 45–64 years, and 65 years and over. Age-adjusted estimates may differ from other age-adjusted estimates based on the same data and presented elsewhere if different age groups are used in the adjustment procedure.
[c]High cholesterol is defined as measured serum total cholesterol of great than or equal to 240 mg/dl or reporting taking cholesterol-lowering medication. Respondents were asked, "Are you now following this advice [from a doctor or health professional] to take prescribed medicine [to lower your cholesterol]" Risk levels for serum total cholesterol have been defined by the Third Report of the National Cholesterol Education Program Expert Panel on Detection, Evaluation, and Treatment of High Blood Cholesterol in Adults.
[d]Age-adjusted to the 2000 standard population using five age groups: 20–34 years, 35–44 years, 45–54 years, 55–64 years, and 65 years and over. Age-adjusted estimates may differ from the age-adjusted estimates based on the same data and presented elsewhere if different age groups are used in the adjustment procedure.
[e]High serum total cholesterol is defined as greater than or equal to 240 mg/dl (6.20 mmll/L). This second measure of cholesterol presented in *Health, United States*, is based solely on measured high serum total cholesterol.
[f]Hypertension is defined as having elevated blood pressue and/or taking antihypertensive medication. Elevated blood pressure is defined as having systolic pressure of at least 140 mmHg or diastolic pressure of at least 90 mmHg. Those with elevated blood pressure may be taking prescribed medicine for high blood pressure. Respondents were asked, "Are you now taking prescribed medicine for your high blood pressure?"
[g]Uncontrolled high blood pressure among persons with hypertentions is defined as measured systolic pressure of at least 140 mmHg or diastolic pressure of at least 90 mmHg, among those with measured high blood pressure or reporting taking antihypertensive medication.
[h]Excludes pregnant women. Overweight is defined as body mass index (BMI) greater than or equal to 25 kg/m[2].
[i]Excludes pregnant women. Obesity is defined as body mass index (BMI) greater than or equal to 30 kg/m[2].
[j]Untreated dental caries refers to untreated coronal caries. Starting with 2005–2006 NHANES data, dental caries data were collected using a simplified examination process. Because of this change in data collection and because estimates from 2003–2004 and earlier years considered whether the teeth were primary or permanent, 2005–2006 estimates and beyond are not comparable with earlier data. In addition, dental caries data are no longer collected on children younger than 5 years of age.

starting at age 75 the prevalence of cardiovascular disease is higher among women than among men of the same age group.

Women are more seriously affected by heart disease than men are because women have smaller arteries, they frequently wait longer to get care, and they are generally

TABLE 5.1

Selected health conditions and risk factors, 1988–94 through 2007–08 [CONTINUED]

[Data are based on interviews and physical examinations of a sample of the civilian noninstitutionalized population]

[k]Obesity is defined as body mass index (BMI) at or above the sex- and age-specific 95th percentile BMI cutoff points from the 2000 Center for Disease Control Growth Charts: United States. Advance data from vital and health statistics; no 314. Starting with *Health, United States, 2010*, the terminology describing height for weight among children changed from previous editions. The term obesity now refers to children who were formerly labeled as overweight. This is a change in terminology only and not in measurement; the previous definition of overweight is now the definition of obesity.
[l]Estimate is for 2005–2008. The 4-year estimate is shown for children because it is more reliable than the 2-year estimates.

SOURCE: "Table 66. Selected Health Conditions and Risk Factors: United States, 1988–1994 through 2007–2008," in *Health, United States, 2010: With Special Feature on Death and Dying*, Centers for Disease Control and Prevention, National Center for Health Statistics, 2011, http://www.cdc.gov/nchs/data/hus/hus10 .pdf#listtables (accessed December 14, 2011)

FIGURE 5.6

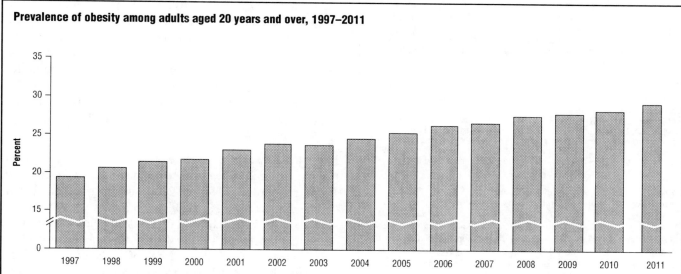

Prevalence of obesity among adults aged 20 years and over, 1997–2011

Notes: Data are based on household interviews of a sample of the civilian noninstitutionalized population. Obesity is defined as a body mass index (BMI) of 30 kg/m² or more. The measure is based on self-reported height (m) and weight (kg). Estimates of obesity are restricted to adults aged 20 and over for consistency with the Healthy People 2020 (3) program. The analyses excluded people with unknown height or weight (about 6% of respondents each year).

SOURCE: "Figure 6.1. Prevalence of Obesity among Adults Aged 20 Years and over: United States, 1997–June 2011," in *Early Release of Selected Estimates Based on Data from the January–June 2011 National Health Interview Survey*, Centers for Disease Control and Prevention, National Center for Health Statistics, December 2011, http://www.cdc.gov/nchs/data/nhis/earlyrelease/201112_06.pdf (accessed December 26, 2011)

older (typically by 10 years) when heart disease strikes. Another reason is that women's early symptoms of heart disease often differ from those of the "classic" heart attack. According to Samantha J. Zbierajewski-Eischeid and Susan J. Loeb, in "Myocardial Infarction in Women: Promoting Symptom Recognition, Early Diagnosis, and Risk Assessment" (*Dimensions of Critical Care Nursing*, vol. 28, no. 1, January–February 2009), symptoms that often occur in women before a heart attack are unusual fatigue, sleep disturbance, shortness of breath, indigestion, and anxiety. Even though many symptoms that may occur during a heart attack are comparable to the symptoms men experience (shortness of breath, weakness, unusual fatigue, cold sweat, and dizziness), women may also experience nausea (with or without vomiting and back pain). Zbierajewski-Eischeid and Loeb also assert that health professionals may fail to identify accurately a heart attack in women.

Lori Mosca et al. note in "Effectiveness-Based Guidelines for the Prevention of Cardiovascular Disease in Women—2011 Update" (*Circulation*, vol. 123, no. 11, March 2011) that there has been considerable progress in the increasing awareness, treatment, and prevention of cardiovascular disease in women since the first women-specific recommendations were published in 1999 by the AHA. The researchers note that public awareness of cardiovascular disease as the leading cause of death among women rose from 30% in 1997 to 54% in 2009. The death rate from coronary heart disease in women declined to 95.7 per 100,000 women in 2007, a third of the rate in 1980. According to Mosca et al., about half of this decline in coronary heart disease deaths is attributed to reducing major risk factors and the other half to treatment, including secondary prevention such as the widespread use of cholesterol-lowering drugs.

FIGURE 5.7

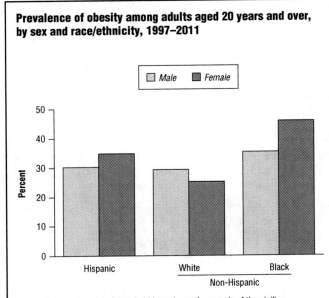

Prevalence of obesity among adults aged 20 years and over, by sex and race/ethnicity, 1997–2011

Notes: Data are based on household interviews of a sample of the civilian noninstitutionalized population. Obesity is defined as a body mass index (BMI) of 30 kg/m² or more. The measure is based on self-reported height (m) and weight (kg). Estimates of obesity are restricted to adults aged 20 and over for consistency with the Healthy People 2020 (3) program. The analyses excluded 3.6% of persons with unknown height or weight. Estimates are age adjusted using the projected 2000 U.S. population as the standard population and using five age groups: 20–24, 25–34, 35–44, 45–64, and 65 and over.

SOURCE: "Figure 6.3. Age-Adjusted Prevalence of Obesity among Adults Aged 20 Years and Over, by Sex and Race/Ethnicity: United States, 1997–June 2011," in *Early Release of Selected Estimates Based on Data from the January–June 2011 National Health Interview Survey*, Centers for Disease Control and Prevention, National Center for Health Statistics, December 2011, http://www.cdc.gov/nchs/data/nhis/earlyrelease/201112_06.pdf (accessed December 26, 2011).

Stroke

Stroke (cerebrovascular disease) is a cardiovascular disease that affects the blood vessels of the central nervous system. When an artery supplying oxygen and nutrients to the brain bursts or becomes clogged with a blood clot, a part of the brain does not receive the oxygen it needs. Without the necessary oxygen, the affected nerve cells die within moments. The parts of the body that are controlled by these nerve cells also become dysfunctional. Because dead brain cells cannot be replaced, the damage done by a stroke is often permanent.

Stroke affects people in different ways. The extent of the resulting damage or loss depends on the type of stroke and the area of the brain that has been damaged. Physicians can often identify the location of a stroke in the brain from the symptoms and deficits that are observed during a neurologic examination, even before an imaging study (computed tomography [CT] or magnetic resonance imaging) confirms the region of the brain affected. The senses, speech, the ability to understand speech, behavioral patterns, thought, and memory are affected most frequently. The most common effect is for one side of the body to become paralyzed or severely weakened. A loss of sensation or vision as the result of the stroke can result in a loss of awareness of the affected parts, so many stroke victims may forget or "neglect" the parts of the body that are weakened or paralyzed. Falls, bumping into objects, or dressing only one side of the body tend to result from this sudden lack of awareness.

INCIDENCE OF STROKE DEATHS IS DECLINING. In *Health, United States, 2010*, the NCHS notes that stroke was the third-leading cause of death in the United States in 2007, following heart disease and cancer, and that 135,952 Americans died of stroke. (See Table 1.12 in Chapter 1.) Lloyd-Jones et al. indicate that each year about 610,000 people suffer a new stroke and 185,000 experience recurrent strokes. The AHA explains in the fact sheet "Older Americans and Cardiovascular Diseases" (December 2011, http://www.heart.org/idc/groups/heart-public/@wcm/@sop/@smd/documents/downloadable/ucm_319574.pdf) that among people aged 60 to 79 years, 7.2% of men and 8.3% of women have had a stroke. Among those aged 80 years and older, 14.5% of men and 14.8% of women have had a stroke.

Lloyd-Jones et al. observe that in 2006 stroke accounted for one in every 18 deaths. The death rate for stroke declined by 33.5% between 1996 and 2006, and the actual number of stroke deaths fell by 18.4%. Figure 5.8 shows that the rate of stroke deaths in people aged 65 years and older declined by one-quarter between 1997 and 2007. Roger et al. report that women have a higher lifetime risk of stroke and on average are older than men when a stroke occurs—at age 75 versus age 71. Because women live longer than men, more women die of stroke each year. In 2008 women accounted for 60.1% of stroke deaths in the United States.

The two blood thinners heparin and warfarin are often used to reduce the chance of blood clots and recurrent strokes, even though these drugs pose some risk of bleeding problems. Clinical trials show that the drugs are safe if their use is closely monitored. Another drug, tissue plasminogen activator (tPA), is a "clot-busting drug" approved specifically for fighting strokes. tPA, which became available in 1996, must be administered within three hours after the onset of a stroke. The drug works to stop the swift advance of damage that is caused by clots shutting off blood flow to the brain, which accounts for four-fifths of strokes. Early detection and immediate treatment are vital for tPA treatment to be optimally effective. The use of statin drugs and regular, low doses of aspirin have also proved effective in preventing stroke.

Aspirin not only helps prevent ischemic stroke (the most common type of stroke; it is usually caused by a clot occluding a blood vessel that supplies the brain) but also helps when given to a person immediately after an ischemic stroke to reduce the risk of suffering another stroke. Aspirin confers protection against stroke by preventing the

FIGURE 5.8

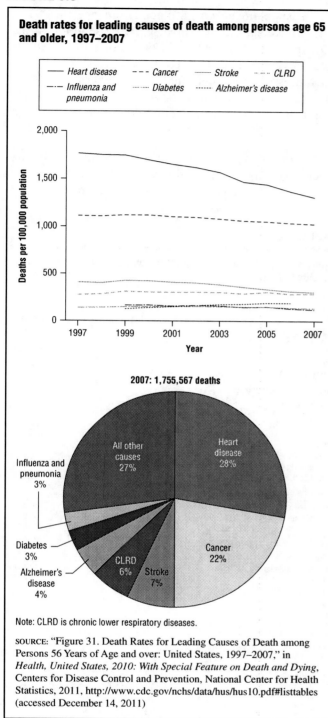

Death rates for leading causes of death among persons age 65 and older, 1997–2007

Note: CLRD is chronic lower respiratory diseases.

SOURCE: "Figure 31. Death Rates for Leading Causes of Death among Persons 56 Years of Age and over: United States, 1997–2007," in *Health, United States, 2010: With Special Feature on Death and Dying*, Centers for Disease Control and Prevention, National Center for Health Statistics, 2011, http://www.cdc.gov/nchs/data/hus/hus10.pdf#listtables (accessed December 14, 2011)

formation of the clots that can block blood vessels. However, aspirin does not help prevent hemorrhagic stroke (another common type of stroke) because this type of stroke is caused by the rupture of a blood vessel in the brain and results in an accumulation of blood.

REHABILITATION FOR STROKE SURVIVORS. Stroke is a leading cause of serious long-term disability. The AHA asserts that stroke accounts for more than half of all patients who are hospitalized for acute brain diseases. According to

Philippe Couillard, Alexandre Y. Poppe, and Shelagh B. Coutts, in "Predicting Recurrent Stroke after Minor Stroke and Transient Ischemic Attack" (*Expert Review of Cardiovascular Therapy*, vol. 7, no. 10, October 2009), the risk of recurrent stroke after even a minor stroke is quite high—10% in the 90 days following the first stroke.

Many survivors lose mental and physical abilities and need expensive, long, and intensive rehabilitation to regain their independence. In some cases independence is not achievable. Stroke can affect most senses and perception, and patients who have had a stroke may find even familiar surroundings incomprehensible. They may be unable to recognize or understand well-known objects or people. The simplest activities become difficult, and depression is a common problem because patients who have had a stroke may feel overwhelmed and develop a sense of despair.

According to Lloyd-Jones et al., the duration of recovery depends on the severity of the stroke. Between 50% and 70% of stroke survivors regain the ability to function independently, whereas 15% to 30% suffer permanent disability. Three months after a stroke, 20% of patients require institutional care. Lloyd-Jones et al. also note a study of sex differences among first-time stroke patients, which showed that women suffered more disability than men—33% of women compared with 27% of men had moderate to severe disability when they were discharged from the hospital.

In *Acute Stroke Management* (August 10, 2011, http://www.emedicine.com/neuro/TOPIC9.HTM), Edward C. Jauch, Brett Kissela, and Brian Stettler explain that according to the Framingham Heart Study (a study of heart health initiated in Framingham, Massachusetts, in 1948 that by 2002 included the grandchildren of the original 5,209 participants), 31% of stroke survivors needed help taking care of themselves, 20% required help walking, and 71% had some type of impaired vocational ability when examined seven years after the occurrence of their stroke. Sixteen percent needed to be institutionalized.

Spontaneous recovery during the initial 30 days after a stroke probably accounts for the highest levels of regained functional ability. However, rehabilitation to reduce dependency and improve physical ability is also vital. The patient's attitude, the skills of the rehabilitation team, and the support and understanding from the patient's family all affect the quality of recovery.

Toby B. Cumming et al. observe in "Very Early Mobilization after Stroke Fast-Tracks Return to Walking: Further Results from the Phase II AVERT Randomized Controlled Trial" (*Stroke*, vol. 42, no. 1, January 2011) that within 12 months of a stroke, one-third of stroke patients will die and another third are left with disability—meaning that they are restricted in performing simple activities of daily living and require some kind of assistance. For many stroke patients, one of the most important goals is to regain or improve walking ability. The researchers compare functional outcomes of patients who receive standard stroke care and those who receive earlier, more intensive treatment (mobilization within 24 hours poststroke and regular physical activity). Cumming et al. find that earlier and more intensive physical activity after stroke improves functional recovery by reducing the time to unassisted walking and improving independence in the activities of daily living.

High Blood Pressure

Blood pressure is a combination of two forces: the heart pumping blood into the arteries and the resistance of small arteries called arterioles to the flow of blood. The greater the resistance, the greater the pressure that is needed by the heart to keep the blood moving. The walls of the arterioles are elastic enough to allow for the expansion and contraction that is caused by the constantly changing rate of blood flow, thus allowing for a steady blood pressure in normal bodies. If the arterioles stay contracted or lose their elasticity as a result of atherosclerosis (commonly known as "hardening of the arteries"), the resistance to blood flow increases and blood pressure rises.

Blood pressure is measured in millimeters of mercury (mm Hg) by an instrument known as a sphygmomanometer. The sphygmomanometer produces two values: the systolic pressure (a measurement of the maximum pressure of the blood flow when the heart contracts or beats) and the diastolic pressure (the minimum pressure of the blood flow between beats). A typical normal range of values may vary, but the more resistance there is to blood flow, the higher the reading. High blood pressure (hypertension) for adults is defined as a systolic pressure equal to or greater than 140 mm Hg and/or a diastolic pressure equal to or greater than 90 mm Hg.

Prehypertension is defined as systolic pressure of 120 mm Hg to 139 mm Hg and diastolic pressure of 80 mm Hg to 89 mm Hg. According to the Agency for Healthcare Research and Quality, in "Prehypertension Accounts for a Substantial Number of Hospitalizations, Nursing Home Admissions, and Premature Deaths" (April 2005, http://archive.ahrq.gov/research/apr05/0405RA10.htm#head10), approximately two-thirds of individuals aged 45 to 64 years and 80% of those aged 65 to 74 years have prehypertension.

Elevated blood pressure causes the heart to work harder than normal and places the arteries under a strain that might contribute to a heart attack, stroke, or atherosclerosis. When the heart works too hard, it can become enlarged and will eventually be unable to function at maximum pumping capacity.

PREVALENCE OF HYPERTENSION. In "Prevalence of Hypertension and Controlled Hypertension—United States, 2005–2008" (*Morbidity and Mortality Weekly Report*, supplement, vol. 60, no. 1, January 14, 2011), Nora L. Keenan and Kimberly A. Rosendorf of the CDC report that in 2005–08, 29.9% of all U.S. adults aged 18 years and older were hypertensive (either had blood pressure readings equal to or greater than 140/90 mm Hg or were taking antihypertensive medication). (See Table 5.2.) Among people with hypertension, the overall prevalence of hypertension control was 43.7%.

According to Keenan and Rosendorf, in 2005–08 hypertension prevalence rose with advancing age and lowered with increasing educational attainment and

TABLE 5.2

Hypertension and controlled hypertension among adults age 18 and older, 2005–08

Characteristic	Hypertension[a] %	Controlled hypertension[b] %
Sex		
Male	30.6	38.6
Female (referent)	28.7	52.0
Age group (yrs), unadjusted[c]		
18–44 (referent)	10.5	37.5
45–64	40.6	48.9
≥65	70.3	45.6
Race/ethnicity		
Mexican American	25.5	31.8
Black, non-Hispanic	42.0	41.2
White, non-Hispanic (referent)	28.8	46.5
Marital status (persons aged ≥20 yrs)		
Never married	34.7	36.5
Married/living with partner (referent)	30.0	44.9
Divorced or separated/widowed	33.0	47.6
Education (persons aged ≥25 yrs)[c]		
<High school	37.3	36.5
High school graduate	35.9	47.2
Some college	33.6	44.6
College graduate or above (referent)	29.6	50.2
Foreign-born status		
Born in United States (referent)	30.8	45.2
Born outside United States	24.9	31.5
Family income, U.S. poverty level,[d] (%)		
<100	32.6	42.4
100–199	32.7	37.3
200–399	30.8	45.2
400–499	28.6	44.5
≥500 (referent)	27.4	47.9
Health insurance status (age ≤64 yrs)[c, e]		
Insured	21.8	47.6
Private insurance	20.2	45.4
Public insurance	32.1	55.5
Uninsured (referent)	20.0	26.4
Veteran status		
Yes	30.6	43.1
No (referent)	29.8	43.6
Diabetes[f]		
Yes	57.3	56.9
No (referent)	28.6	41.7
Obesity[g]		
Yes	39.8	47.5
No (referent)	25.8	39.8

TABLE 5.2

Hypertension and controlled hypertension among adults age 18 and older, 2005–08 [CONTINUED]

Characteristic	Hypertension[a] %	Controlled hypertension[b] %
Disability[h]		
Yes	39.3	54.1
No (referent)	29.3	41.1
Total	**29.9**	**43.7**

Note: Age adjusted to the 2000 U.S. standard population. Hypertension is age adjusted to the following seven age groups: 18–29, 30–39, 40–49, 50–59, 60–69, 70–79, and ≥80 yrs. Hypertension control and data by diabetes status are age adjusted to the following five age groups: 18–49, 50–59, 60–69, 70–79, and ≥80 yrs.

[a]Systolic blood pressure (SBP) ≥140 mm Hg, diastolic blood pressure (DBP) ≥90 mm Hg, or taking high blood pressure medicine.

[b]SBP <140 mm Hg and DBP <90 mm Hg among persons with hypertension.

[c]p < 0.05, test of trend for hypertension prevalence; not significant for controlled hypertension.

[d]Family income: income of all persons within a household who are related to each other by blood, marriage, or adoption. Poverty level: family income relative to family size and age of the members adjusted for inflation by using the poverty thresholds developed by the U.S. Bureau of the Census.

[e]Private health insurance: private health insurance or Medigap insurance. Public health insurance: Medicare, Medicaid, State Children's Health Insurance Program, military health care, state-sponsored health plan, or other government insurance.

[f]Persons with diabetes: those who have ever been told by a health-care professional that they have diabetes. Persons without diabetes: those who have never been told by a health-care professional that they have diabetes or have never been told that they have borderline diabetes.

[g]Obesity: body mass index ≥30 kg/m^2 based on measured weight and height.

[h]Disability: inability to work at a job or business because of a physical, mental, or emotional problem; limitation caused by difficulty remembering or periods of confusion; limitation in any activity because of a physical, mental, or emotional problem; or use of special equipment (e.g., a cane, a wheelchair, a special bed, or a special telephone).

SOURCE: Nora L. Keenan and Kimberly A. Rosendorf, "Table. Age-Adjusted Percentage of Hypertension and Controlled Hypertension among Adults Aged ≥18 Years, by Selected Demographic and Health Characteristics—National Health and Nutrition Examination Survey, United States, 2005–2008," in "Prevalence of Hypertension and Controlled Hypertension—United States, 2005–2008," *Morbidity and Mortality Weekly Report*, supplement, vol. 60, no. 1, January 14, 2011, http://www.cdc.gov/mmwr/pdf/other/su6001.pdf (accessed December 27, 2011)

income level. (See Table 5.2.) Non-Hispanic African-Americans (42%) had higher levels of hypertension than non-Hispanic whites (28.8%) and Mexican-Americans (25.5%), and adults born in the United States (30.8%) had higher levels of hypertension than foreign-born adults (24.9%). People with diabetes (57.3%) had a significantly higher prevalence of hypertension than those without diabetes (28.6%). Similarly, more people who were obese (39.8%) had hypertension, compared with those who were not obese (25.8%). Adults under the age of 64 years with public insurance (32.1%) were more likely to be hypertensive than those with private insurance (20.2%) and those without insurance (20%).

TREATMENT. In almost all cases, hypertension is treatable. A variety of medications, including diuretics, which rid the body of excess fluid and salt, can lower blood pressure.

Diet and lifestyle changes are also essential to control hypertension. Some people with only mildly elevated blood pressure need only to reduce or eliminate salt in their diet.

Blood pressure in overweight or obese people often declines when they lose weight. Heavy drinkers often see improved blood pressure when they abstain from alcohol or drink less. Similarly, smokers and people who use chewing tobacco are advised to quit because tobacco use causes an immediate spike in blood pressure and can also cause arterial narrowing, which increases blood pressure. Some people find exercise, stress management techniques, and relaxation therapy helpful. When people are aware of the problem and follow prescribed treatments, hypertension can be controlled and need not be fatal. However, patients often stop taking high blood pressure medication once their hypertension is controlled. This poses a serious danger; it is essential that patients continue to take the medication even if they feel perfectly well.

CANCER

Cancer is a large group of diseases that are characterized by the uncontrolled growth and spread of abnormal cells. These cells may grow into masses of tissue called tumors. Tumors made up of cells that are not cancerous are called benign tumors. The tumors consisting of cancer cells are called malignant tumors. The dangerous aspect of cancer is that cancer cells invade and destroy normal tissue.

The spread of cancer cells occurs either by a local growth of the tumor or by some of the cells becoming detached and traveling through the blood and lymph systems to start additional tumors in other parts of the body. Metastasis (the spread of cancer cells) may be confined to a region of the body, but if left untreated (and often despite treatment), the cancer cells can spread throughout the entire body, causing death. The rapid, invasive, and destructive nature of cancer makes it, arguably, the most feared of all diseases, even though it was second to heart disease as the leading cause of death in the United States in 2007. (See Table 1.12 in Chapter 1.)

What Causes Cancer, Who Gets Cancer, and Who Survives?

Cancer may be caused by both external factors (chemicals, radiation, and viruses) and internal factors (hormones, immune conditions, and inherited mutations). These factors act together or in sequence to begin or promote cancer.

No one is immune to cancer. Because the incidence increases with age, most cases are found among adults in midlife or older. However, in *Health, United States, 2010*, the NCHS reports that in 2007 cancer was the second-leading cause of death in the United States among children aged five to 14 years. (See Table 1.14 in Chapter 1.) The American Cancer Society (ACS) estimates in *Cancer Facts and Figures, 2011* (2011, http://www.cancer.org/acs/groups/content/@epidemiologysurveilance/documents/document/acspc-029771.pdf) that about one out of two men and one

out of three women in the United States will have some type of cancer at some point during their lifetime.

The ACS indicates that in 2011, 1.6 million new cancer cases were diagnosed and 571,950 people died of cancer. In the United States cancer causes one out of every four deaths. Even though the five-year survival rate for all cancers diagnosed between 1996 and 2006 was 68%, up from 50% between 1975 and 1977, the death rates for many forms of cancer have remained fairly steady since the 1930s. Three exceptions are stomach, uterine, and lung cancer. During the 1930s stomach cancer and uterine cancer had some of the highest death rates, but they have since declined to some of the lowest death rates. Meanwhile, the lung cancer death rate increased dramatically from 1930 up until 1990, especially for men, and then began to decline.

The improved rates of survival are largely attributable to earlier diagnosis and improved treatment. Just 50 years ago fewer than one out of four patients treated for cancer were still living after five years. Approximately 11.7 million Americans have a history of cancer. Many of these individuals are considered "cured," meaning that there is no evidence of the disease, and survivors have a life expectancy that is comparable to people who have never had cancer.

Research reveals that long-term survivors of childhood cancers are at an increased risk for subsequent health problems or limitations in physical performance and are likely to have difficulty with certain activities of daily living. In the editorial "Survivors of Childhood Cancer" (*BMJ*, December 8, 2009), Meriel Jenney and Gill Levitt observe that the numbers of children who survive cancer are increasing but that some may suffer lifelong problems as a result of the disease or its treatment. For example, Jenney and Levitt report that childhood cancer survivors are more likely than their siblings to report heart problems in young adult life.

Many childhood cancer survivors have endocrine conditions (disorders of the glands that secrete hormones into the bloodstream). Briana C. Patterson et al. review in "Endocrine Health Problems Detected in 519 Patients Evaluated in a Pediatric Cancer Survivor Program" (*Journal of Clinical Endocrinology and Metabolism*, December 21, 2011) the medical records of 519 pediatric and young adult cancer survivors. The researchers identified 480 endocrine conditions such as problems with weight and gonadal (related to the ovaries or testes) function in over half (58%) of the cancer survivors.

BEHAVIORAL AND ENVIRONMENTAL RISK FACTORS CONTRIBUTE TO CANCER DEATHS. In "Causes of Cancer in the World: Comparative Risk Assessment of Nine Behavioural and Environmental Risk Factors" (*Lancet*, vol. 366, no. 9499, November 19, 2005), Goodarz Danaei et al. collaborated with more than 100 scientists around the world in 2001 to estimate mortality for 12 types of cancer that are linked to certain risk factors. They find that of the 7 million cancer deaths worldwide, 35% were attributable to nine potentially modifiable behavioral and environmental risk factors: overweight and obesity, low fruit and vegetable intake, physical inactivity, smoking, alcohol consumption, unsafe sex, urban air pollution, indoor smoke from household use of coal, and contaminated injections in health care settings.

Worldwide, the nine risk factors caused 1.6 million cancer deaths among men and 830,000 cancer deaths among women. Smoking alone was estimated to have caused 21% of deaths from cancer worldwide. Smoking, which is linked to lung, mouth, stomach, pancreatic, and bladder cancers, was the biggest avoidable risk factor, followed by alcohol consumption and low fruit and vegetable intake. In high-income countries the nine risk factors caused 760,000 cancer deaths; smoking, alcohol consumption, and overweight and obesity were the most important causes of cancer in these nations.

In low- and middle-income regions the nine risk factors caused nearly 1.7 million cancer deaths; smoking, alcohol consumption, and low fruit and vegetable intake were the leading risk factors for these deaths. The sexual transmission of the human papillomavirus (HPV) was the leading risk factor for uterine cancer in women in low- and middle-income countries, particularly in sub-Saharan Africa and South Asia, mainly because access to cervical cancer screening is limited.

Danaei et al. conclude that "these results clearly show that many globally important types of cancer are preventable by changes in lifestyle behaviors and environmental interventions. To win the war against cancer we must focus not just on advances in biomedical technologies, but also on technologies and policies that change the behaviors and environments that cause those cancers."

Michael J. Thun et al. of the ACS observe in "The Global Burden of Cancer: Priorities for Prevention" (*Carcinogenesis*, vol. 31, no. 1, January 2010) that despite decreasing cancer death rates in high-resource countries such as the United States, the number of cancer cases and deaths is projected to more than double worldwide during the coming 20 to 40 years. By 2030 it is projected that there will be approximately 26 million new cancer cases and 17 million cancer deaths per year. Thun et al. advocate intensified efforts to control and limit international tobacco use, which is the single largest preventable cause of cancer worldwide, and increased availability of vaccines against hepatitis B (HBV) and HPV. (Chronic infection with HBV is associated with liver cancer and chronic infection with HPV is associated with cancer of the uterine cervix, the opening of the uterus into the vagina.)

The Seven Warning Signs of Cancer

In "Signs and Symptoms of Cancer" (January 6, 2010, http://www.cancer.org/Cancer/CancerBasics/signs-and-symptoms-of-cancer), the ACS identifies the general signs and symptoms that may be associated with cancer, such as fever, unexplained weight loss, fatigue, pain and skin changes such as hyperpigmentation (darker looking skin), jaundice (yellow-tinged eyes and skin), erythema (reddened skin), itching, and excessive hair growth. The ACS also lists the following symptoms or changes as possible signs of cancer and indications to see a physician:

- Change in bowel or bladder habits
- A sore that does not heal
- White patches inside the mouth or white spots on the tongue
- Unusual bleeding or discharge
- Thickening or lump in breast or elsewhere
- Indigestion or difficulty swallowing
- Obvious change in wart or mole
- Persistent cough or hoarseness

Could More Americans Be Saved?

The ACS estimates in *Cancer Facts and Figures, 2011* that many more lives could be saved with early detection and treatment. Regular screening can detect cancers of the breast, oral cavity, colon, rectum, cervix, prostate, and skin at early stages, when treatment is more likely to be successful. For example, 90% of female breast cancer patients currently survive five years or more, up from 63% during the early 1960s. With early detection, the ACS points out that for women who are diagnosed with localized breast cancer (cancer that has not spread to lymph nodes or other locations outside the breast), the five-year survival rate is 98%. Likewise, protecting skin from sunlight would prevent many of the more than 3 million skin cancers found annually.

In 2009 the U.S. Preventive Services Task Force (USPSTF) issued new mammogram guidelines for breast cancer screening. The USPSTF calls for screening mammograms every two years beginning at the age of 50 for women with average risk of breast cancer and advises against teaching women self-examination. The ACS and many other health organizations, including the American College of Surgeons and the Mayo Clinic, continue to recommend an annual screening mammogram beginning at the age of 40. Even though there is not yet consensus about when to begin mammography screening or the optimal frequency of screening, there is widespread agreement that mammography screening as well as other cancer screens, such as Papanicolaou tests (also called Pap smear or Pap test) to detect changes that could lead to cervical cancer, do save lives.

According to Table 5.3, the percentage of women aged 40 years and older who reported that they had received a mammogram within the past two years rose between 1987 and 2000, then stabilized at about 70% until 2003. In 2005 the percentage of women who were screened for breast cancer dropped to 66.6% and then increased slightly to 67.1% in 2008. A higher percentage of women aged 50 to 64 years (74.2%) than those aged 40 to 49 years (61.5%) reported having had a mammogram within the past two years. Table 5.4 shows that the percentage of women aged 18 years and older who reported receiving a Pap test to screen for cervical cancer within the past three years rose until 2000 but by 2008 had fallen slightly to 75.6%.

Cancer among African-Americans

African-Americans are more likely to be diagnosed with cancer and to die from the disease than any other racial or ethnic population. Table 5.5 shows that the rate of cancer deaths among African-American males in 2007 was 282.3 per 100,000 population, compared with 215.1 per 100,000 population among white men. According to the ACS, in *Cancer Facts and Figures, 2011*, most of these differences are not likely due to genetics; they are more likely due to social, cultural, behavioral, and environmental factors. Examples of social and economic inequities include a lack of health insurance, transportation, or access to quality, affordable health care that prevents or delays testing and timely treatment.

Gender and Cancer

Men and women are each more prone to certain types of cancer—most obviously, the cancers of the reproductive system, such as ovarian and cervical cancer in women and prostate or testicular cancer in men. Breast cancer also occurs mainly in women, although some men do die from this disease.

Similarly, cancer claims more males than females. In 2007 there were 217.5 cancer deaths per 100,000 males, compared with 151.3 cancer deaths per 100,000 females. (See Table 5.5.) The cancer death rates were higher among males of all ages.

Lung Cancer

The ACS estimates in *Cancer Facts and Figures, 2011* that 221,130 new cases of lung cancer were diagnosed in 2011. The incidence of lung cancer increased until 1991, after which it declined slightly. The incidence of new cases of lung cancer in men declined from a high of 102.1 per 100,000 in 1984 to 71.8 per 100,000 in 2007.

Lung cancer was estimated to claim 156,940 lives in 2011, accounting for 27% of all cancer deaths. Each year since 1987 more women have died of lung cancer than breast cancer, which had been the leading cause of

TABLE 5.3

Use of mammography by selected age groups, selected years 1987–2008

[Data are based on household interviews of a sample of the civilian noninstitutionalized population]

Characteristic	1987	1990	1993	1994	1999	2000	2003	2005	2008
	Percent of women having a mammogram within the past 2 years[a]								
40 years and over, age-adjusted[b, c]	29.0	51.7	59.7	61.0	70.3	70.4	69.5	66.6	67.1
40 years and over, crude[b]	28.7	51.4	59.7	60.9	70.3	70.4	69.7	66.8	67.6
50 years and over, age-adjusted[b, c]	27.3	49.8	59.7	60.9	72.1	73.7	72.4	68.2	70.3
50 years and over, crude[c]	27.4	49.7	59.7	60.6	71.9	73.6	72.4	68.4	70.5
Age									
40–49 years	31.9	55.1	59.9	61.3	67.2	64.3	64.4	63.5	61.5
50–64 years	31.7	56.0	65.1	66.5	76.5	78.7	76.2	71.8	74.2
65 years and over	22.8	43.4	54.2	55.0	66.8	67.9	67.7	63.8	65.5
65–74 years	26.6	48.7	64.2	63.0	73.9	74.0	74.6	72.5	72.6
75 years and over	17.3	35.8	41.0	44.6	58.9	61.3	60.6	54.7	57.9
Race[d]									
40 years and over, crude:									
White only	29.6	52.2	60.0	60.6	70.6	71.4	70.1	67.4	67.9
Black or African American only	24.0	46.4	59.1	64.3	71.0	67.8	70.4	64.9	68.0
American Indian or Alaska Native only	*	43.2	49.8	65.8	63.0	47.4	63.1	72.8	62.7
Asian only	*	46.0	55.1	55.8	58.3	53.5	57.6	54.6	66.1
Native Hawaiian or other Pacific Islander only	—	—	—	—	*	*	*	*	*
2 or more races	—	—	—	—	70.2	69.2	65.3	63.7	55.2
Hispanic origin and race[d]									
40 years and over, crude:									
Hispanic or Latina	18.3	45.2	50.9	51.9	65.7	61.2	65.0	58.8	61.2
Not Hispanic or Latina:	29.4	51.8	60.3	61.5	70.7	71.1	70.1	67.5	68.3
White only	30.3	52.7	60.6	61.3	71.1	72.2	70.5	68.3	68.7
Black or African American only	23.8	46.0	59.2	64.4	71.0	67.9	70.5	65.2	68.3
Age, Hispanic origin, and race[d]									
40–49 years:									
Hispanic or Latina	15.3	45.1	52.6	47.5	61.6	54.1	59.4	54.2	54.1
Not Hispanic or Latina:									
White only	34.3	57.0	61.6	62.0	68.3	67.2	65.2	65.5	64.1
Black or African American only	27.8	48.4	55.6	67.2	69.2	60.9	68.2	62.1	59.5
50–64 years:									
Hispanic or Latina	23.0	47.5	59.2	60.1	69.7	66.5	69.4	61.5	71.3
Not Hispanic or Latina:									
White only	33.6	58.1	66.2	67.5	77.9	80.6	77.2	73.5	74.1
Black or African American only	26.4	48.4	65.5	63.6	75.0	77.7	76.2	71.6	76.7
65 years and over:									
Hispanic or Latina	*	41.1	35.7	48.0	67.2	68.3	69.5	63.8	59.0
Not Hispanic or Latina:									
White only	24.0	43.8	54.7	54.9	66.8	68.3	68.1	64.7	66.1
Black or African American only	14.1	39.7	56.3	61.0	68.1	65.5	65.4	60.5	66.4
Age and percent of poverty level[e]									
40 years and over, crude:									
Below 100%	14.6	30.8	41.1	44.2	57.4	54.8	55.4	48.5	51.4
100%–199%	20.9	39.1	47.5	48.6	59.5	58.1	60.8	55.3	55.8
200%–399%	29.7	53.3	63.2	65.0	69.1	68.8	69.9	67.2	64.4
400% or more	42.9	68.7	74.1	74.1	79.8	81.5	77.7	76.6	79.0
40–49 years:									
Below 100%	18.6	32.2	36.1	43.0	51.3	47.4	50.6	42.5	46.6
100%–199%	18.4	39.0	47.8	47.6	52.8	43.6	54.0	49.8	46.5
200%–399%	31.2	55.2	63.0	64.5	63.0	60.2	63.0	61.8	56.8
400% or more	44.1	68.9	69.6	69.9	77.4	75.8	71.6	73.6	72.5
50–64 years:									
Below 100%	14.6	29.9	47.3	46.2	63.3	61.7	58.3	50.4	57.5
100%–199%	24.2	39.8	47.0	49.0	64.9	68.3	64.0	58.8	58.9
200%–399%	29.7	56.2	66.1	69.6	74.8	75.1	74.1	70.7	69.8
400% or more	44.7	71.6	78.7	78.0	83.4	86.9	84.9	80.6	84.3

cancer deaths for women for more than 40 years. For men, lung cancer is also the leading cause of cancer-related deaths.

The main risk factor for lung cancer is cigarette smoking, especially a long history of smoking (20 years or more). In addition, exposure to certain industrial

TABLE 5.3

Use of mammography by selected age groups, selected years 1987–2008 [CONTINUED]

[Data are based on household interviews of a sample of the civilian noninstitutionalized population]

Characteristic	1987	1990	1993	1994	1999	2000	2003	2005	2008
65 years and over:	Percent of women having a mammogram within the past 2 years[a]								
Below 100%	13.1	30.8	40.4	43.9	57.6	54.8	57.0	52.3	49.1
100%–199%	19.9	38.6	47.6	48.8	60.2	60.3	62.8	56.1	59.4
200%–399%	27.7	47.4	60.3	61.0	70.0	71.1	72.3	68.6	65.0
400% or more	34.7	61.2	71.3	73.0	76.7	81.9	73.0	72.6	78.3

*Estimates are considered unreliable.
—Data not available.
[a]Questions concerning use of mammography differed slightly on the National Health Interview Survey across the years for which data are shown.
[b]Includes all other races not shown separately, unknown poverty level in 1987, unknown health insurance status, unknown education level, and unknown disability status.
[c]Estimates for women 40 years of age and over are age-adjusted to the year 2000 standard population using four age groups: 40–49 years, 50–64 years, 65–74 years, and 75 years and over. Estimates for women 50 years of age and over are age-adjusted using three age groups.
[d]The race groups, white, black, American Indian or Alaska Native, Asian, Native Hawaiian or other Pacific Islander, and 2 or more races, include persons of Hispanic and non-Hispanic origin. Persons of Hispanic origin may be of any race. Starting with 1999 data, race-specific estimates are tabulated according to the 1997 Revisions to the Standards for the Classification of Federal Data on Race and Ethnicity and are not strictly comparable with estimates for earlier years. The five single-race categories plus multiple-race categories shown in the table conform to the 1997 Standards. Starting with 1999 data, race-specific estimates are for persons who reported only one racial group; the category 2 or more races includes persons who reported more than one racial group. Prior to 1999, data were tabulated according to the 1977 Standards with four racial groups and the Asian only category included Native Hawaiian or other Pacific Islander. Estimates for single-race categories prior to 1999 included persons who reported one race or, if they reported more than one race, identified one race as best representing their race. Starting with 2003 data, race responses of other race and unspecified multiple race were treated as missing, and then race was imputed if these were the only race responses. Almost all persons with a race response of other race were of Hispanic origin.
[e]Percent of poverty level is based on family income and family size and composition using U.S. Census Bureau poverty thresholds. Poverty level was unknown for 11% of women 40 years of age and over in 1987. Missing family income data were imputed for 1997 and beyond.
Notes: Data starting in 1997 are not strictly comparable with data for earlier years due to the 1997 questionnaire redesign. Data for additional years are available. Data have been revised and differ from previous editions of *Health, United States.*

SOURCE: Adapted from "Table 86. Use of Mammography among Women 40 Years of Age and over, by Selected Characteristics: United States, Selected Years 1987–2008," in *Health, United States, 2010: With Special Feature on Death and Dying,* Centers for Disease Control and Prevention, National Center for Health Statistics, 2011, http://www.cdc.gov/nchs/data/hus/2010/086.pdf (accessed December 14, 2011)

---

substances, such as asbestos, organic chemicals, and radon, can increase the risk of developing the disease.

Passive, or involuntary or secondhand smoking (inhaling other people's smoke), also increases the risk for nonsmokers. Research shows that the risk to a nonsmoking woman who is married to a smoker is 30% greater than for a woman with a nonsmoking spouse. In "Health Effects of Exposure to Secondhand Smoke" (November 30, 2011, http://www.epa.gov/smokefree/healtheffects.html), the U.S. Environmental Protection Agency claims that an estimated 3,000 nonsmokers die each year from secondhand-smoke-induced lung cancer. The agency added secondhand smoke to its list of known carcinogens in 1993.

Lowell Dale explains in "What Is Third-Hand Smoke, and Why Is It a Concern?" (July 1, 2011, http://www.mayoclinic.com/health/third-hand-smoke/AN01985) that thirdhand smoke, the residue of nicotine and other toxic chemicals in tobacco that coats indoor surfaces such as walls, carpet, drapes, furniture, and bedding, has been identified as a health hazard. Thirdhand smoke, which can interact with other indoor pollutants to form cancer-causing compounds, poses a risk to both the skin and lungs.

The ACS explains that early diagnosis of lung cancer is difficult. By the time a tumor is visible on x-rays, it is often in the advanced stages. However, if an individual stops smoking before cellular changes occur, damaged

tissues often return to normal. New diagnostic tests such as low-dose spiral CT scans, which provide detailed three-dimensional images of the lungs, and laboratory procedures that can detect molecular markers for cancer in sputum have demonstrated an ability to diagnose lung cancer earlier than conventional tests, and research to evaluate their effects on survival rates is under way. The National Lung Screening Trial (http://www.cancer.gov/clinicaltrials/noteworthy-trials/nlst), a clinical trial to determine the effectiveness of lung cancer screening in high-risk people (people who smoked at least a pack of cigarettes per day for 30 years), reports 20% fewer lung cancer deaths among current and former heavy smokers who were screened with spiral CT, compared with standard chest x-ray. However, this detection method may not be useful in the general population because this study considered only subjects with a history of heavy smoking. Furthermore, the risks that are associated with screening, including radiation exposure from multiple CT scans and unnecessary lung biopsy and surgery, may outweigh the benefits in the general population. The treatment options for lung cancer include surgery, radiation therapy, and chemotherapy (anticancer drugs).

Colon and Rectal Cancer

The ACS reports in *Cancer Facts and Figures, 2011* that in 2011 an estimated 101,340 cases of colon cancer and 39,870 cases of rectal cancer were diagnosed and that

TABLE 5.4

Use of Pap smears by selected age groups, selected years 1987–2008

[Data are based on household interviews of a sample of the civilian noninstitutionalized population]

Characteristic	1987	1993	1994	1999	2000	2003	2005	2008
	Percent of women having a Pap smear within the past 3 years[a]							
18 years and over, age-adjusted[b, c]	74.1	77.7	76.8	80.8	81.3	79.2	77.9	75.6
18 years and over, crude[b]	74.4	77.7	76.8	80.8	81.2	79.0	77.7	75.1
Age								
18–44 years	83.3	84.6	82.8	86.8	84.9	83.9	83.6	81.8
18–24 years	74.8	78.8	76.6	76.8	73.5	75.1	74.5	70.5
25–44 years	86.3	86.3	84.6	89.9	88.5	86.8	86.8	85.7
45–64 years	70.5	77.2	77.4	81.7	84.6	81.3	80.6	78.8
45–54 years	75.7	82.1	81.9	83.8	86.3	83.6	83.4	81.0
55–64 years	65.2	70.6	71.0	78.4	82.0	77.8	76.8	76.0
65 years and over	50.8	57.6	57.3	61.0	64.5	60.8	54.9	50.0
65–74 years	57.9	64.7	64.9	70.0	71.6	70.1	66.3	61.6
75 years and over	40.4	48.0	47.3	50.8	56.7	51.1	42.7	37.5
Race[d]								
18 years and over, crude:								
White only	74.1	77.3	76.2	80.6	81.3	78.7	77.7	74.9
Black or African American only	80.7	82.7	83.5	85.7	85.1	84.0	81.1	80.1
American Indian or Alaska Native only	85.4	78.1	73.5	92.2	76.8	84.8	75.2	69.4
Asian only	51.9	68.8	66.4	64.4	66.4	68.3	64.1	65.1
Native Hawaiian or other Pacific Islander only	—	—	—	*	*	*	*	*
2 or more races	—	—	—	86.9	80.0	81.6	86.2	77.1
Hispanic origin and race[d]								
18 years and over, crude:								
Hispanic or Latina	67.6	77.2	74.4	76.3	77.0	75.4	75.5	75.4
Not Hispanic or Latina	74.9	77.8	77.0	81.3	81.7	79.5	78.0	75.1
White only	74.7	77.3	76.5	81.0	81.8	79.3	78.1	74.9
Black or African American only	80.9	82.7	83.8	86.0	85.1	83.8	81.2	80.0
Age, Hispanic origin, and race[d]								
18–44 years:								
Hispanic or Latina	73.9	80.9	80.6	77.0	78.1	75.9	76.5	77.9
Not Hispanic or Latina:								
White only	84.5	85.3	82.9	88.7	86.6	85.8	85.8	83.8
Black or African American only	89.1	88.0	89.1	90.8	88.5	88.6	86.4	83.5
45–64 years:								
Hispanic or Latina	57.7	75.8	70.1	79.5	77.8	77.9	78.4	78.2
Not Hispanic or Latina:								
White only	71.2	77.2	77.5	81.9	85.9	81.4	81.4	79.0
Black or African American only	76.2	80.3	82.2	84.6	85.7	84.7	80.5	82.1
65 years and over:								
Hispanic or Latina	41.7	57.1	43.8	63.7	66.8	64.6	60.0	52.6
Not Hispanic or Latina:								
White only	51.8	57.1	58.2	60.5	64.2	60.7	54.1	49.0
Black or African American only	44.8	61.2	59.5	64.5	67.2	59.6	60.1	58.7
Age and percent of poverty level[e]								
18 years and over, crude:								
Below 100%	64.3	70.3	68.8	73.6	72.0	70.5	68.7	68.9
100%–199%	68.2	71.2	68.8	72.5	73.4	71.4	69.0	65.0
200%–399%	77.6	80.6	80.1	80.6	80.2	78.6	77.9	72.5
400% or more	83.6	85.1	85.4	87.6	89.1	86.6	85.7	84.4
18–44 years:								
Below 100%	77.1	77.0	78.9	79.7	77.1	77.1	76.2	76.5
100%–199%	80.4	81.9	78.2	84.0	79.4	79.5	78.1	75.5
200%–399%	84.8	86.6	84.5	86.7	86.1	84.0	85.5	82.6
400% or more	88.9	91.3	88.7	91.1	89.8	89.5	88.7	87.0
45–64 years:								
Below 100%	53.6	66.5	62.0	73.1	73.6	66.0	65.9	66.2
100%–199%	60.4	64.8	66.2	70.4	76.1	71.4	69.6	65.6
200%–399%	71.0	79.5	80.3	79.9	80.0	80.8	79.3	75.3
400% or more	79.1	83.9	84.0	87.4	91.5	87.5	87.4	87.1

an estimated 49,380 people died of the diseases. The incidence of colorectal cancer has been decreasing since the mid-1980s, from 66.3 cases per 100,000 population in 1985 to 45.3 cases per 100,000 population in 2007.

When colorectal cancer is detected early, the ACS indicates that the five-year survival rate is 90%. However, only 39% of this type of cancer is found at this stage. If the malignancy has spread regionally, the five-year survival rate drops to 70%.

TABLE 5.4

Use of Pap smears by selected age groups, selected years 1987–2008 [CONTINUED]

[Data are based on household interviews of a sample of the civilian noninstitutionalized population]

Characteristic	1987	1993	1994	1999	2000	2003	2005	2008
65 years and over:	Percent of women having a Pap smear within the past 3 years[a]							
Below 100%	33.2	47.4	44.0	51.9	53.7	52.6	44.4	41.6
100%–199%	50.4	55.7	51.5	54.7	61.0	55.4	49.5	43.5
200%–399%	58.0	59.7	63.7	64.0	65.1	62.4	56.8	45.8
400% or more	65.2	67.5	76.2	70.4	75.4	70.2	64.6	65.7

—Data not available.
*Estimates are considered unreliable.
[a]Questions concerning use of Pap smears differed slightly on the National Health Interview Survey across the years for which data are shown.
[b]Includes all other races not shown separately, unknown poverty level in 1987, unknown health insurance status, unknown education level, and unknown disability status.
[c]Estimates are age-adjusted to the year 2000 standard population using five age groups: 18–44 years, 45–54 years, 55–64 years, 65–74 years, and 75 years and over. Age-adjusted estimates in this table may differ from other age-adjusted estimates based on the same data and presented elsewhere if different age groups are used in the adjustment procedure.
[d]The race groups, white, black, American Indian or Alaska Native, Asian, Native Hawaiian or other Pacific Islander, and 2 or more races, include persons of Hispanic and non-Hispanic origin. Persons of Hispanic origin may be of any race. Starting with 1999 data, race-specific estimates are tabulated according to the 1997 Revisions to the Standards for the Classification of Federal Data on Race and Ethnicity and are not strictly comparable with estimates for earlier years. The five single-race categories plus multiple-race categories shown in the table conform to the 1997 Standards. Starting with 1999 data, race-specific estimates are for persons who reported only one racial group; the category 2 or more races includes persons who reported more than one racial group. Prior to 1999, data were tabulated according to the 1977 Standards with four racial groups and the Asian only category included Native Hawaiian or other Pacific Islander. Estimates for single-race categories prior to 1999 included persons who reported one race or, if they reported more than one race, identified one race as best representing their race. Starting with 2003 data, race responses of other race and unspecified multiple race were treated as missing, and then race was imputed if these were the only race responses. Almost all persons with a race response of other race were of Hispanic origin.
[e]Percent of poverty level is based on family income and family size and composition using U.S. Census Bureau poverty thresholds. Missing family income data were imputed for 1993 and beyond.
Notes: Data starting in 1997 are not strictly comparable with data for earlier years due to the 1997 questionnaire redesign. Data for additional years are available.

SOURCE: Adapted from "Table 87. Use of Pap Smears among Women 18 Years of Age and over, by Selected Characteristics: United States, Selected Years 1987–2008," in *Health, United States, 2010: With Special Feature on Death and Dying*, Centers for Disease Control and Prevention, National Center for Health Statistics, 2011, http://www.cdc.gov/nchs/data/hus/2010/087.pdf (accessed December 14, 2011)

Colon cancer occurs most often in people without any known risk factors. However, people with a family history of polyps in the colon or rectum and people who have suffered from ulcerative colitis and other diseases of the bowel are considered to be at a greater risk for developing the disease. Other significant risk factors may be physical inactivity, obesity, diabetes, smoking, heavy alcohol consumption, and a diet high in fat and low in fiber.

The ACS recommends a variety of screening tests to detect bowel cancer in its early stages. A digital rectal examination, performed by a physician during a routine office visit, is recommended annually for those older than 40 years of age. For people older than age 50, an annual stool test for fecal occult blood (hidden blood) is recommended, along with flexible sigmoidoscopy (examination of the lower colon and rectum using a hollow, lighted tube) every five years or as often as recommended by the physician. The ACS also recommends an imaging procedure called a double-contrast barium enema, which provides a complete radiologic examination of the colon, every five years for people older than 50 years of age and a screening colonoscopy (examination of the entire colon) every 10 years or as often as recommended by the physician. Even though it is a more costly screening test, some people prefer a virtual colonoscopy, which uses x-rays and computers to produce images of the entire length of the colon.

Despite overwhelming evidence that screening and early detection save lives, many adults do not receive even

the simplest of the colon cancer screening tests. The CDC asserts in "Colorectal Cancer Screening Rates" (July 5, 2011, http://www.cdc.gov/cancer/colorectal/statistics/screening_rates.htm) that if everyone aged 50 years or older had regular screening tests and all precancerous polyps were removed, as many as 60% of deaths from colorectal cancer could be prevented.

The most common treatment for cancer of the bowel is surgery to remove the diseased area, in combination with radiation. A colostomy (an opening in the abdomen to allow for waste elimination) is seldom necessary for patients with colon cancer but may be required for patients with rectal cancer. The ACS reports that few patients with rectal cancer require a permanent colostomy if the cancer is detected in the early stages. Of those who do require a permanent colostomy, most go on to lead normal, active lives. Chemotherapeutic agents that are used to treat metastatic (spreading) colon and rectal cancer include the drugs oxaliplatin with 5-fluorouracil followed by leucovorin and bevacizumab, which block the growth of blood vessels to the tumor, and cetuximab and panitumumab, both of which block the effects of hormone-like factors that promote cancer cell growth.

Breast Cancer

Breast cancer is the most common form of cancer among women. According to the ACS, in *Cancer Facts and Figures, 2011*, an estimated 230,480 new cases of

TABLE 5.5

Death rates for cancer by sex, age, ethnicity and race, selected years 1950–2007

[Data are based on death certificates]

Sex, race, Hispanic origin, and age	1950[a,b]	1960[a,b]	1970[b]	1980[b]	1990[b]	2000[c]	2006[c]	2007[c]
All persons				Deaths per 100,000 resident population				
All ages, age-adjusted[d]	193.9	193.9	198.6	207.9	216.0	199.6	180.7	178.4
All ages, crude	139.8	149.2	162.8	183.9	203.2	196.5	187.0	186.6
Under 1 year	8.7	7.2	4.7	3.2	2.3	2.4	1.8	1.7
1–4 years	11.7	10.9	7.5	4.5	3.5	2.7	2.3	2.2
5–14 years	6.7	6.8	6.0	4.3	3.1	2.5	2.2	2.4
15–24 years	8.6	8.3	8.3	6.3	4.9	4.4	3.9	3.9
25–34 years	20.0	19.5	16.5	13.7	12.6	9.8	9.0	8.5
35–44 years	62.7	59.7	59.5	48.6	43.3	36.6	31.9	30.8
45–54 years	175.1	177.0	182.5	180.0	158.9	127.5	116.3	114.3
55–64 years	390.7	396.8	423.0	436.1	449.6	366.7	321.2	315.4
65–74 years	698.8	713.9	754.2	817.9	872.3	816.3	727.2	715.5
75–84 years	1,153.3	1,127.4	1,169.2	1,232.3	1,348.5	1,335.6	1,263.8	1,256.3
85 years and over	1,451.0	1,450.0	1,320.7	1,594.6	1,752.9	1,819.4	1,606.1	1,590.2
Male								
All ages, age-adjusted[d]	208.1	225.1	247.6	271.2	280.4	248.9	220.1	217.5
All ages, crude	142.9	162.5	182.1	205.3	221.3	207.2	196.6	197.0
Under 1 year	9.7	7.7	4.4	3.7	2.4	2.6	1.8	1.8
1–4 years	12.5	12.4	8.3	5.2	3.7	3.0	2.5	2.3
5–14 years	7.4	7.6	6.7	4.9	3.5	2.7	2.5	2.4
15–24 years	9.7	10.2	10.4	7.8	5.7	5.1	4.6	4.5
25–34 years	17.7	18.8	16.3	13.4	12.6	9.2	8.6	8.2
35–44 years	45.6	48.9	53.0	44.0	38.5	32.7	27.4	26.4
45–54 years	156.2	170.8	183.5	188.7	162.5	130.9	119.0	117.5
55–64 years	413.1	459.9	511.8	520.8	532.9	415.8	363.6	358.5
65–74 years	791.5	890.5	1,006.8	1,093.2	1,122.2	1,001.9	870.4	854.3
75–84 years	1,332.6	1,389.4	1,588.3	1,790.5	1,914.4	1,760.6	1,631.3	1,617.4
85 years and over	1,668.3	1,741.2	1,720.8	2,369.5	2,739.9	2,710.7	2,248.7	2,249.2
Female								
All ages, age-adjusted[d]	182.3	168.7	163.2	166.7	175.7	167.6	153.6	151.3
All ages, crude	136.8	136.4	144.4	163.6	186.0	186.2	177.6	176.5
Under 1 year	7.6	6.8	5.0	2.7	2.2	2.3	1.8	1.6
1–4 years	10.8	9.3	6.7	3.7	3.2	2.5	2.1	2.2
5–14 years	6.0	6.0	5.2	3.6	2.8	2.2	2.0	2.3
15–24 years	7.6	6.5	6.2	4.8	4.1	3.6	3.1	3.2
25–34 years	22.2	20.1	16.7	14.0	12.6	10.4	9.5	8.9
35–44 years	79.3	70.0	65.6	53.1	48.1	40.4	36.4	35.2
45–54 years	194.0	183.0	181.5	171.8	155.5	124.2	113.7	111.3
55–64 years	368.2	337.7	343.2	361.7	375.2	321.3	281.8	275.2
65–74 years	612.3	560.2	557.9	607.1	677.4	663.6	605.9	597.6
75–84 years	1,000.7	924.1	891.9	903.1	1,010.3	1,058.5	1,012.5	1,007.4
85 years and over	1,299.7	1,263.9	1,096.7	1,255.7	1,372.1	1,456.4	1,305.5	1,276.7
White male[e]								
All ages, age-adjusted[d]	210.0	224.7	244.8	265.1	272.2	243.9	217.9	215.1
All ages, crude	147.2	166.1	185.1	208.7	227.7	218.1	208.7	208.8
25–34 years	17.7	18.8	16.2	13.6	12.3	9.2	8.6	8.1
35–44 years	44.5	46.3	50.1	41.1	35.8	30.9	26.7	25.9
45–54 years	150.8	164.1	172.0	175.4	149.9	123.5	113.6	112.0
55–64 years	409.4	450.9	498.1	497.4	508.2	401.9	352.9	346.7
65–74 years	798.7	887.3	997.0	1,070.7	1,090.7	984.3	862.0	845.4
75–84 years	1,367.6	1,413.7	1,592.7	1,779.7	1,883.2	1,736.0	1,631.3	1,617.4
85 years and over	1,732.7	1,791.4	1,772.2	2,375.6	2,715.1	2,693.7	2,258.3	2,253.2
Black or African American male[e]								
All ages, age-adjusted[d]	178.9	227.6	291.9	353.4	397.9	340.3	284.9	282.3
All ages, crude	106.6	136.7	171.6	205.5	221.9	188.5	172.3	172.9
25–34 years	18.0	18.4	18.8	14.1	15.7	10.1	10.0	9.5
35–44 years	55.7	72.9	81.3	73.8	64.3	48.4	36.5	34.0
45–54 years	211.7	244.7	311.2	333.0	302.6	214.2	182.2	178.0
55–64 years	490.8	579.7	689.2	812.5	859.2	626.4	542.9	544.1
65–74 years	636.5	938.5	1,168.9	1,417.2	1,613.9	1,363.8	1,156.5	1,139.5
75–84 years[f]	853.5	1,053.3	1,624.8	2,029.6	2,478.3	2,351.8	1,979.1	1,936.9
85 years and over	—	1,155.2	1,387.0	2,393.9	3,238.3	3,264.8	2,543.3	2,637.1

TABLE 5.5

Death rates for cancer by sex, age, ethnicity and race, selected years 1950–2007 [CONTINUED]

[Data are based on death certificates]

Sex, race, Hispanic origin, and age	1950[a, b]	1960[a, b]	1970[b]	1980[b]	1990[b]	2000[c]	2006[c]	2007[c]
American Indian or Alaska Native male[e]				Deaths per 100,000 resident population				
All ages, age-adjusted[d]	—	—	—	140.5	145.8	155.8	135.5	139.4
All ages, crude	—	—	—	58.1	61.4	67.0	76.1	83.3
25–34 years	—	—	—	*	*	*	*	0.0
35–44 years	—	—	—	*	22.8	21.4	15.1	16.0
45–54 years	—	—	—	86.9	86.9	70.3	74.5	78.3
55–64 years	—	—	—	213.4	246.2	255.6	222.8	264.5
65–74 years	—	—	—	613.0	530.6	648.0	583.5	565.5
75–84 years	—	—	—	936.4	1,038.4	1,152.5	1,016.8	984.5
85 years and over	—	—	—	1,471.2	1,654.4	1,584.2	1,161.0	1,271.2
Asian or Pacific Islander male[e]								
All ages, age-adjusted[d]	—	—	—	165.2	172.5	150.8	126.7	130.2
All ages, crude	—	—	—	81.9	82.7	85.2	84.5	89.0
25–34 years	—	—	—	6.3	9.2	7.4	6.9	6.5
35–44 years	—	—	—	29.4	27.7	26.1	19.6	18.8
45–54 years	—	—	—	108.2	92.6	78.5	70.2	73.4
55–64 years	—	—	—	298.5	274.6	229.2	197.2	190.0
65–74 years	—	—	—	581.2	687.2	559.4	459.9	470.7
75–84 years	—	—	—	1,147.6	1,229.9	1,086.1	942.3	1,014.5
85 years and over	—	—	—	1,798.7	1,837.0	1,823.2	1,439.0	1,427.4
Hispanic or Latino male[e, g]								
All ages, age-adjusted[d]	—	—	—	—	174.7	171.7	143.4	141.4
All ages, crude	—	—	—	—	65.5	61.3	60.4	61.6
25–34 years	—	—	—	—	8.0	6.9	6.1	6.3
35–44 years	—	—	—	—	22.5	20.1	16.0	17.4
45–54 years	—	—	—	—	96.6	79.4	71.4	74.2
55–64 years	—	—	—	—	294.0	253.1	224.8	221.9
65–74 years	—	—	—	—	655.5	651.2	574.8	560.3
75–84 years	—	—	—	—	1,233.4	1,306.4	1,098.4	1,072.6
85 years and over	—	—	—	—	2,019.4	2,049.7	1,440.1	1,417.9
White, not Hispanic or Latino male[g]								
All ages, age-adjusted[d]	—	—	—	—	276.7	247.7	223.4	220.8
All ages, crude	—	—	—	—	246.2	244.4	239.9	240.6
25–34 years	—	—	—	—	12.8	9.7	9.3	8.6
35–44 years	—	—	—	—	36.8	32.3	28.9	27.7
45–54 years	—	—	—	—	153.9	127.2	118.7	116.8
55–64 years	—	—	—	—	520.6	412.0	363.4	357.6
65–74 years	—	—	—	—	1,109.0	1,002.1	883.0	867.3
75–84 years	—	—	—	—	1,906.6	1,750.2	1,662.9	1,652.8
85 years and over	—	—	—	—	2,744.4	2,714.1	2,300.2	2,300.4
White female[e]								
All ages, age-adjusted[d]	182.0	167.7	162.5	165.2	174.0	166.9	153.6	151.2
All ages, crude	139.9	139.8	149.4	170.3	196.1	199.4	190.1	188.8
25–34 years	20.9	18.8	16.3	13.5	11.9	10.1	9.1	8.6
35–44 years	74.5	66.6	62.4	50.9	46.2	38.2	34.9	33.9
45–54 years	185.8	175.7	177.3	166.4	150.9	120.1	109.5	107.1
55–64 years	362.5	329.0	338.6	355.5	368.5	319.7	279.1	271.8
65–74 years	616.5	562.1	554.7	605.2	675.1	665.6	611.5	602.3
75–84 years	1,026.6	939.3	903.5	905.4	1,011.8	1,063.4	1,023.0	1,017.7
85 years and over	1,348.3	1,304.9	1,126.6	1,266.8	1,372.3	1,459.1	1,317.5	1,291.6
Black or African American female[e]								
All ages, age-adjusted[d]	174.1	174.3	173.4	189.5	205.9	193.8	176.1	174.9
All ages, crude	111.8	113.8	117.3	136.5	156.1	151.8	147.7	148.2
25–34 years	34.3	31.0	20.9	18.3	18.7	13.5	12.5	12.0
35–44 years	119.8	102.4	94.6	73.5	67.4	58.9	50.8	48.5
45–54 years	277.0	254.8	228.6	230.2	209.9	173.9	158.7	156.1
55–64 years	484.6	442.7	404.8	450.4	482.4	391.0	356.9	352.5
65–74 years	477.3	541.6	615.8	662.4	773.2	753.1	672.9	681.0
75–84 years[f]	605.3	696.3	763.3	923.9	1,059.9	1,124.0	1,065.3	1,071.7
85 years and over	—	728.9	791.5	1,159.9	1,431.3	1,527.7	1,324.4	1,265.2

invasive breast cancer in women and 57,650 new cases of in situ breast cancer as well as 2,140 new cases of breast cancer in men were diagnosed in 2011. (In situ, or noninvasive, breast cancer is confined to the milk-ducts or glands, whereas invasive forms of breast cancer spread to surrounding breast tissue.) An estimated 39,970

TABLE 5.5

Death rates for cancer by sex, age, ethnicity and race, selected years 1950–2007 [CONTINUED]

[Data are based on death certificates]

Sex, race, Hispanic origin, and age	1950[a, b]	1960[a, b]	1970[b]	1980[b]	1990[b]	2000[c]	2006[c]	2007[c]
American Indian or Alaska Native female[e]				Deaths per 100,000 resident population				
All ages, age-adjusted[d]	—	—	—	94.0	106.9	108.3	108.3	102.1
All ages, crude	—	—	—	50.4	62.1	61.3	76.8	75.0
25–34 years	—	—	—	*	*	*	*	0.0
35–44 years	—	—	—	36.9	31.0	23.7	25.4	20.3
45–54 years	—	—	—	96.9	104.5	59.7	72.8	75.6
55–64 years	—	—	—	198.4	213.3	200.9	193.8	190.3
65–74 years	—	—	—	350.8	438.9	458.3	469.8	444.3
75–84 years	—	—	—	446.4	554.3	714.0	756.8	712.1
85 years and over	—	—	—	786.5	843.7	983.2	684.8	639.5
Asian or Pacific Islander female[e]								
All ages, age-adjusted[d]	—	—	—	93.0	103.0	100.7	92.2	90.0
All ages, crude	—	—	—	54.1	60.5	72.1	77.8	78.2
25–34 years	—	—	—	9.5	7.3	8.1	7.3	6.0
35–44 years	—	—	—	38.7	29.8	28.9	24.7	24.0
45–54 years	—	—	—	99.8	93.9	78.2	73.5	70.0
55–64 years	—	—	—	174.7	196.2	176.5	160.2	162.2
65–74 years	—	—	—	301.9	346.2	357.4	330.9	308.8
75–84 years	—	—	—	522.1	641.4	650.1	602.4	601.2
85 years and over	—	—	—	800.0	971.7	988.5	878.4	875.2
Hispanic or Latina female[e, g]								
All ages, age-adjusted[d]	—	—	—	—	111.9	110.8	100.4	98.6
All ages, crude	—	—	—	—	60.7	58.5	59.7	59.9
25–34 years	—	—	—	—	9.7	7.8	8.5	8.9
35–44 years	—	—	—	—	34.8	30.7	27.9	26.5
45–54 years	—	—	—	—	100.5	84.7	78.1	75.5
55–64 years	—	—	—	—	205.4	192.5	174.4	175.6
65–74 years	—	—	—	—	404.8	410.0	370.2	364.4
75–84 years	—	—	—	—	663.0	716.5	665.9	665.7
85 years and over	—	—	—	—	1,022.7	1,056.5	884.9	814.2
White, not Hispanic or Latina female[g]								
All ages, age-adjusted[d]	—	—	—	—	177.5	170.0	157.6	155.3
All ages, crude	—	—	—	—	210.6	220.6	214.7	213.7
25–34 years	—	—	—	—	11.9	10.5	9.2	8.4
35–44 years	—	—	—	—	47.0	38.9	35.9	35.2
45–54 years	—	—	—	—	154.9	123.0	113.0	110.9
55–64 years	—	—	—	—	379.5	328.9	288.5	280.6
65–74 years	—	—	—	—	688.5	681.0	631.3	622.2
75–84 years	—	—	—	—	1,027.2	1,075.3	1,044.4	1,040.1
85 years and over	—	—	—	—	1,385.7	1,468.7	1,336.7	1,315.2

—Data not available.

*Rates based on fewer than 20 deaths are considered unreliable and are not shown.

0.0 Quantity more than zero but less than 0.05.

[a]Includes deaths of persons who were not residents of the 50 states and the District of Columbia (D.C.).

[b]Underlying cause of death was coded according to the 6th Revision of the International Classification of Diseases (ICD) in 1950, 7th Revision in 1960, 8th Revision in 1970, and 9th Revision in 1980–1998.

[c]Starting with 1999 data, cause of death is coded according to ICD-10.

[d]Age-adjusted rates are calculated using the year 2000 standard population. Prior to 2003, age-adjusted rates were calculated using standard million proportions based on rounded population numbers. Starting with 2003 data, unrounded population numbers are used to calculate age-adjusted rates.

[e]The race groups, white, black, Asian or Pacific Islander, and American Indian or Alaska Native, include persons of Hispanic and non-Hispanic origin. Persons of Hispanic origin may be of any race. Death rates for the American Indian or Alaska Native and Asian or Pacific Islander populations are known to be underestimated.

[f]In 1950, rate is for the age group 75 years and over.

[g]Prior to 1997, excludes data from states lacking an Hispanic-origin item on the death certificate.

Notes: Starting with *Health, United States, 2003*, rates for 1991–1999 were revised using intercensal population estimates based on the 2000 census. Rates for 2000 were revised based on 2000 census counts. Rates for 2001 and later years were computed using 2000-based postcensal estimates. Age groups were selected to minimize the presentation of unstable age-specific death rates based on small numbers of deaths and for consistency among comparison groups. Starting with 2003 data, some states allowed the reporting of more than one race on the death certificate. The multiple-race data for these states were bridged to the single-race categories of the 1977 Office of Management and Budget standards for comparability with other states. Data for additional years are available.

SOURCE: "Table 32. Death Rates for Malignant Neoplasms, by Sex, Race, Hispanic Origin, and Age: United States, Selected Years 1950–2007," in *Health, United States, 2010: With Special Feature on Death and Dying*, Centers for Disease Control and Prevention, National Center for Health Statistics, 2011, http://www.cdc.gov/nchs/data/hus/2010/032.pdf (accessed December 14, 2011)

people died from breast cancer in 2011. The disease ranks second in terms of cancer deaths in women, after lung cancer.

Both the incidence of breast cancer and deaths from the disease have been declining since 2000. According to the ACS, the declining incidence is due to earlier detection and improved treatment; however, the dramatic decrease of 7% between 2002 and 2003 has been attributed to the sharply decreased use of hormone replacement therapy, which has been linked to increased breast cancer risk.

The five-year survival rates for cancers of the breast are encouraging. The ACS reports that if the cancer is localized, the survival rate is 98%—up from 80% during the 1950s. If the cancer is undetected and has spread regionally, however, the survival rate decreases to 84%, and for women whose cancer has spread to distant parts of the body, the survival rate is only 23%.

The precise causes of breast cancer are still unknown. The disease is most common in women older than the age of 50, and the risks are higher among women with a family history of breast cancer, those who have never had children, and women who gave birth to their first baby after the age of 30. Other factors that may contribute to increased risk for breast cancer include having a longer-than-average menstrual history (menstruation beginning at an early age and ending late in life), being obese after menopause, consuming alcohol, and eating a high-fat diet.

CHOICES OF TREATMENT. Breast cancer treatment remains a subject of continuing medical debate. If a breast contains cancerous tissue, the patient and her physician have four standard treatment options: surgery, radiation therapy, chemotherapy, or hormone therapy. Treatment choices depend on the location and size of the tumor, the stage of the cancer (whether the cancer has spread within the breast or to other parts of the body affects staging), and the size of the breast. A small, contained tumor can be removed in a procedure commonly called a lumpectomy (removal of the tumor, or "lump") and a lymph node dissection (microscopic examination of lymph nodes to detect cancer cells), followed by radiation therapy to the whole breast. If the cancer is more advanced and invasive, removing the breast (mastectomy) and usually the adjoining lymph nodes, combined with chemotherapy or hormone therapy, may be the most effective treatment.

Favorable outcomes for women with early stage breast cancer who undergo breast conserving therapy (lumpectomy, usually with radiation therapy) have been confirmed in many studies. For example, in "Long-Term Outcomes after Breast Conservation Therapy for Early Stage Breast Cancer in a Community Setting" (*Breast Journal*, vol. 12, no. 2, March–April 2006), Susan A. McClosky et al. compare cancer survival and recurrence rates of 744 breast cancer patients over the course of eight years and conclude that breast conserving therapy in place of mastectomy is "an accepted option for patients with early stage breast cancer." In *Cancer Facts and Figures, 2011*, the ACS

confirms that numerous studies show that the long-term survival rates after lumpectomy plus radiation therapy are similar to the survival rates after mastectomy for women whose cancer has not spread.

Some treatments are standard (the treatment used currently), and some treatments are being tested in clinical trials. A clinical trial is a research study that is designed to help improve already-existing treatments or obtain information about the safety and efficacy of new treatments for patients with cancer. If a clinical trial shows that a new treatment is better than the standard treatment, the new treatment may become the standard treatment.

Sentinel lymph node (SLN) biopsy is a form of treatment that was tested in two large clinical trials that compared SLN biopsy with conventional axillary lymph node dissection. The trials were conducted by the National Surgical Adjuvant Breast and Bowel Project and the American College of Surgeons Oncology Group—which are networks of institutions and physicians across the country that jointly conduct trials under the sponsorship of the National Cancer Institute. SLN biopsy is a surgical procedure involving the removal of the sentinel lymph node (the first lymph node the cancer is likely to spread to from the tumor) during surgery. Either a radioactive substance or a blue dye (in some cases both) is injected near the tumor. This flows through the lymph ducts to the lymph nodes. The first lymph node to receive the substance or dye is removed for biopsy. If cancer cells are not found, no more lymph nodes may need to be removed. After the SLN biopsy, the surgeon performs a lumpectomy or mastectomy to remove the tumor.

Peer and professionally facilitated support groups are available to help patients deal with the emotional consequences and physical side effects of breast cancer treatment. Significant advances and techniques have made breast reconstruction possible—frequently during or immediately following surgery.

GENETIC RESEARCH. Physicians have known for some time that a predisposition to some forms of breast cancer is inherited. For this reason, physicians have been searching for the gene or genes responsible so that they can test patients and provide more careful monitoring for those who are at risk. In 1994 doctors identified the BRCA1 gene, and in late 1995 they isolated the BRCA2 gene.

Kelly A. Metcalfe of the University of Toronto explains in "Oophorectomy for Breast Cancer Prevention in Women with BRCA1 or BRCA2 Mutations" (*Future Medicine*, vol. 5, no. 1, January 2009) that if a woman with a family history of breast cancer inherits a defective form of either BRCA1 or BRCA2, she has an estimated 80% to 90% risk of developing breast cancer. Researchers also think that the two genes are linked to ovarian, prostate, and colon cancer and that BRCA2 likely plays some role in breast cancer in men. Scientists suspect that the two genes may also participate in some way in the development of breast cancer in women with no family history of the disease. In *Cancer Facts and Figures, 2011*, the ACS reports that only 5% to 10% of all cases of breast cancer are attributable to defects in BRCA1 and BRCA2. Variations of other genes are also associated with an increased risk for breast cancer.

In "Which Role for EGFR Therapy in Breast Cancer?" (*Frontiers in Bioscience*, no. 4, January 1, 2012), Vito Lorusso et al. indicate that other forms of breast cancer are driven by copies of the genes EGFR and HER2 and are expressed in up to 30% of the new cases of the disease in the United States each year. HER2/neu is an aggressive form of cancer with increased rates of recurrence and poor survival in node-positive breast cancer patients. The HER2 gene produces a protein on the surface of cells that serves as a receiving point for growth-stimulating hormones.

Trastuzumab, a genetically engineered antibody drug that became available in 1998, increases the benefits of chemotherapy by shrinking tumors and slowing the progression of HER2/neu. By 2012 promising therapies included treatment with the anti-HER2/neu antibody trastuzumab (for patients with high levels of the HER2 protein) and aromatase inhibitors. Clinical trials of trastuzumab in combination with other chemotherapeutic agents were conducted in 2009 and 2010. One such study was conducted by Andrew M. Wardley et al. In "Randomized Phase II Trial of First-Line Trastuzumab Plus Docetaxel and Capecitabine Compared with Trastuzumab Plus Docetaxel in HER2-Positive Metastatic Breast Cancer" (*Journal of Clinical Oncology*, vol. 28, no. 6, February 2010), Wardley et al. find the combination of trastuzumab and docetaxel with or without capecitabine effective therapy for HER2-positive locally advanced or metastatic breast cancer. Many breast tumors are "estrogen sensitive," meaning the hormone estrogen helps them to grow. Aromatase inhibitors help block the growth of these tumors by lowering the amount of estrogen in the body. In 2012 there were three aromatase inhibitors approved by the FDA: anastrozole, exemestane, and letrozole.

Breast cancer genetic research is rapidly evolving. However, Abhik Mukherjee and Emad A. Rakha observe in "Integrating Breast Cancer Genetics into Clinical Practice" (*Women's Health*, vol. 8, no. 1, January 2012) that despite the fact that remarkable strides have been made in breast cancer genetics, the new information and understanding have not yet been translated into patient care. Mukherjee and Rakha opine that in the future genetics and genomics will allow individualized and patient-tailored therapies.

Skin Cancer

According to the ACS, in *Cancer Facts and Figures, 2011*, more than 3 million unreported cases of nonmelanoma (basal cell or squamous cell) cancers occur annually. The majority of these cancers are easily cured, especially if they are detected and treated early. The ACS estimates that 70,230 new cases of malignant melanoma, a far more serious form of skin cancer, were diagnosed in 2011.

The ACS reports that there were an estimated 11,980 deaths from skin cancer (8,790 from malignant melanoma) in 2011. Melanoma can spread to other parts of the body quickly, but if it is detected early and properly treated, it is highly curable. The five-year survival rate for localized malignant melanoma is 98%, and the five-year survival rates for regional and distant stage diseases are 62% and 16%, respectively.

Simple precautions can prevent most skin cancers. According to the ACS, avoiding the sun between 10 a.m. and 4 p.m. (when the ultraviolet rays are the strongest), using sunscreen with a sun protection factor of 15 or higher, and wearing protective clothing decrease the risk of skin cancer considerably.

Prostate Cancer

The ACS indicates in *Cancer Facts and Figures, 2011* that an estimated 240,890 American men were diagnosed with prostate cancer in 2011. Approximately 33,720 men died from the disease, making it the second-leading cause of cancer death in men, exceeded only by lung cancer. The probability of developing prostate cancer increases with advancing age.

During the late 1980s prostate-specific antigen (PSA) screening became available to test for the disease. This is a blood test that measures a protein that is made by prostate cells. PSA blood tests are reported in nanograms per milliliter (ng/mL). Results are considered to be normal if the reading is under 4 ng/mL; borderline results are between 4 and 10 ng/mL; and any reading of more than 10 ng/mL is high. The higher the reading, the more likely prostate cancer is present. However, normal levels increase with age, and older men with higher readings are frequently found to have no prostate cancer. For example, PSA levels greater than or equal to 2.5 ng/mL are considered to be abnormally high for men younger than the age of 49 years, whereas PSA levels greater than or equal to 4.5 ng/mL are considered to be abnormally high for men between the ages of 60 and 69 years.

Roger Chou et al. report in "Screening for Prostate Cancer: A Review of the Evidence for the U.S. Preventive Services Task Force" (*Annals of Internal Medicine*, vol. 155, no. 11, December 2011) that in October 2011 the USPSTF recommended against routine PSA screening. The revised recommendation was based on a USPSTF review of the scientific evidence, which failed to support the premise that

"PSA-based early detection of prostate cancer prolongs lives." Furthermore, the USPSTF concluded that PSA-based screening may result in harm, specifically, overdiagnosis and overtreatment of prostate tumors that would not cause illness or death. Despite the USPSTF recommendation, the ACS opines that there is not enough data to "recommend for or against routine testing for early prostate cancer detection with the PSA test." As such, the ACS recommends that a PSA blood test and a digital rectal examination should be offered once a year to men aged 50 years and older with a life expectancy of at least 10 years. African-American men and men who have a first-degree relative who had prostate cancer should begin receiving these tests at age 40 to 45 because they are at a higher risk of developing the disease. The ACS reports that in 2009 two large clinical trials were conducted to help determine the efficacy of PSA testing and they produced conflicting results. One of the studies, which was conducted in Europe, reported a lower risk of death from prostate cancer among men receiving PSA screening, whereas the other study, which was conducted in the United States, did not.

The controversy about using the PSA test to screen for prostate cancer continued at the close of 2011 and was documented in a series of opinion pieces in the December 2011 issue of the *Journal of the American Medical Association* (vol. 306, no. 24). Writing in support of the USPSTF recommendation, H. Gilbert Welch of the Dartmouth Institute for Health Policy and Clinical Practice in Hanover, New Hampshire, states in "Making the Call" that "the United States now needs the medical profession to make more calls like this. The nation also needs the profession to communicate the nuances of medicine. Most tests and treatment are neither unambiguously good nor unambiguously bad. Instead, their effect is modified by how they are used." In "Missing the Mark on Prostate-Specific Antigen Screening," David C. Miller and Brent K. Hollenbeck of the University of Michigan disagree with Welch, writing, "Clinicians must preserve the ability to detect aggressive prostate cancer while these tumors are still at an early stage.... At the present time, PSA screening is the best tool available to achieve this objective, even if it means some men may experience morbidity and mortality associated with diagnosis and treatment."

PROSTATE CANCER TREATMENTS. In *Cancer Facts and Figures, 2011*, the ACS explains that prostate cancer may be treated in several ways, depending on the age of the patient, the severity of the cancer, and any other medical conditions the patient may have. Radiation and surgery may be used if the disease is in an early stage. Hormone therapy (which shrinks the tumor, thus relieving pain and other symptoms for a long period), chemotherapy, and radiation may be used alone or in combination if the cancer has spread, and these methods may be effective as supplements to treatments during early stages. "Watchful

waiting" (close observation with no treatment) may also be appropriate in patients who are older or who have less aggressive tumors.

A radical prostatectomy is the removal of the prostate and some of the tissue surrounding the gland. This is done when the cancer has not spread outside the gland. Radiation therapy kills cancer cells and shrinks tumors and may be used before or after prostate surgery. Impotence (erectile dysfunction) and urinary incontinence occur slightly more often when radiation is used following surgery. Radiation therapy can also cause damage to the rectum.

Therapy to reduce hormone (testosterone) levels may be prescribed to limit prostate cancer cell growth. Patients may be given drugs such as luteinizing hormone-releasing hormone agonists, which decrease the amount of testosterone in the body, or antiandrogens, which block the activity of testosterone. These cause cancer cells to shrink because testosterone promotes the growth of prostate cancer cells.

Transurethral resection relieves the blockage of urinary flow that is caused by cancer of the prostate gland. This procedure is often performed to relieve symptoms of urinary obstruction caused by the tumor. Chemotherapy is used to treat prostate cancer if it returns after being treated with other types of treatment. For men who have less aggressive tumors, are older than 70 years of age, or have coexisting illnesses, many physicians will use a watch-and-wait approach before suggesting active treatment.

Men with advanced prostate cancer that no longer responds to hormones may be candidates for immunization with a cancer vaccine known as sipuleucel-T. The vaccine entails removing immune cells from the man's body, exposing them to prostate proteins, and then reinfusing them to combat the prostate cancer cells. In 2010 cabazitaxel, a new chemotherapy drug, was approved to treat metastatic prostate cancer that fails to respond to other treatments.

Because more than 90% of all prostate cancers are detected in the local and regional stages, the five-year relative survival rate for patients whose tumors are diagnosed at these stages approaches 100%. The ACS reports that since the mid-1980s the five-year survival rate for all stages combined has increased from 69% to almost 100%.

RESPIRATORY DISEASES AND LUNG HEALTH

The lungs are especially vulnerable to airborne particles, such as viruses, bacteria, tobacco smoke, pollen, fungi, and air pollution. Workers who are exposed to certain airborne hazards—cotton fibers, asbestos, and coal, metal, and silica dust—can also develop serious lung diseases. Pneumoconiosis is the general term for occupationally induced lung diseases.

Asthma

According to the CDC, in "Asthma" (January 27, 2012, http://www.cdc.gov/nchs/fastats/asthma.htm), an estimated 18.7 million American adults had asthma in 2010. In *Summary Health Statistics for U.S. Children: National Health Interview Survey, 2010* (December 2011, http://www.cdc.gov/nchs/data/series/sr_10/sr10_250.pdf), the NCHS indicates that asthma is the most common chronic illness among children. In 2010 an estimated 7 million children younger than 18 years of age had asthma.

People with asthma experience acute attacks of wheezing and shortness of breath. This difficulty in breathing is caused by a sudden narrowing of the bronchial tubes. Usually, it is not life threatening, but asthma often limits activities and can be extremely serious for the very young and the very old.

The incidence of asthma has increased dramatically since the 1980s in the United States and in other industrialized nations as a result of lifestyle changes and living conditions in modern society. Exposure to air pollutants including tobacco smoke, ozone, and diesel exhaust may be contributing to this increased incidence. Indoor exposures to allergens may also contribute to the increase in asthma because many indoor environments have been made more air tight to improve energy efficiency. Other factors implicated in the rise in asthma include the increased incidence of obesity, decreased physical activity, change in diet, decreased exposure to microbes during early life, and increased viral respiratory infections such as those that are contracted by children in day care settings. Even though children appear to be the population most at risk, new cases are also occurring in adults, particularly older adults.

RACIAL, AGE, AND GENDER DISPARITIES. The CDC explains in "Healthy Youth! Health Topics: Asthma" (March 18, 2011, http://www.cdc.gov/HealthyYouth/asthma/index.htm) that in 2005–07 non-Hispanic African-American children and Puerto Rican children had higher rates of asthma and asthma-related problems than non-Hispanic white children in the United States. In 2011 the asthma prevalence rates continued to be highest among African-Americans under 15 years old. (See Figure 5.9.)

In 2011 asthma was more prevalent in children under the age of 15 years, and boys were more likely to have asthma than girls. (See Figure 5.10.) However, in all other age groups the prevalence was higher among females than among males.

CAUSES OF ASTHMA ATTACKS. Even though the specific cause of asthma is not known, the disease appears to be associated with allergic reactions, heredity, and environment. Many environmental factors can trigger an asthma attack in susceptible individuals. Indoor and outdoor pollution do not cause the disease, but pollutants such as ozone,

FIGURE 5.9

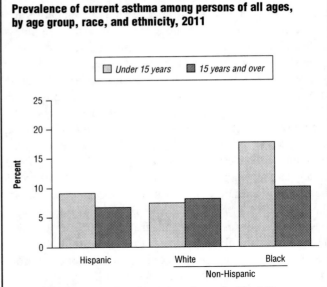

Prevalence of current asthma among persons of all ages, by age group, race, and ethnicity, 2011

Notes: Data are based on household interviews of a sample of the civilian noninstitutionalized population. Information on current asthma is self-reported by adults aged 18 and over. For children under age 18, the information is collected from an adult family member, usually a parent, who is knowledgeable about the child's health. The analyses excluded 0.2% of persons with unknown current asthma status.

SOURCE: "Figure 15.6. Sex-Adjusted Prevalence of Current Asthma among Persons of All Ages, by Age Group and Race/Ethnicity: United States, January–June 2011," in *Early Release of Selected Estimates Based on Data from the January–June 2011 National Health Interview Survey*, Centers for Disease Control and Prevention, National Center for Health Statistics, December 2011, http://www.cdc.gov/nchs/data/nhis/earlyrelease/201112_15.pdf (accessed December 26, 2011)

sulfur dioxide, nitrogen dioxide, and tobacco smoke can trigger an episode of asthma. Allergens such as pollen and dust mites can also provoke asthma attacks.

MANAGING ASTHMA SYMPTOMS. In "Managing Asthma in Primary Care: Putting New Guideline Recommendations into Context" (*Mayo Clinic Proceedings*, vol. 84, no. 8, August 2009), Michael E. Wechsler of Harvard Medical School notes that many people with asthma are unable to effectively manage their symptoms. Wechsler avers that "many patients overestimate their level of disease control, often tolerating substantial asthma symptoms and having low expectations about the degree of control that is possible." Patients may mistakenly assume that symptoms and resulting reduced activity or disability are the natural and unavoidable consequences of the disease. Wechsler contends that patients and physicians must learn to recognize exactly what constitutes good control of asthma symptoms and advises physicians to adhere to treatment guidelines that were issued in 2007 by the National Asthma Education and Prevention Program, which emphasize how to manage asthma more effectively with an increased focus on achieving and maintaining good asthma control over time.

FIGURE 5.10

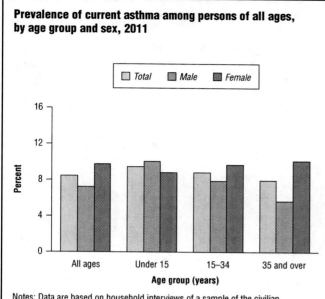

Prevalence of current asthma among persons of all ages, by age group and sex, 2011

Legend: Total, Male, Female

Y-axis: Percent (0, 4, 8, 12, 16)

X-axis: Age group (years) — All ages, Under 15, 15–34, 35 and over

Notes: Data are based on household interviews of a sample of the civilian noninstitutionalized population. Information on current asthma is self-reported by adults aged 18 and over. For children under age 18, the information is collected from an adult family member, usually a parent, who is knowledgeable about the child's health. The analyses excluded 0.2% of persons with unknown current asthma status.

SOURCE: "Figure 15.5. Prevalence of Current Asthma among Persons of All Ages, by Age Group and Sex: United States, January–June 2011," in *Early Release of Selected Estimates Based on Data from the January–June 2011 National Health Interview Survey*, Centers for Disease Control and Prevention, National Center for Health Statistics, December 2011, http://www.cdc.gov/nchs/data/nhis/earlyrelease/201112_15.pdf (accessed December 26, 2011)

Chronic Obstructive Pulmonary Disease

Chronic obstructive pulmonary diseases (COPD; also referred to as chronic lower respiratory diseases), which include emphysema and chronic bronchitis, are progressive diseases that cause the obstruction of airflow. The American Lung Association estimates in "Understanding COPD" (2012, http://www.lungusa.org/lung-disease/copd/about-copd/understanding-copd.html) that between 12 million and 24 million people suffer from COPD. The National Heart Lung and Blood Institute reports that in 2007 COPD was the fourth-leading cause of death in the United States. (See Figure 5.1.) In *Health, United States, 2011*, the NCHS states that deaths attributable to COPD have increased sharply. In 1980, 56,050 people died from COPD; by 2007 the number had more than doubled to 127,924. (See Table 1.12 in Chapter 1.)

CHRONIC BRONCHITIS. Bronchitis is an inflammation of the lining of the bronchi, tubes that connect the trachea (windpipe) to the lungs. When the bronchi are inflamed and infected, less air is able to flow to and from the lungs, and mucus forms and is coughed up. Acute bronchitis is usually brief in duration and follows the flu or a cold. Chronic bronchitis, however, lingers for months or even years and is characterized by a persistent mucus-producing cough. It is a long-term disease that is characterized by breathlessness and wheezing.

In 2010 nearly 9.9 million adults over the age of 18 years had chronic bronchitis. (See Table 5.6.) The NCHS indicates in "Summary Health Statistics for U.S. Adults: National Health Interview Survey, 2010" (*Vital and Health Statistics*, series 10, no. 252, January 2012) that in all age, sex, and race categories, people who smoke cigarettes are far more likely to develop chronic bronchitis than nonsmokers. Workers whose jobs involve inhaling large amounts of dust and irritating fumes are also more likely to get the disease. When air pollution becomes excessive, symptoms intensify.

Antibiotics and bronchodilator drugs are useful treatments, but even more important is the need to eliminate the sources of respiratory irritation. This could mean quitting smoking or avoiding polluted air, fumes, and dust. Chronic bronchitis is often the forerunner of emphysema.

EMPHYSEMA. Emphysema is a severe disease of the lungs that usually develops gradually. The air sacs on the walls of the lungs slowly lose their elasticity, and stale air becomes trapped in the lungs, which become overly inflated. This interferes with the normal exchange of oxygen and carbon dioxide. People with emphysema often feel as if they are drowning in a sea of air. In its late stage, emphysema also affects the heart, because the flow of blood from the lungs is disrupted by changes caused by the disease. The heart has to pump harder to compensate for the disease and may become enlarged. Death often results from heart failure. Approximately 4.3 million adults over the age of 18 years had emphysema in 2010. (See Table 5.6.)

DIABETES

Diabetes is a disease that affects the body's use of food, causing levels of blood glucose (sugar in the blood) to become too high. Normally, the body converts sugars, starches, and proteins into a form of sugar called glucose. The blood then carries glucose to all the cells throughout the body. In the cells, with the help of the hormone insulin, the glucose is either converted into energy for use immediately or stored for the future. Beta cells of the pancreas, a small organ located behind the stomach, manufacture insulin. The process of turning food into energy via glucose is important because the body depends on glucose for every function.

Because diabetes deprives body cells of the glucose that is needed to function properly, several complications can develop to threaten the lives of diabetics further. The healing process of the body is slowed or impaired, and the risk of infection increases. Complications of diabetes include higher risk and rates of heart disease; circulatory problems, especially in the legs, which often are severe enough to require surgery or even amputation; diabetic

TABLE 5.6

Frequency of selected respiratory diseases among persons 18 and older, by selected characteristics, 2010

			Selected respiratory conditions[a]				
			Asthma				Chronic
Selected characteristic	All persons aged 18 years and over	Emphysema	Ever had	Still has	Hay fever	Sinusitis	bronchitis
			Number in thousands[b]				
Total[c]	229,505	4,314	29,057	18,734	17,937	29,821	9,883
Sex							
Male	110,929	2,248	11,869	6,418	7,513	11,021	3,399
Female	118,576	2,066	17,188	12,316	10,424	18,800	6,484
Age							
18–44 years	110,615	361	15,020	8,902	6,656	11,584	3,265
45–64 years	80,198	1,703	9,723	6,704	8,638	13,025	4,247
65–74 years	21,291	1,153	2,492	1,849	1,684	3,240	1,279
75 years and over	17,401	1,097	1,822	1,279	958	1,973	1,092
Race							
One race[d]	226,314	4,214	28,406	18,235	17,600	29,309	9,656
White	185,330	3,822	22,837	14,528	14,969	24,261	8,324
Black or African American	27,807	281	4,285	2,950	1,802	3,929	1,115
American Indian or Alaska Native	1,795	†	234	202	87	238	*73
Asian	11,096	*88	1,014	546	724	862	137
Two or more races[e]	284	—	*36	†	†	†	†
Native Hawaiian or other Pacific Islander	3,191	*100	651	499	336	511	227
Black or African American, white	625	†	150	*112	*42	*63	*32
American Indian or Alaska Native, white	1,394	*61	299	239	163	316	*125
Hispanic or Latino origin[f] and race							
Hispanic or Latino	32,094	231	3,289	2,224	1,440	2,783	878
Mexican or Mexican American	19,712	112	1,686	1,173	804	1,545	509
Not Hispanic or Latino	197,411	4,083	25,768	16,510	16,497	27,038	9,005
White, single race	156,119	3,600	19,926	12,552	13,659	21,752	7,525
Black or African American, single race	26,689	279	4,118	2,841	1,744	3,833	1,074
Education[g]							
Less than a high school diploma	28,159	1,239	3,264	2,307	1,441	3,272	1,756
High school diploma or GED[h]	53,058	1,308	5,451	3,877	3,491	6,950	2,720
Some college	56,710	1,099	7,927	5,449	5,112	8,802	2,723
Bachelor's degree or higher	61,185	582	7,410	4,267	6,627	8,735	1,802
Family income[i]							
Less than $35,000	74,281	2,321	10,397	7,267	4,519	9,108	4,544
$35,000 or more	141,904	1,700	17,479	10,709	12,426	19,107	4,770
$35,000–$49,999	31,868	652	3,999	2,572	2,421	4,268	1,226
$50,000–$74,999	38,780	499	4,656	2,929	2,817	5,237	1,346
$75,000–$99,999	26,379	261	2,944	1,820	2,350	3,152	924
$100,000 or more	44,877	289	5,880	3,389	4,838	6,451	1,274
Poverty status[j]							
Poor	28,677	653	4,398	3,102	1,532	3,159	1,795
Near poor	36,390	1,194	4,900	3,262	2,420	4,502	1,951
Not poor	145,271	2,025	17,673	10,944	12,703	19,845	5,281
Health insurance coverage[k]							
Under 65 years:							
Private	123,257	819	15,657	9,396	11,225	17,387	4,061
Medicaid	18,030	466	3,229	2,450	1,141	2,181	1,380
Other	8,012	426	1,318	1,014	973	1,467	777
Uninsured	40,684	353	4,446	2,667	1,897	3,435	1,274
65 years and over:							
Private	20,579	1,141	2,204	1,563	1,492	2,973	1,116
Medicare and Medicaid	2,633	245	558	447	163	479	314
Medicare only	12,633	641	1,235	907	804	1,396	678
Other	2,406	171	300	193	183	325	201
Uninsured	379	†	†	†	—	†	†
Marital status							
Married	124,307	2,156	13,676	8,600	11,010	16,873	4,684
Widowed	13,676	747	1,751	1,266	864	2,010	1,146
Divorced or separated	26,083	812	3,908	2,857	2,190	4,231	1,576
Never married	49,249	303	7,446	4,577	3,095	5,049	1,791
Living with a partner	15,915	296	2,236	1,422	771	1,600	675

retinopathy, a condition that can cause blindness; kidney disease that may require dialysis; dental problems; and problems with pregnancy. Close attention to preventive health care such as regular eye, dental, and foot examinations and tight control of blood sugar levels have been shown to prevent some of the consequences of diabetes.

TABLE 5.6

Frequency of selected respiratory diseases among persons 18 and older, by selected characteristics, 2010 [CONTINUED]

Selected characteristic	All persons aged 18 years and over	Selected respiratory conditions[a]						
		Emphysema	Asthma		Hay fever	Sinusitis	Chronic bronchitis
			Ever had	Still has			
Place of residence[l]		Number in thousands[b]						
Large MSA	121,307	1,594	15,236	9,540	9,583	14,667	4,520
Small MSA	71,921	1,564	9,314	6,068	5,867	9,624	3,363
Not in MSA	36,277	1,157	4,507	3,125	2,487	5,530	2,000
Region							
Northeast	40,577	759	5,110	3,487	3,390	4,892	1,632
Midwest	53,316	1,298	6,542	4,363	3,791	6,994	2,602
South	81,721	1,607	9,965	6,342	5,932	13,083	3,972
West	53,891	650	7,441	4,541	4,824	4,851	1,678
Sex and ethnicity							
Hispanic or Latino, male	16,529	124	1,331	810	599	1,048	312
Hispanic or Latina, female	15,565	108	1,958	1,414	841	1,735	566
Not Hispanic or Latino:							
White, single race, male	75,723	1,848	8,286	4,317	5,886	7,994	2,644
White, single race, female	80,396	1,753	11,639	8,236	7,773	13,757	4,881
Black or African American, single race, male	11,959	170	1,547	901	635	1,422	313
Black or African American, single race, female	14,730	109	2,571	1,941	1,110	2,411	760

†Estimates with a relative standard error greater than 50% are replaced with a dagger and are not shown.
*Estimates preceded by an asterisk have a relative standard error greater than 30% and less than or equal to 50% and should be used with caution as they do not meet standards of reliability or precision.
—Quantity zero.
[a]Respondents were asked in two separate questions if they had ever been told by a doctor or other health professional that they had emphysema or asthma. Respondents who had been told they had asthma were asked if they still had asthma. Respondents were asked in three separate questions if they had been told by a doctor or other health professional in the past 12 months that they had hay fever, sinusitis, or bronchitis. A person may be represented in more than one column.
[b]Unknowns for the columns were not included in the frequencies but they are included in the "All persons aged 18 years and over" column. The numbers in this table are rounded.
[c]Includes other races not shown separately and persons with unknown education, family income, poverty status, health insurance, and marital status characteristics.
[d]In accordance with the 1997 standards for federal data on race and Hispanic or Latino origin, the category "One race" refers to persons who indicated only a single race group. Persons who indicated a single race other than the groups shown are included in the total for "One race," but not shown separately due to small sample sizes. Therefore, the frequencies for the category "One race" will be greater than the sum of the frequencies for the specific groups shown separately. Persons of Hispanic or Latino origin may be of any race or combination of races. The tables in this report use the 1997 Office of Management and Budget race and Hispanic origin terms, and the text uses shorter versions of these terms for conciseness. For example, the category "One race, Black or African American" in the tables is referred to as "black persons" in the text.
[e]Refers to all persons who indicated more than one race group. Only two combinations of multiple race groups are shown due to small sample sizes for other combinations. Therefore, the frequencies for the category "Two or more races" will be greater than the sum of the frequencies for the specific combinations shown separately. Persons of Hispanic or Latino origin may be of any race or combination of races.
[f]Persons of Hispanic or Latino origin may be of any race or combination of races. Similarly, the category "Not Hispanic or Latino" refers to all persons who are not of Hispanic or Latino origin, regardless of race.
[g]Shown only for persons aged 25 years and over.
[h]GED is General Educational Development high school equivalency diploma.
[i]The categories "Less than $35,000" and "$35,000 or more" include both persons reporting dollar amounts and persons reporting only that their incomes were within one of these two categories. The indented categories include only those persons who reported dollar amounts. Because of the different income questions used in 2007 and beyond, income estimates may not be comparable with those from earlier years.
[j]Based on family income and family size using the U.S. Census Bureau's poverty thresholds for the previous calendar year. "Poor" persons are defined as below the poverty threshold. "Near poor" persons have incomes of 100% to less than 200% of the poverty threshold. "Not poor" persons have incomes that are 200% of the poverty threshold or greater. Because of the different income questions used in 2007 and beyond, poverty ratio estimates may not be comparable with those from earlier years.
[k]Based on a hierarchy of mutually exclusive categories. Persons with more than one type of health insurance were assigned to the first appropriate category in the hierarchy. Persons under age 65 years and those aged 65 years and over were classified separately due to the predominance of Medicare coverage in the older population. The category "Private" includes persons who had any type of private coverage either alone or in combination with other coverage. For example, for persons aged 65 years and over, "Private" includes persons with only private or private in combination with Medicare coverage. The category "Uninsured" includes persons who had no coverage as well as those who had only Indian Health Service coverage or had only a private plan that paid for one type of service such as accidents or dental care.
[l]MSA is metropolitan statistical area. Large MSAs have a population size of 1 million or more; small MSAs have a population size of less than 1 million. "Not in MSA" consists of persons not living in a metropolitan statistical area.
Note: Estimates are based on household interviews of a sample of the civilian noninstitutionalized population.

SOURCE: "Table 3. Frequencies of Selected Respiratory Diseases among Persons 18 Years of Age and over, by Selected Characteristics: United States, 2010," in "Summary Health Statistics for U.S. Adults: National Health Interview Survey, 2010," *Vital and Health Statistics*, series 10, no. 252, January 2012, http://www.cdc.gov/nchs/data/series/sr_10/sr10_252.pdf (December 29, 2011)

The types of diabetes, the populations that are at risk of developing the disease, the complications of diabetes, and the measures to prevent the development of diabetes and its complications are described in Chapter 2.

Warning Signs of Prediabetes and Diabetes

To determine whether someone has prediabetes or diabetes, a fasting plasma glucose test or an oral glucose tolerance test (OGTT) is done in the doctor's office. A fasting blood glucose level between 100 and 125 mg/dL signals prediabetes, and a fasting blood glucose level of 126 mg/dL or higher signals diabetes. With the OGTT, a patient fasts overnight, then drinks a solution that is rich in glucose. The patient's blood glucose level is then measured at one-hour intervals, commonly over two to five hours, to determine the rate at which the glucose is consumed. A diagnosis of prediabetes is made when the two-hour blood glucose level is between 140 and 199 mg/dL, and diabetes is diagnosed when the level is 200 mg/dL or higher.

The symptoms of type 1 diabetes usually occur suddenly. These include excessive thirst, frequent urination, weight loss, weakness and fatigue, nausea and vomiting, and irritability. The symptoms of type 2 diabetes generally appear gradually. These may include any of the symptoms seen in type 1 diabetes, plus recurring infections that are slow to heal, drowsiness, blurred vision, numbness in the hands or feet, and itching.

Prevalence of Diabetes

Between 1997 and 2010 there was an increase in diagnosed diabetes among U.S. adults aged 18 years and older, and in 2011 there was a slight decrease. (See Figure 5.11.) In 2011 a physician or other health professional had diagnosed 8.8% of the U.S adult population aged 18 years and older with diabetes. The prevalence of diabetes increases with age among men and women, with the highest rates among older adults—people aged 65 years and older. In all age categories except for ages 18 to 44 years, the prevalence of diagnosed diabetes in 2011 was higher in men than in women. (See Figure 5.12.) The prevalence of diagnosed diabetes was higher among non-Hispanic African-Americans (12.1%) and Hispanics (12.1%) than among non-Hispanic whites (7.1%). (See Figure 5.13.)

People who are older than the age of 40 years, overweight, have a family history of diabetes, and are physically inactive are at greater risk of developing type 2 diabetes. There is an increased prevalence of diabetes with age. The percentage of people over the age of 65 years (19.8%) who were diagnosed with diabetes in 2011 was nearly eight times as high as for people aged 18 to 44 years (2.5%). (See Figure 5.12.)

Causes of Diabetes

The causes of both type 1 and type 2 diabetes are unknown, but a family history of diabetes increases the risk for both types, which strongly suggests a genetic component in the genesis of the disease. Some scientists believe that a flaw in the body's immune system may be a factor in type 1 diabetes. Other researchers believe that physical inactivity and the resulting poor cardiovascular fitness is a risk factor for developing diabetes.

In type 2 diabetes heredity may be a factor, but because the pancreas continues to produce insulin, the disease is considered to be more of a problem of insulin resistance, in which the body is not using the hormone efficiently. In people who are prone to type 2 diabetes, being overweight can set off the disease because excess fat prevents insulin from working correctly. Maintaining a healthy weight and keeping physically fit can usually prevent type 2 diabetes. To date, type 1 diabetes cannot be prevented.

FIGURE 5.11

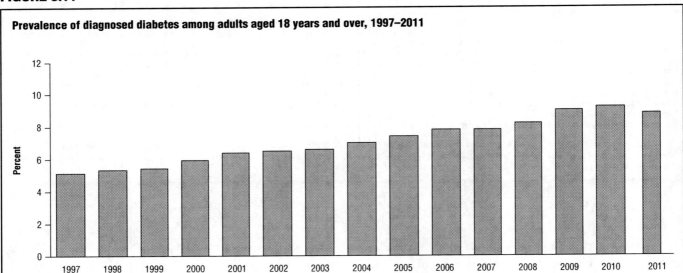

Prevalence of diagnosed diabetes among adults aged 18 years and over, 1997–2011

Notes: Data are based on household interviews of a sample of the civilian noninstitutionalized population. Prevalence of diagnosed diabetes is based on self-report of ever having been diagnosed with diabetes by a doctor or other health professional. Persons reporting "borderline" diabetes status and women reporting diabetes only during pregnancy were not coded as having diabetes in the analyses. The analyses excluded persons with unknown diabetes status (about 0.1% of respondents each year).

SOURCE: "Figure 14.1. Prevalence of Diagnosed Diabetes among Adults Aged 18 Years and over: United States, 1997–June 2011," in *Early Release of Selected Estimates Based on Data from the January–June 2011 National Health Interview Survey*, Centers for Disease Control and Prevention, National Center for Health Statistics, December 2011, http://www.cdc.gov/nchs/data/nhis/earlyrelease/201112_14.pdf (accessed December 26, 2011)

FIGURE 5.12

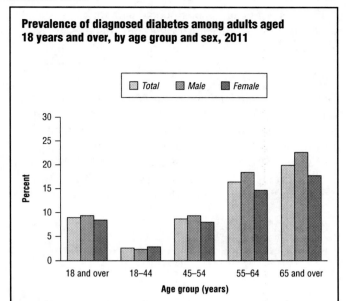

Prevalence of diagnosed diabetes among adults aged 18 years and over, by age group and sex, 2011

Notes: Data are based on household interviews of a sample of the civilian noninstitutionalized population. Prevalence of diagnosed diabetes is based on self-report of ever having been diagnosed with diabetes by a doctor or other health professional. Persons reporting "borderline" diabetes status and women reporting diabetes only during pregnancy were not coded as having diabetes in the analyses. The analyses excluded 0.1% of persons with unknown diabetes status.

SOURCE: "Figure 14.2. Prevalence of Diagnosed Diabetes among Adults Aged 18 Years and over, by Age Group and Sex: United States, 2011," in *Early Release of Selected Estimates Based on Data from the January–June 2011 National Health Interview Survey*, Centers for Disease Control and Prevention, National Center for Health Statistics, December 2011, http://www.cdc.gov/nchs/data/nhis/earlyrelease/201112_14.pdf (accessed December 26, 2011)

FIGURE 5.13

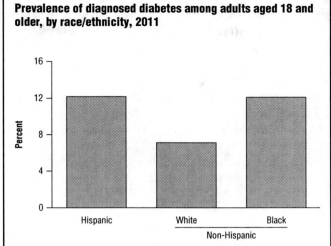

Prevalence of diagnosed diabetes among adults aged 18 and older, by race/ethnicity, 2011

Notes: Data are based on household interviews of a sample of the civilian noninstitutionalized population. Prevalence of diagnosed diabetes is based on self-report of ever having been diagnosed with diabetes by a doctor or other health professional. Persons reporting "borderline" diabetes status and women reporting diabetes only during pregnancy were not coded as having diabetes in the analyses. The analyses excluded 0.1% of persons with unknown diabetes status. Estimates are age-sex-adjusted using the projected 2000 U.S. population as the standard population and using four age groups: 18–44, 45–54, 55–64, and 65 and over.

SOURCE: "Figure 14.3. Age-Sex-Adjusted Prevalence of Diagnosed Diabetes among Adults Aged 18 Years and over, by Race/Ethnicity: United States, January–June 2011," in *Early Release of Selected Estimates Based on Data from the January–June 2011 National Health Interview Survey*, Centers for Disease Control and Prevention, National Center for Health Statistics, December 2011, http://www.cdc.gov/nchs/data/nhis/earlyrelease/201112_14.pdf (accessed December 26, 2011)

"Diabesity" and "Double Diabetes"

The recognition of obesity-dependent diabetes prompted scientists and physicians to coin a new term to describe this condition: diabesity. The term was first used during the 1990s and has gained widespread acceptance. Even though diabesity is attributed to the same causes as type 2 diabetes—insulin resistance and pancreatic cell dysfunction—researchers are beginning to link the inflammation that is associated with obesity to the development of diabetes and cardiovascular disease.

In *Diabesity: The Obesity-Diabetes Epidemic That Threatens America—And What We Must Do to Stop It* (2005), Francine Ratner Kaufman, the former director of the Center for Endocrinology, Diabetes, and Metabolism at the Children's Hospital in Los Angeles, asserts that the diabesity epidemic "imperils human existence as we now know it." Kaufman predicts that based on current trends, more than one-third of American children born in 2000 will develop diabetes during their lifetime. She cautions that unless drastic measures are taken to reverse or slow this trend, by 2020 there will be a 72% increase in the number of diabetics in the United States.

Elbert S. Huang et al. predict in "Projecting the Future Diabetes Population Size and Related Costs for the U.S." (*Diabetes Care*, vol. 32, no. 12, December 2009) that between 2009 and 2034 the number of Americans with diagnosed and undiagnosed diabetes will nearly double, from 23.7 million to 44.1 million. Huang et al. caution that "without significant changes in public or private strategies, this population and cost growth are expected to add a significant strain to an overburdened health care system."

Another recently recognized and increasingly prevalent problem is posed by patients who are diagnosed with both type 1 and type 2 diabetes simultaneously. Called "double diabetes," it has been diagnosed in both children and adults. It occurs when children with type 1 diabetes who rely on insulin injections to control their diabetes gain weight and develop the insulin resistance that is the hallmark of type 2 diabetes. Among adults who have been diagnosed with type 2 diabetes, those who fail to respond to conventional treatment have been found to also suffer from the type 1, insulin-dependent form of the disease.

In "Double Diabetes: A Mixture of Type 1 and Type 2 Diabetes in Youth" (*Endocrine Involvement in Developmental Syndromes*, vol. 14, 2009), Paolo Pozzilli and

Chiara Guglielmi of the University Campus Bio-Medico in Rome, Italy, observe that there was an increase in type 1 diabetes, especially in children younger than five years old, during the previous decade that may be attributed to changes in environmental factors, rather than to genetic factors. They assert that the marked increase in the incidence of type 2 diabetes in children and adolescents is very likely the result of the increase in obesity and sedentary lifestyle that is occurring in developed countries. Pozzilli and Guglielmi opine that the "current classification of diabetes should be revised taking into account this new form of diabetes which [is] called double diabetes or hybrid diabetes."

Deaths Resulting from Diabetes

The risk of death among people with diabetes is about twice that of their age peers without diabetes. In 2007 diabetes was the seventh-leading cause of death in the United States. (See Figure 5.1.) The NCHS notes in *Health, United States, 2010* that 71,382 people died from it in 2007. (See Table 1.12 in Chapter 1.) In "National Diabetes Statistics, 2011," the National Institute of Diabetes and Digestive and Kidney Diseases asserts that diabetes is likely to be underreported as a cause of death. The institute notes that only about 35% to 40% of the deceased with diabetes had diabetes listed on their death certificates, and just 10% to 15% had it listed as the underlying cause of death.

CHAPTER 6
DEGENERATIVE DISEASES

Degenerative diseases are noninfectious disorders that are characterized by progressive disability. Patients can often live for years with their diseases. Even though they may not die from degenerative diseases, patients' symptoms usually grow more disabling, and they often succumb to complications of their disorders.

ARTHRITIS

The word *arthritis* literally means joint inflammation, and it is applied to more than 100 related diseases that are known as rheumatic diseases. When a joint (the point where two bones meet) becomes inflamed, swelling, redness, pain, and loss of motion occur. In the most serious forms of the disease, the loss of motion can be physically disabling.

Normally, inflammation is the body's response to an injury or a disease. It causes pain, redness, swelling, and warmth in the inflamed body part. Once the injury is healed or the disease is cured, the inflammation stops. In arthritis, however, the inflammation does not subside. Instead, it becomes part of the problem, damaging healthy tissues. This generates more inflammation and more damage, and the painful cycle continues. The damage can change the shape of bones and other tissues of the joints, making movement difficult and painful.

Types of Arthritis

More than 100 types of arthritis have been identified, but four major types affect large numbers of Americans:

- Osteoarthritis—the most common type of arthritis, osteoarthritis generally affects people as they grow older. Sometimes called degenerative arthritis, it causes the breakdown of bones and cartilage (connective tissue that attaches to bones) and usually causes pain and stiffness in the fingers, knees, feet, hips, and back. The Arthritis Foundation notes in "What Is Osteoarthritis?" (2012, http://www.arthritis.org/what-is-osteoarthritis.php) that osteoarthritis affects about 27 million Americans.

- Fibromyalgia—fibromyalgia affects the muscles and connective tissues and causes widespread pain, fatigue, sleep problems, and stiffness. Fibromyalgia also causes "tender points" that are more sensitive to pain than other areas of the body. According to the National Fibromyalgia Association, in "About Fibromyalgia" (2011, http://fmaware.org/site/PageServera6cc.html?pagename=fibromyalgia_affected), about 10 million Americans, mostly women, have this condition.

- Rheumatoid arthritis—rheumatoid arthritis is caused by a flaw in the body's immune system that results in inflammation and swelling in joint linings, followed by damage to bone and cartilage in the hands, wrists, feet, knees, ankles, shoulders, or elbows. The Arthritis Foundation reports in "Who Gets Rheumatoid Arthritis?" (2012, http://www.arthritis.org/who-gets-rheumatoid-arthritis.php) that 1.3 million Americans, mostly women, have this form of arthritis.

- Gout—gout is an inflammation of a joint that is caused by an accumulation of uric acid (a natural substance) in the joint, usually the big toe, knee, or wrist. The uric acid forms crystals in the affected joint, causing severe pain and swelling. According to the Arthritis Foundation, in "Gout" (2012, http://www.arthritis.org/disease-center.php?disease_id=42), about 6.1 million Americans have had at least one gout attack. A gout attack lasts from days to two weeks. More men than women are affected.

Other Inflammatory and Autoimmune Disorders

Another less common, but potentially life-threatening, form of rheumatic disease is systemic lupus erythematosus (SLE; also called lupus), an inflammatory autoimmune disease (the immune system mistakenly attacks the body's own tissues) that attacks skin, joints, blood, and the kidneys. The Centers for Disease Control and Prevention

(CDC) reports in the fact sheet "Eliminate Disparities in Lupus" (May 14, 2008, http://www.cdc.gov/omhd/AMH/factsheets/lupus.htm) that SLE occurs more frequently among women than among men (nine out of 10 people diagnosed with lupus are women) and that death rates from SLE are three times higher for African-Americans than for whites. U.S. prevalence estimates vary from about 322,000 to more than 1.5 million. Generally diagnosed in women of childbearing age, the symptoms of SLE include:

- Painful or swollen joints, muscle pain, and fatigue

- Fever, weight loss, hair loss, and skin rashes

- Cold, pale, or blue fingers, also known as Raynaud's phenomenon

- Swollen legs or glands

- Nephritis (inflammation of the kidneys)

- Pleuritis (inflammation of the lungs) that may produce chest pain or increase the risk of developing pneumonia

- Myocarditis, endocarditis, or pericarditis (inflammation of the heart muscle, the heart valves, and the membrane around the heart, respectively) and vasculitis (inflammation of blood vessels)

As with other inflammatory and autoimmune disorders, each patient experiences the disease differently. SLE symptoms ranging from mild to severe flare up and subside throughout the course of the illness. Some patients with SLE also experience headaches, vision disturbances, strokes, or behavior changes as a result of the effects of the disease on the central nervous system.

No cure exists for SLE, and treatment aims to relieve symptoms and reduce the potential for organ damage and complications. Most patients receive corticosteroid hormones, such as prednisone and dexamethasone, which rapidly reduce inflammation. Patients with SLE are also treated with nonsteroidal anti-inflammatory drugs (NSAIDs) such as ibuprofen, naproxen, and indomethacin along with other drugs to combat pain, swelling, and fever. Drugs that were originally used to treat malaria are also used to treat the fatigue, joint pain, rashes, and pleuritis that result from SLE.

Many chronic degenerative diseases, especially autoimmune diseases, are thought to occur when a genetically susceptible individual encounters an environmental trigger. For example, some researchers believe viruses may be the environmental triggers for diseases such as SLE and scleroderma (an illness in which skin and internal organs thicken and harden).

Prevalence of Arthritis

Arthritis is a common problem. In "Arthritis Related Statistics" (October 20, 2010, http://www.cdc.gov/arthritis/data_statistics/arthritis_related_stats.htm), the CDC's National Center for Chronic Disease Prevention and Health Promotion reports that in 2010 an estimated 50 million U.S. adults

TABLE 6.1

Projected prevalence of physician-diagnosed arthritis among adults aged 18 and older, selected years 2015–30

Year	Estimated number of adults with doctor-diagnosed arthritis (in 1,000s)		
	Men	Women	Total
2015	21,732	33,993	55,725
2020	23,164	36,244	59,409
2025	24,622	38,587	63,209
2030	26,053	40,915	66,969

SOURCE: Adapted from "Projected Prevalence of Doctor-Diagnosed Arthritis, US Adults Aged 18+ Years, 2005–2030," in *NHIS Arthritis Surveillance—Text Description*, Centers for Disease Control and Prevention, National Center for Chronic Disease Prevention and Health Promotion, Division of Adult and Community Health, October 20, 2010, http://www.cdc.gov/arthritis/data_statistics/national_nhis_text.htm#1 (accessed December 30, 2011)

had been diagnosed with arthritis. By 2030 the total number in the United States is expected to increase to 67 million adults suffering from some form of arthritis. (See Table 6.1.)

The CDC indicates in "Arthritis: Meeting the Challenge—At a Glance 2011" (February 16, 2011, http://www.cdc.gov/chronicdisease/resources/publications/aag/pdf/2011/Arthritis-AAG-2011-508.pdf) that arthritis is the leading cause of disability among Americans. Nearly 21 million adults report activity limitations because of arthritis each year. Among all adults aged 18 to 64 years, about 6.9 million say they have arthritis that limits their ability to work, and among the 23 million adults in this age group who have arthritis, one out of three experiences work limitations that are attributable to arthritis. Arthritis-attributable activity limitations increase with weight—over four out of 10 (44.8%) obese adults with arthritis reported activity limitations in 2010. (See Figure 6.1.)

The Arthritis Foundation observes in "Arthritis Prevalence: A Nation in Pain" (2008, http://www.arthritis.org/media/newsroom/media-kits/Arthritis_Prevalence.pdf) that arthritis is a more frequent cause of activity limitation than heart disease, cancer, or diabetes.

In "The Heavy Burden of Arthritis in the U.S." (August 10, 2011, http://www.arthritis.org/media/newsroom/Arthritis_Prevalence_Fact_Sheet_5-31-11.pdf), the Arthritis Foundation indicates that about half of all people older than age 65 will experience some form of arthritis during their lifetime. Even though some think of it as only an older person's disease, it can also affect children. The Arthritis Foundation indicates that arthritis is one of the most common childhood diseases in the United States. About 300,000 children and teenagers suffer from arthritis.

Developments in Arthritis Research

As researchers learn more about inflammation and the body's immune system, they come closer to finding

FIGURE 6.1

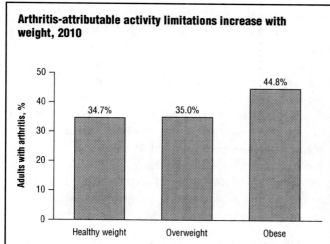

Arthritis-attributable activity limitations increase with weight, 2010

SOURCE: "Arthritis-Attributable Activity Limitations Increase with Weight," in *Arthritis: Meeting the Challenge—At a Glance 2011,* Centers for Disease Control and Prevention, National Center for Chronic Disease Prevention and Health Promotion, 2011, http://www .cdc.gov/chronicdisease/resources/publications/aag/pdf/2011/Arthritis-AAG-2011-508.pdf (accessed December 30, 2011)

new drugs that can relieve the pain of arthritis and block the degenerative process of these diseases. Researchers are investigating ways to improve treatment with the body's own biologic response modifiers (products that modify immune responses). They expect that these substances can be used to control the destructive processes of autoimmune diseases without weakening the whole immune system.

In "Rejuvenating the Immune System in Rheumatoid Arthritis" (*Nature Reviews Rheumatology*, vol. 5, October 2009), Cornelia M. Weyand et al. explain that in rheumatoid arthritis the aging process of the immune system is accelerated. This was thought to be a consequence of chronic inflammatory activity. However, recent research indicates that impaired ability to repair damaged deoxyribonucleic acid (DNA) may be involved. This finding suggests pursuing treatments that are aimed at resetting the immune systems of patients with rheumatoid arthritis to help restore their ability to repair broken or defective DNA.

Medications that are used to help relieve the symptoms of joint pain, stiffness, and swelling include NSAIDs, aspirin, analgesics, and corticosteroids. These drugs may be used in combination. Among recent advances are more effective pain-relief drugs with fewer adverse side effects than those already on the market. One of the problems with NSAIDs, the most widely used class of drugs for osteoarthritis, is the potential to irritate the stomach and cause ulcers.

Disease-modifying antirheumatic drugs (DMARDs) help reduce joint inflammation. They are generally effective but take as long as three to four months to produce benefits, so they must be started as early as possible to help prevent joint deformities and disability later in life.

Doctors often prescribe an additional medication, such as a corticosteroid or an NSAID, to help control pain and inflammation while the DMARD starts to work.

DMARDs include low doses of methotrexate, leflunomide, penicillamine, sulfasalazine, auranofin (also known as oral gold), gold sodium thiomalate (also known as injectable gold), minocycline, azathioprine, hydroxychloroquine sulfate (and other antimalarials), cyclosporine, and biologic agents. DMARDs are used most often for rheumatoid arthritis, but some DMARDs can also be used for juvenile rheumatoid arthritis, ankylosing spondylitis, psoriatic arthritis, and SLE.

Other therapies are also available. For instance, patients with moderate to severe rheumatoid arthritis who have not responded well to DMARDs may try Prosorba therapy. This involves drawing blood, separating plasma from red blood cells, and treating plasma through a Prosorba column (a cylinder the size of a soup can that holds a sandlike substance coated with protein A, a molecule that binds antibodies). The treated plasma is then rejoined with red blood cells and returned to the body. Treatments are given in 12 weekly sessions that last about two and a half hours each. The therapy works in much the same way that dialysis does. It cleans and filters the blood, removing the autoantibodies (self-attacking) that may contribute to causing painful, swollen joints. It may take as long as four months for patients to feel the benefits of the therapy.

Patients with osteoarthritis of the knee may be treated with joint fluid therapy, called viscosupplements, which act to lubricate the knee joint to relieve pain and ease motion. Along with medical therapies, regular exercise, weight control, and other self-care measures considerably reduce the incidence and effects of the disease.

Setbacks in Arthritis Drug Treatment

In 1999 two new drugs, celecoxib and rofecoxib, were marketed to physicians and directly to consumers as potent painkillers for arthritis sufferers. Celecoxib was marketed as Celebrex and rofecoxib as Vioxx, among other brand names. The drugs, called COX-2 inhibitors, are NSAIDs and were heralded as superior to conventional NSAIDs because they provided the same pain-relieving effects as aspirin and NSAIDs but with less chance of causing ulcers and intestinal bleeding. Almost immediately after their introduction, the drugs joined the ranks of the nation's best-selling prescription pharmaceuticals.

However, in November 2001 the first reports of increased heart disease among patients taking rofecoxib were issued, and in April 2002 the U.S. Food and Drug Administration (FDA) required Merck and Co., the pharmaceutical company that makes rofecoxib, to inform the public about the potential for increased risk of heart attack and stroke. That same year a third COX-2 inhibitor, called valdecoxib, was introduced by the drug company Pfizer Inc.

When the study "Risk of Acute Myocardial Infarction and Sudden Cardiac Death in Patients Treated with COX-2 Selective and Non-selective NSAIDs" (http://www.fda.gov/downloads/Drugs/DrugSafety/PostmarketDrugSafetyInformationforPatientsandProviders/ucm106880.pdf) by David J. Graham et al. was released in September 2004, it revealed that patients taking rofecoxib were twice as likely to suffer from stroke and heart attack as nonusers, and Merck withdrew the product from the market. Less than three months later the FDA asked Pfizer to add a black-box warning to the valdecoxib label alerting doctors and consumers to the increased risk of heart attack and stroke. (A black-box warning is the strongest form of warning the FDA can request.) In December 2004 the National Cancer Institute terminated a colon polyp study because of an increased cardiovascular risk in celecoxib users, and the National Institutes of Health halted a study of Alzheimer's disease because it suggested that the NSAID naproxen also increased the risk for heart attack and stroke. At the close of 2004 the FDA formally exhorted limited and cautious use of COX-2 inhibitors and traditional NSAIDs.

In February 2005 the FDA reversed its determination about naproxen, stating that it was not associated with increased cardiovascular risk and recommended that COX-2 drugs remain on the market. By April 2005 the FDA asked Pfizer to take valdecoxib off the market, and manufacturers of over-the-counter (nonprescription) and prescription NSAIDs, as well as celecoxib, were asked to change their labels to reflect the increased risk.

Merck weathered lawsuits from former Vioxx users or their survivors as well as legal action from its investors, who accused the company of misleading them about the risks that were associated with the use of Vioxx. In November 2009 lawyers representing Merck addressed the U.S. Supreme Court in an effort to overturn a decision by the U.S. Court of Appeals for the Third Circuit to allow a class-action securities lawsuit brought by the shareholders who lost value after Merck withdrew Vioxx from the market. Merck's representatives contended that information was made public beginning as early as 2001 that risks associated with Vioxx were becoming evident. In April 2010 the U.S. Supreme Court ruled that the shareholders' lawsuit arising from Merck's alleged misrepresentations of Vioxx was not time-barred by a statute of limitations and could proceed. The case was returned to a lower court in New Jersey, Merck's U.S. headquarters.

In April 2011 the FDA approved two new arthritis drugs: toclizumab for juvenile arthritis (in January 2010 this drug was approved for treatment of rheumatoid arthritis in adults) and a combination of ibuprofen and famatodine for rheumatoid arthritis and osteoarthritis.

OSTEOPOROSIS

Osteoporosis is a skeletal disorder that is characterized by compromised bone strength, which predisposes affected individuals to increased risk of fracture. In "Detecting Osteoporosis: Having a Bone Density Test" (2012, http://www.nof.org/aboutosteoporosis/detectingosteoporosis/bmdtest), the National Osteoporosis Foundation defines osteoporosis as about 25% bone loss compared with a healthy young adult, or, on a bone density test, 2.5 standard deviations below normal. Even though some bone loss occurs naturally with advancing age, the stooped posture (kyphosis) and loss of height (greater than 1 to 2 inches [2.5 to 5.1 cm]) experienced by many older adults result from vertebral fractures that are caused by osteoporosis.

Bone density builds during childhood growth and reaches its peak in early adulthood. From then on, bone loss gradually increases, outpacing the body's natural ability to replace bone. The denser bones are during the growth years, the less likely they will be to develop osteoporosis. A proper diet, especially one that contains foods rich in calcium and vitamin D long before the visible symptoms of osteoporosis appear, is vitally important.

Screening tests for bone density can identify people who are in need of additional testing. Often performed at health fairs, such tests are also known as peripheral tests and measure bone density in the lower arm, wrist, finger, or heel. Peripheral bone density tests may be performed using:

- Peripheral dual energy x-ray absorptiometry—this is a portable machine that uses very low doses of radiation to measure the density of bones in the arms or legs

- Quantitative ultrasound—this technique assesses mineral bone density without using radiation

- Peripheral quantitative computed tomography—this technique is often used to measure bone density and strength in the wrist

An online fracture risk assessment tool called FRAX helps health care practitioners determine who will benefit from bone density screening or testing. FRAX calculates an individual's fracture risk or the risk of breaking a bone in 10 years.

Bone density testing is generally performed using dual energy x-ray absorptiometry to measure bone density in the hip and spine. The painless test takes less than 15 minutes and uses very little radiation. Bone density testing is generally recommended for women aged 65 years and older, men aged 70 years and older, anyone who breaks a bone after the age of 50 years, and postmenopausal women under the age of 65 years and men aged 50 to 69 years with risk factors for osteoporosis (e.g., a family history of osteoporosis, people with low bone density known as osteopenia, and so on).

Osteoporosis worsens with age, leaving its sufferers at risk of broken hips or other bones, curvature of the spine, and other disabilities. According to the National Osteoporosis Foundation, in "Fast Facts" (2012, http://www.nof.org/node/40), an estimated 8 million women (non-Hispanic white women are disproportionately affected) and 2 million men have the disease; another 34 million are considered at risk of developing the condition. In severe cases the disease may cause patients to experience spontaneous (without external causes) fractures, generally in the vertebrae of the spine.

The National Institute of Arthritis and Musculoskeletal and Skin Diseases (NIAMS) reports that like other chronic conditions that disproportionately affect older adults, the prevalence of bone disease and fractures is projected to increase markedly as the population ages. In "Preventing Falls and Related Fractures" (January 2011, http://www.niams.nih.gov/Health_Info/Bone/Osteoporosis/Fracture/prevent_falls.asp), NIAMS reports that more than 90% of hip fractures are associated with osteoporosis. Older adults who have a hip fracture are 5% to 20% more likely to die in the year following the fracture than their age peers, and among people living independently before a hip fracture, as many as 25% will remain in long-term care institutions a year after their fractures.

The 1994 discovery of a gene linked to bone density was hailed as the most important finding in osteoporosis research in a decade. Two forms of the gene, B and b, exist. People with two b genes, one from each parent, have the highest bone density and are the least likely to develop osteoporosis, whereas those with one of each, the Bb genotype, have intermediate bone density. People with two B genes have the lowest bone density and the highest risk of osteoporosis. Women with the BB genotype may be four times as likely to experience hip fractures as those with the bb genotype.

The article "The Latest Osteoporosis Research" (*Arthritis Today*, May–June 2007) notes that researchers in Iceland identified the bone morphogenetic protein-2 gene in 2003 and that researchers were actively formulating a simple test to identify children at risk for osteoporosis in later life. The test would allow doctors to prescribe an increased intake of calcium, vitamin D, and protein during the growth years for these children, thus preventing or delaying the onset of osteoporosis. Although by early 2012 this specific genetic test was not yet available commercially, it and others were being developed and refined. It is also hoped that tests such as these will pave the way for effective gene therapy to prevent osteoporosis.

According to the press release "Interleukin Genetics Launches Bone Health Genetic Test" (http://www.ilgenetics.com/content/news-events/newsDetail.jsp/q/news-id/209), in December 2009 Interleukin Genetics introduced the Bone Health Genetic Test that detects genetic patterns associated with the development of osteoporosis. The test analyzes gene variations that are associated with an increased risk for spinal fracture and low bone mineral density.

Table 6.2 summarizes the factors that predispose a person to osteoporosis and fractures. Apart from genetics, the risk factors—nutrition, physical activity (especially weight-bearing exercise), and choosing not to smoke—are all modifiable.

Treatment of Osteoporosis

The primary goal of therapy is to prevent fractures. Nonpharmacologic (without medicine) preventive measures that help prevent osteoporosis include diet modification (an increase in the intake of calcium and vitamin D), exercise programs, and fall-prevention strategies. These may include subtle lifestyle changes such as wearing rubber-soled shoes for better traction, installing grab bars in bathtubs and showers, and keeping floors clear of clutter. Current pharmacologic (medication) therapies improve bone mass and reduce fracture risk.

At the turn of the 21st century the typical treatment for postmenopausal women with osteoporosis, or those who were at risk for the disease, was hormone replacement therapy (HRT), often combined with daily doses of calcium and regular weight-bearing exercise, such as walking and exercising with weights. This treatment slows the advance of the disease and helps prevent fractures and disability. However, serious side effects of HRT were recognized in 2002, including increased risks of cardiovascular disease and certain types of cancer, so many women discontinued HRT treatment. For some women at heightened risk for

TABLE 6.2

Causes of bone loss and fractures in osteoporosis

Failure to develop a strong skeleton

Genetics—limited growth or abnormal bone composition
Nutrition—calcium, phosphorous and vitamin D deficiency, poor general nutrition
Lifestyle—lack of weight-bearing exercise, smoking

Loss of bone due to excessive breakdown (resorption)

Decreased sex hormone production
Calcium and vitamin D deficiency, increased parathyroid hormone
Excess production of local resorbing factors

Failure to replace lost bone due to impaired formation

Loss of ability to replenish bone cells with age
Decreased production of systemic growth factors
Loss of local growth factors

Increased tendency to fall

Loss of muscle strength
Slow reflexes and poor vision
Drugs that impair balance

SOURCE: "Table 2-2. Causes of Bone Loss and Fractures in Osteoporosis," in *Bone Health and Osteoporosis: A Report of the Surgeon General 2004*, U.S. Department of Health and Human Services, Public Health Service, Office of the Surgeon General, 2004, http://www.surgeongeneral.gov/library/bonehealth/chapter_2.html (accessed December 31, 2011)

osteoporosis who also have fewer risk factors for cardiovascular disease, HRT remains a treatment option.

One of the goals of osteoporosis treatment is to maintain bone health by preventing bone loss and by building new bone. Another is to minimize the risk and impact of falls because they can cause fractures. Figure 6.2 shows the pyramid for prevention and treatment of osteoporosis. At its base is nutrition, with adequate intake of calcium, vitamin D, and other minerals; physical exercise; and preventive measures to reduce the risk of falls. The second layer of the pyramid involves identifying drugs (e.g., aluminum-coated antacids, some antiseizure medications, and steroids) and diseases (e.g., thyroid disease) that can cause osteoporosis. The peak of the pyramid involves drug therapy for osteoporosis.

There are two primary types of drugs that are used to treat osteoporosis. Antiresorptive agents act to reduce bone loss, and anabolic agents act to build bone. Antiresorptive therapies include use of bisphosphonates, estrogen, selective estrogen receptor modulators, and calcitonin. Antiresorptive therapies reduce bone loss, stabilize the architecture of the bone, and decrease bone turnover. In 2005 the FDA approved two bisphosphonates (alendronate and risedronate) for the prevention or treatment of osteoporosis and one anabolic agent (a synthetic form of parathyroid hormone known as teriparatide that is administered by injection). In 2010 the FDA approved denosumab, another injected agent, for postmenopausal women with osteoporosis who are at high risk for fractures. Denosumab is a monoclonal antibody that binds to a protein involved in the formation, function, and survival of osteoclasts, the cells that are responsible for bone resorption.

In the press release "FDA Drug Safety Communication: Safety Update for Osteoporosis Drugs, Bisphosphonates, and Atypical Fractures" (October 13, 2010 http://www.fda.gov/drugs/drugsafety/ucm229009.htm), the FDA cautions physicians and users of bisphosphonates about the risk of atypical fractures of the thigh. Atypical femur fractures are fractures in the bone just below the hip joint in the long part of the thighbone. These fractures occur very rarely, accounting for less than 1% of all hip and femur fractures. Even though it is not yet known whether bisphosphonates cause these fractures, these unusual femur fractures have been reported primarily in patients taking bisphosphonates. The FDA is continuing its ongoing safety review of bisphosphonate use and the occurrence of atypical femur fractures. The agency requires that this new information be included in the Warnings and Precautions section of the labels of all bisphosphonate products that are approved for the prevention or treatment of osteoporosis.

EXERCISE IMPROVES BONE HEALTH IN OLDER ADULTS. Evidence that exercise has measurable positive effects on bone structure continues to mount. Silvia Tolomio et al. find in "Short-Term Adapted Physical Activity Program Improves Bone Quality in Osteopenic/Osteoporotic Postmenopausal Women" (*Journal of Physical Activity and Health*, vol. 5, no. 6, November 2008) that bone structure in postmenopausal women who were diagnosed with bone loss was improved by an exercise program that included aerobic, balance, and strength training. Comparing a group of patients who participated in a 20-week supervised exercise program with a control group of patients who did not perform the activities, the researchers note that the exercises improved both limb strength and bone density, two factors that contribute to the ability to prevent falls and fractures.

In "Effects of Exercise on Bone Density and Falls Risk Factors in Post-menopausal Women with Osteopenia: A Randomised Controlled Trial" (*Journal of Science and Medicine in Sport*, vol. 15, no. 2, March 2012), Karen L. Bolton et al. explain that they followed postmenopausal

FIGURE 6.2

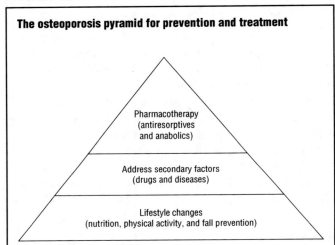

The osteoporosis pyramid for prevention and treatment

Pharmacotherapy
(antiresorptives
and anabolics)

Address secondary factors
(drugs and diseases)

Lifestyle changes
(nutrition, physical activity, and fall prevention)

Note: **The base of the pyramid:** The first step in the prevention and treatment of osteoporosis and the prevention of fractures is to build a foundation of nutrition and lifestyle measures that maximize bone health. The diet should not only be adequate in calcium and vitamin D, but should have a healthy balance of other nutrients. A weight-bearing exercise program should be developed. Cigarette smoking and excessive alcohol use must be avoided. In the older individual, at high risk for fractures, the changes in lifestyle would include a plan not only to maximize physical activity, but also to minimize the risk of falls. The use of hip protectors can be considered in some high-risk patients. Diseases that increase the risk of falls by causing visual impairment, postural hypotension (a drop in blood pressure on standing, which leads to dizziness), or poor balance should be treated. Drugs that cause bone loss or increase the risk of falls should be avoided or given at the lowest effective dose.
The second level of the pyramid: The next step is to identify and treat diseases that produce secondary osteoporosis or aggravate primary osteoporosis. These measures are the foundation upon which specific pharmacotherapy is built and should never be forgotten.
The third level of the pyramid: If there is sufficiently high risk of fracture to warrant pharmacotherapy, the patient is usually started on antiresorptives. Anabolic agents are used in individuals in whom antiresorptive therapy is not adequate to prevent bone loss or fractures.

SOURCE: "Figure 9-1. The Osteoporosis Pyramid for Prevention and Treatment," in *Bone Health and Osteoporosis: A Report of the Surgeon General 2004*, U.S. Department of Health and Human Services, Public Health Service, Office of the Surgeon General, 2004, http://www.surgeongeneral.gov/library/bonehealth/chapter_9.html (accessed December 31, 2011)

women with osteopenia (low bone mineral density) who were enrolled in an exercise program that met three times per week for 52 weeks and compared their health-related quality of life and bone mineral density to a control group of women who did not exercise. The researchers find that the participants who exercised had small increases in bone mineral density, endurance, and health-related quality of life. In contrast, those who did not exercise experienced a slight loss of bone mineral density.

MULTIPLE SCLEROSIS

Multiple sclerosis (MS) is a chronic, degenerative, and often intermittent disease of the central nervous system. It eventually destroys the myelin protein sheaths that surround and insulate nerve fibers in the brain and spinal cord. Myelin is a fatty substance that aids the flow of electrical impulses from the brain through the spinal cord. These nerve impulses control all conscious and unconscious movements. In MS the myelin sheath disintegrates and is replaced by hard sclerotic plaques (scar tissue) that distort or prevent the flow of electrical impulses along the nerves to various parts of the body.

MS usually appears in young adulthood and is common enough to have earned the title "the great crippler of young adults." Many problems and symptoms are associated with the disease, but the major problem is lost mobility. Symptoms can range from mild problems, such as numbness and muscle weakness, to uncontrollable tremors, slurred speech, loss of bowel and bladder control, memory lapses, and paralysis. Even though almost all parts of the nervous system may become involved, the spinal cord is the most vulnerable. Wild mood swings, from euphoria to depression, are another manifestation of the disease. The disease is not fatal in itself, but it weakens its victims and makes them far more susceptible to infection.

The disease is called "multiple" because it usually affects many parts of the nervous system and is often characterized by relapses followed by periods of partial and sometimes complete recovery. Therefore, it is multiple both in how it affects the body and in how often it strikes.

Prevalence

In "Who Gets MS" (2012, http://www.nationalmssociety .org/about-multiple-sclerosis/what-we-know-about-ms/who-gets-ms/index.aspx), the National Multiple Sclerosis Society estimates that 400,000 people in the United States have been diagnosed with MS and that every week approximately 200 people are newly diagnosed with the disease. The disease is most often diagnosed in patients between the ages of 20 and 50 years old. A possible clue to the cause of MS is that it is more common in cold, damp climates. In Europe it is found most often in the Scandinavian countries, the Baltic region, northern Germany, and Great Britain. It is rare in the Mediterranean countries, China, and Japan, and among Native Americans. It is also rare among African-Americans. White females are affected twice as often as males. In the United States most cases are found in the northern areas, and it is more common in Canada than in the southern United States.

Diagnosing MS

The diagnosis of MS is generally made after a thorough history and physical examination and the results of diagnostic tests are evaluated. Among the tests are magnetic resonance imaging (MRI; this provides a detailed view of the brain), spinal tap (to examine spinal fluid for signs of the disease), and evoked potentials (which measure how quickly and accurately a person's nervous system responds to certain stimulation). No single test can detect MS; several must be done and compared.

The neurologic examination for MS focuses on detecting hyperactive (as opposed to normal) reflexes and balance and gait disturbances. An eye examination evaluates damage to the optic nerve. Even though some cases of MS are readily diagnosed by physicians based on the history and physical examination, most physicians confirm the diagnosis by using an imaging study to document evidence of plaques in at least two locations of the central nervous system.

Causes of MS

The exact cause of MS is unknown. Many theories about its cause have been proposed—genetics, gender, or exposure to environmental triggers such as viruses, trauma, or heavy metals—but none have been proven. The most widely accepted theory is that damage to myelin results from an abnormal response by the body's immune system. Normally, the immune system defends the body against foreign invaders such as viruses or bacteria. However, in an autoimmune disease the body attacks its own tissue. Some believe that MS is an autoimmune disease in which myelin is attacked.

The National Multiple Sclerosis Society explains in "What Causes MS?" (2012, http://www.nationalmssociety .org/about-multiple-sclerosis/what-we-know-about-ms/what-causes-ms/index.aspx) that like other diseases, genetic factors, in a complex interplay with environmental influences such as exposure to viruses, very likely play a significant role in determining who develops MS. Close relatives of people with MS—such as children, siblings, or a nonidentical twin—have a higher chance of developing the disease than do people without relatives with MS, and an identical twin of someone with MS has a one in four chance of developing the disease. If genes were the sole determinant, an identical twin of someone with MS would have a 100% chance of developing the disease. Given that the risk is only one out of four reveals that other factors, such as geography, ethnicity, and viral infection, are probably necessary to trigger the development of the disease. Because MS is two to three times more common in women than in men, it is also possible that hormones play a role in determining susceptibility to MS.

Treatment of MS

No known specific treatment halts the disease process. Once nerve fibers have been destroyed, they cannot recover their function. Current methods of treatment include powerful immune-suppressant drugs that often leave patients vulnerable to secondary infections. In "Treatments" (http://www.nationalmssociety.org/about-multiple-sclerosis/what-we-know-about-ms/treatments/index.aspx), the National Multiple Sclerosis Society explains that as of February 2012 the FDA had approved eight disease-modifying medications for use in relapsing forms of MS: six are injected and two are given by intravenous infusion in a medical facility.

The National Multiple Sclerosis Society recommends that people who are diagnosed with the disease should start drug treatment immediately, before symptoms worsen. The society recommends prompt treatment with medication, because it appears that patients who receive early treatment will probably have fewer disabling symptoms than those who do not.

The drugs to treat MS are beta-interferon products that act by reducing the inflammation of MS lesions and reducing the accumulation of the lesions. All have demonstrated effectiveness in reducing the number and severity of relapses. Two other medications, glatiramer acetate and mitoxantrone, are also used to treat MS. Glatiramer acetate is believed to work by suppressing the immune system's attacks on myelin. Mitoxantrone reduces the activity of white blood cells that attack myelin and is generally prescribed for patients with worsening MS.

Exacerbations, or flare-ups, of the disease, which may last from a few days to several months, are commonly treated with high doses of corticosteroids (to reduce inflammation). Rehabilitation programs help people with MS maintain fitness and pace themselves to conserve their energy during their daily activities. People with MS are advised to build general resistance and avoid fatigue and exposure to extremes in temperature. Physical therapy and psychotherapy are useful in helping patients and their families cope with the limitations that are caused by MS. Other therapy programs provide strategies to maintain independence, to use assistive technologies in the workplace, and to adjust to changes in speech, swallowing, and cognitive abilities.

PARKINSON'S DISEASE

Parkinsonism refers not to a particular disease but to a condition that is marked by a characteristic set of symptoms affecting more than 1 million people in the United States in 2012, according to the National Parkinson Foundation in "Parkinson's Disease Overview" (http://www.parkinson.org/Parkinson-s-Disease.aspx). Both men and women are affected, and the probability of developing Parkinson's disease (PD) increases with advancing age. PD usually strikes people older than age 62, but an estimated 10% of patients are 40 years old or younger.

PD is caused by the progressive deterioration of about half a million brain cells in the portion of the brain that controls certain types of muscle movement. These cells secrete dopamine, a neurotransmitter (chemical messenger). Dopamine's function is to allow nerve impulses to move smoothly from one nerve cell to another. These nerve cells, in turn, transmit messages to the muscles of the body to begin movement. When the normal supply of dopamine is reduced, the messages are not correctly sent, and the symptoms of PD appear.

The four early warning signs of PD are tremors, muscle stiffness, unusual slowness, and a stooped posture. Medications can control initial symptoms, but as time goes on they become less effective. As the disease worsens, patients develop tremors, causing them to fall or jerk uncontrollably. (The jerky body movements that patients with PD experience are known as dyskinesias.) At other times rigidity sets in, rendering patients unable to move. About one-third of patients also develop dementia, an impairment of cognition (thought processes).

Treatment of PD

The management of PD is individualized and includes drug therapy and a program that stresses daily exercise. Medication and therapy may modify the progression of PD. Exercise can often reduce the rigidity of muscles, prevent weakness, and improve the ability to walk.

The main goal of drug treatment is to restore the chemical balance between dopamine and another neurotransmitter, acetylcholine. The standard treatment for most patients is levodopa (L-dopa), which was first approved for use in 1970. L-dopa is a compound that the body converts into dopamine to replace it in the body and help alleviate symptoms. (Without dopamine, signals from the brain cannot "transmit" properly to the body, and movement is impaired.) However, treatment with L-dopa does not slow the progressive course of the disease or even delay the changes in the brain that PD produces, and it may produce some unpleasant side effects because of its change to dopamine before reaching the brain. Simultaneously administering substances that inhibit this change allows a higher concentration of L-dopa to reach the brain and considerably decreases the side effects.

Along with L-dopa and other drugs called dopamine agonists, which mimic the action of dopamine, four other classes of drugs are used to treat the symptoms of PD, including anticholinergics, COMT inhibitors, MAO-B inhibitors, and amantadine, which was initially developed as an antiviral drug. Anticholinergics work to relieve tremor and rigidity. COMT inhibitors act by prolonging the effectiveness of a dose of L-dopa by preventing its breakdown. MAO-B inhibitors slow the breakdown of dopamine in the brain. Amantadine has demonstrated effectiveness in reducing dyskinesias.

In "Surgical Treatment Options" (2012, http://www.parkinson.org/Parkinson-s-Disease/Treatment/Surgical-Treatment-Options), the National Parkinson Foundation explains that surgical treatment is only used for PD patients who have exhausted medical treatment and remain symptomatic. Even though it can be an effective treatment option for different symptoms of PD, only symptoms that previously improved on L-dopa have the potential to improve after the surgery.

Genetic Link to PD

Two studies, Suzanne Lesage et al.'s "LRRK2 G2019S as a Cause of Parkinson's Disease in North African Arabs" and Laurie J. Ozelius et al.'s "LRRK2 G2019S as a Cause of Parkinson's Disease in Ashkenazi Jews" (both published in New England Journal of Medicine, vol. 354, no. 4, January 26, 2006), describe the discovery of a single genetic mutation on a gene called leucine-rich repeat kinase 2 (LRRK2) that accounts for as many as 30% of all cases of PD in Arabs, North Africans, and Jews. People with the mutation make an abnormal version of a protein called dardarin (a form of the Basque word for tremor) in which a single amino acid—number 2019—is glycine instead of serine. This finding may help direct the development of a drug that modifies the impact of this mutation to prevent or substantially delay onset of the disease.

Subsequent studies, such as Jeanne C. Latourelle et al.'s "Genomewide Association Study for Onset Age in Parkinson Disease" (BMC Medical Genetics, September 22, 2009), find that in addition to the identification of five single genes that are associated with PD, there are multiple genes and gene interactions that increase susceptibility to PD. The researchers note that the age at which PD begins is also a highly heritable trait. This finding is especially important because by identifying the genes that are related to the age of onset, it may be possible to identify ways to delay the onset of PD symptoms. Effectively postponing disease onset could reduce the prevalence of PD.

Experimental Therapies

GENE THERAPY. As of 2012 the use of gene therapy for PD patients remained highly experimental. The therapy entails inserting a beneficial gene into brain cells using technology developed by RheoGene, a University of Pittsburgh Medical Center affiliate, that allows researchers to turn the gene on or off as needed, which is an important safety feature if the proteins it produces have some

unanticipated, harmful effect. It also permits researchers to custom-tailor the activity of the gene based on the individual needs of each patient.

One of the genes that is inserted produces glial cell line–derived neurotrophic factor (GDNF), a protein that appears to strengthen brain cells and helps prevent the death of sick cells. In animal studies GDNF has been shown to stop the progression of the disease and perhaps even reverse it. The challenge has been to find a way to deliver the growth factor.

Chad W. Christine et al. report in "Safety and Tolerability of Putaminal AADC Gene Therapy for Parkinson's Disease" (Neurology, vol. 73, no. 20, November 17, 2009) the promising results of a small (12 patient) clinical trial of gene therapy for PD that proved to be safe, well tolerated, and effective. The therapy subdued overactive circuitry in the brain by stimulating increased production of GABA, an amino acid that acts as an inhibitory neurotransmitter (neurochemical that transmits nerve impulses), without the untoward side effects that are associated with L-dopa treatment. However, the method of administration was problematical and in some patients the therapy produced the undesirable side effect of bleeding in the brain.

In 2011 the first successful rigorous clinical study of gene therapy for PD was completed. The results were published by Peter A. LeWitt et al. in "AAV2-GAD Gene Therapy for Advanced Parkinson's Disease: A Double-Blind, Sham-Surgery Controlled, Randomised Trial" (Lancet Neurology, vol. 10, no. 4, April 2011). The researchers report that patients who received a gene therapy called NLX-P101 via infusion into a region of the brain that is involved in motor function experienced "a significant reduction in the motor symptoms of Parkinson's, including tremor, rigidity and difficulty initiating movement." Half of the patients receiving gene therapy achieved dramatic symptom improvements, compared with just 14% of untreated patients in the control group. Patients receiving gene therapy had nearly twice the improvement in motor score, 23.1%, compared with a 12.7% improvement in the control group.

ELECTRODE IMPLANTS. Another procedure being tested is the use of electrical implants. Electrodes are surgically implanted in the brain and connected to a battery-operated device, which is also implanted in the body. The device allows patients to "turn off" the tremors that prevent them from performing the activities of daily living such as pouring a glass of milk and feeding themselves. One shortcoming is that the device's batteries must be surgically replaced every three to five years.

Brian Parent et al. find in "The Relevance of Age and Disease Duration for Intervention with Subthalamic Nucleus Deep Brain Stimulation Surgery in Parkinson Disease" (Journal of Neurosurgery, vol. 114, no. 4, April

2011) that younger patients with a shorter duration of PD fare better than older patients because early use of the electrode implants seems to maximize the benefits of this surgical procedure. Furthermore, the researchers observe that older patients with dyskinesias also have significant improvement and that the procedure "can offer relief from this common consequence of long-term levodopa use."

STEM CELL RESEARCH. In August 2001 researchers and patients hoping to benefit from treatment based on this promising area of scientific study were partially relieved when President George W. Bush (1946–) announced that federal funds could be used to conduct stem cell research on existing stem cell lines. His decision banned the creation or use of new embryos for federally funded experimental purposes. This meant that federal funds were available to researchers in this field, but it placed significant limits on the scope of research eligible for federal support.

Junying Yu et al. report in "Induced Pluripotent Stem Cell Lines Derived from Human Somatic Cells" (*Science*, vol. 318, no. 5858, December 21, 2007) that they created stem cells without using embryos by turning human skin cells into stem cells capable of growing into any of the 220 types of tissue in the body. This accomplishment was seen as not only effectively overcoming any ethical and legal arguments about stem cell research but also improving the odds of clinical efficacy because immune rejection is unlikely to pose a problem using stem cells made this way.

According to the White House, in the press release "Removing Barriers to Responsible Scientific Research Involving Human Stem Cells" (http://www.whitehouse .gov/the_press_office/Removing-Barriers-to-Responsible-Scientific-Research-Involving-Human-Stem-Cells), in March 2009 President Barack Obama (1961–) relaxed limitations on stem cell research through an executive order that allowed support for "responsible, scientifically worthy human stem cell research, including human embryonic stem cell research." By March 2010 Francis S. Collins (1950–), the director of the National Institutes of Health, noted in the editorial "At NIH, Moving Ahead on Stem Cell Research" (*Washington Post*, March 20, 2010) that the number of cell lines available for research studies had doubled to 44 and that more than 100 additional lines had been submitted to the National Institutes of Health for approval. According to Collins, the new policy "allows for a continually growing number of stem cell lines to be considered and ensures that research will be conducted ethically and responsibly."

The excitement and optimism about human embryonic stem cells centers on the capacity of these cells to renew themselves and develop into specialized cell types. Unlike other cells that have predetermined roles and functions, such as heart or brain cells, stem cells can develop into nearly all the specialized cells of the body—with the potential to replace cells for the nervous system, heart, pancreas, kidneys, skin, bone, or blood.

Research is under way that uses stem cells to treat neurologic disorders by replacing diseased or malfunctioning cells in the brain and spinal cord. The results of this research could have life-changing consequences for people suffering from PD, MS, Alzheimer's disease, and spinal cord injuries. Other research focuses on developing organs and tissues for transplantation, because there is an urgent need for donor organs. Still other researchers are looking at ways to induce stem cells to become insulin-producing cells of the pancreas to treat diabetes.

By 2012 fetal cell transplantation had been used to ease the symptoms of PD patients for more than a decade. In "Using Stem Cells and iPS Cells to Discover New Treatments for Parkinson's Disease" (*Parkinsonism and Related Disorders*, vol. 18, suppl. 1, January 2012), Oliver Cooper, Penny Hallett, and Ole Isacson state that human pluripotent stem cells offer an opportunity to replace specific types of degenerating neurons. Induced pluripotent stem cell-derived neurons (cells that are artificially derived from adult cells and behave like natural pluripotent stem cells—they are able to differentiate into specialized cell types and self-renew to generate more stem cells) may also be used to translate the genetic basis for an individual's risk of developing PD into clinically meaningful information.

ALZHEIMER'S DISEASE

Alzheimer's disease (AD) is a progressive, degenerative disease that affects the brain and results in severely impaired memory, thinking, and behavior. According to the Alzheimer's Association, in *2011 Alzheimer's Disease Facts and Figures* (February 2011, http://www.alz .org/downloads/Facts_Figures_2011.pdf), in 2011 it was the sixth-leading cause of death among American adults and the fifth-leading cause of death for those aged 65 years and older. Approximately 5.4 million Americans were afflicted with AD in 2011. The overwhelming majority of AD sufferers (5.2 million, or 96%) were aged 65 years and older. AD usually begins after age 60, and risk goes up with age. Four percent of people with AD are under the age of 65 years, 6% are aged 65 to 74 years, 45% are aged 75 to 84 years, and the remaining 45% are aged 85 years and older. The number of people with the disease doubles every five years beyond age 65. An estimated 16% of women aged 71 years and older have AD (or other dementia), compared with 11% of men of the same age range. Women have a higher lifetime risk of developing the disease because, on average, they live longer than men.

The German physician Alois Alzheimer (1864–1915) first described the disease in 1907, after he had cared for a patient with an unusual mental illness. Alzheimer observed anatomic changes in his patient's brain and described them as abnormal clumps and tangled bundles of fibers. Nearly a century later these abnormal findings, now described as amyloid plaques and neurofibrillary tangles, along with abnormal clusters of proteins in the brain, are recognized as the characteristic markers of AD.

Suspected Causes

AD is not a normal consequence of healthy aging, and researchers continue to seek its cause. Like most other chronic, progressive diseases, it is believed to be influenced by some combination of genetic and nongenetic factors.

Researchers have identified different patterns of inheritance, ages of onset (when symptoms begin), genes, chromosomes, and proteins that are linked to the development of AD. Mutations in at least four genes, situated on chromosomes 1, 14, 19, and 21, and possibly as many as 14 genes are thought to be involved in the disease.

The first genetic breakthrough—the discovery that a mutation in a single gene could cause this progressive neurological illness—was reported in 1991 by Alison Goate et al. in "Segregation of a Missense Mutation in the Amyloid Precursor Protein Gene with Familial Alzheimer's Disease" (*Nature*, vol. 349, no. 6311, February 21, 1991). The researchers identified the defect in the gene that directs cells to produce a substance called amyloid protein. Goate et al. found that low levels of the brain chemical acetylcholine contribute to the formation of plaques, the hard deposits of amyloid protein that accumulate in the brain tissue of AD patients. In healthy people, these protein fragments are broken down and excreted. Because amyloid protein is found in cells throughout the body, the question is: Why and how does it become a deadly substance in the brain cells of some people and not others?

In 1995 three more genes linked to AD were identified. One gene is linked to a rare, devastating form of early-onset AD, which occurs as early as the third decade of life. When defective, this gene may prevent brain cells from correctly processing a substance called beta amyloid precursor protein. The second gene, which is also involved in the production of beta amyloid, is associated with another early-onset form of AD that strikes people younger than age 65.

The third gene, known as apolipoprotein E (apoE), was initially linked to AD in 1993, but its role in the body was not immediately identified. Researchers have since discovered that the gene regulates lipid metabolism within the organs and helps redistribute cholesterol. In the brain, apoE plays a key role in repairing nerve tissue that has been injured. There are three forms (alleles) of the gene: apoE-2, apoE-3, and apoE-4. Between one-half and one-third of all AD patients have at least one apoE-4 gene, whereas only 15.5% of the general population carries an apoE-4 gene. In 1998 Marion R. Meyer et al. noted in "APOE Genotype Predicts When—Not Whether—One Is Predisposed to Develop Alzheimer Disease" (*Nature*

Genetics, vol. 19, no. 4, August 1998) that the apoE-4 gene does not determine whether an individual will develop the disease; instead, it appears to affect when AD will strike—the age when AD symptoms are likely to begin. The National Institute on Aging (September 27, 2011, http://www.nia.nih.gov/newsroom/1998/02/26-national-alzheimers-disease-centers-collaborate-study-utility-genetic-testing) confirms that even though this gene occurs in 40% of people who develop late-onset AD, one-third of people with AD do not have the form of apoE-4 gene that is associated with AD.

Also in 1998 Deborah Blacker et al. found in "Alpha-2 Macroglobulin Is Genetically Associated with Alzheimer Disease" (*Nature Genetics*, vol. 19, no. 4, August 1998) that A2M-2, another gene variant, appears to affect whether a person will develop AD. An estimated one-third of Americans may carry this gene, potentially tripling their risk of developing late-onset AD, compared with their siblings with the normal version of the A2M gene.

Between 2009 and 2010 three additional genes—CR1, CLU, and BIN1—that may increase the risk for AD were identified. In 2011, six more genes were identified (MS4A, CD2AP, CD33, EPHA1, BIN1, and ABCA7) to increase the risk for late-onset AD. The identification of new genes that are associated with AD improves understanding of the causes of the disease and informs drug discovery.

Symptoms of AD

AD begins slowly. The symptoms include difficulty with memory and a loss of cognition. The patient with AD may also experience confusion; language problems, such as trouble finding words; impaired judgment; disorientation in place and time; and changes in mood, behavior, and personality. How quickly these changes occur varies from person to person, but eventually the disease leaves its victims unable to care for themselves. In their terminal stages, patients with AD require care 24 hours per day. They no longer recognize family members or themselves, and they need help with daily activities such as eating, dressing, bathing, and using the toilet. Eventually, they may become incontinent, blind, and unable to communicate. Finally, their bodies may "forget" how to breathe or make the heart beat. Many patients die from pneumonia.

Testing for AD

A complete physical, psychiatric, and neurologic evaluation can usually produce a diagnosis of AD that is about 90% accurate. For many years the only sure way to diagnose the disease was to examine brain tissue under a microscope, which was not possible while the AD victim was still alive. An autopsy of someone who has died of AD reveals a characteristic pattern that is the hallmark of the disease: tangles of fibers (neurofibrillary tangles) and clusters of degenerated nerve endings (neuritic plaques) in areas of the brain that are crucial for memory and intellect. Also, the cortex of the brain is shrunken.

In October 2000 John C. Mazziotta of the University of California, Los Angeles, School of Medicine reported in "Window on the Brain" (*Archives of Neurology*, vol. 57, no. 10) that the use of MRI techniques could measure the volume of brain tissue in areas of the brain that are used for memory, organizational ability, and planning. In addition, the use of these measurements could accurately identify people with AD and predict which people would develop AD. That same year, in "Using Serial Registered Brain Magnetic Resonance Imaging to Measure Disease Progression in Alzheimer Disease: Power Calculations and Estimates of Sample Size to Detect Treatment Effects" (*Archives of Neurology*, vol. 57, no. 3, March 2000), Nick C. Fox et al. reported using MRI to identify parts of the brain that are affected by AD before symptoms appear and to measure brain atrophy to monitor the progression of AD.

In 2005 Dimitra G. Georganopoulou et al. announced in "Nanoparticle-Based Detection in Cerebral Spinal Fluid of a Soluble Pathogenic Biomarker for Alzheimer's Disease" (*Proceedings of the National Academy of Sciences*, vol. 102, no. 7, February 15, 2005) the development of yet another diagnostic test that detects small amounts of protein in spinal fluid. Called a bio-barcode assay, the test is as much as a million times more sensitive than other tests. Originally used to identify a marker for prostate cancer, the test is used to detect a protein in the brain called amyloid-beta-derived diffusible ligand (ADDL). ADDLs are small soluble proteins. To detect them the researchers used nanoscale particles that had antibodies specific to ADDL.

In "Finding Alzheimer's before a Mind Fails" (*New York Times*, December 26, 2007), Denise Grady reports on a test that uses a special type of dye called Pittsburgh Compound B that enables positron emission tomography (PET) scans (imaging studies) to identify amyloid deposits in the brain. Such testing can help establish the diagnosis by distinguishing Alzheimer's from other kinds of dementia and can help physicians monitor the progress of the disease and the effects of drug treatment.

In 2009 a new test debuted that accurately detects AD in its earliest stages, before the onset of memory problems and other symptoms of cognitive impairment. Leslie M. Shaw et al. explain in "Cerebrospinal Fluid Biomarker Signature in Alzheimer's Disease Neuroimaging Initiative Subjects" (*Annals of Neurology*, vol. 65, no. 4, April 2009) that the test measures the concentration of specific biomarkers, in this case proteins (tau protein and amyloid beta42 polypeptide) in spinal fluid that can indicate AD. The researchers report that subjects with low concentrations of amyloid beta42 and high levels of tau in their spinal fluid were more likely to develop AD.

The test had an 87% accuracy rate when predicting which subjects would be diagnosed with AD.

The results of research published in "Pittsburgh Compound B Imaging and Prediction of Progression from Cognitive Normality to Symptomatic Alzheimer Disease" (*Archives of Neurology*, vol. 66, no. 12, December 14, 2009) suggest that people with no symptoms of dementia may be at risk for developing AD if they have abnormal levels of beta amyloid. A study conducted by John C. Morris et al. of the Alzheimer's Disease Research Center in St. Louis, Missouri, used imaging studies including PET scans and MRI to detect levels of beta amyloid protein in the living brain and measure brain volume. The researchers find that the level of beta amyloid is associated with shrinkage in many parts of the brain and over time, with declining ability to perform well on memory and thinking tests.

In 2010 John L. Woodard et al. reported that the combination of a test for the apoE-4 gene and a functional MRI (fMRI shows how areas of the brain are activated during mental processes) effectively predicted near-term cognitive decline. In "Prediction of Cognitive Decline in Healthy Older Adults Using fMRI" (*Journal of Alzheimer's Disease*, vol. 21, no. 3, January 2010), the researchers indicate that in 75% of study subjects the genetic test and fMRI accurately predicted which healthy older adults would experience cognitive decline within 18 months of testing.

Researchers continue to look at other biological markers, such as blood tests, and at neuropsychological tests, which measure memory, orientation, judgment, and problem solving, to see if they can accurately predict whether healthy, unaffected older adults will develop AD or whether those with mild cognitive impairment will go on to develop AD. However, the availability of tests raises ethical and practical questions about patients' desires or needs to know their risk of developing AD. Is it helpful or useful to predict a condition that is not yet considered preventable or curable?

Treatments for AD

As of 2012 there was still no cure or prevention for AD, and treatment focused on managing symptoms. Medication can reduce some of the symptoms, such as agitation, anxiety, unpredictable behavior, and depression. Physical exercise and good nutrition are important, as is a calm and highly structured environment. The object is to help the patient with AD maintain as much comfort, normalcy, and dignity as possible.

In 2012 there were five FDA-approved prescription drugs for the treatment of AD. The first four drugs to be approved were cholinesterase inhibitors, which are drugs designed to prevent the breakdown of acetylcholine. Cholinesterase inhibitors keep levels of the chemical messenger high, even while the cells that produce the messenger continue to become damaged or die. About half of the people who take cholinesterase inhibitors see modest improvement in cognitive symptoms. Until 1997 tacrine was the nation's only AD medication, but tacrine is rarely prescribed today because of associated side effects, including possible liver damage. However, there are three other cholinesterase inhibitors currently used that produce some delay in the deterioration of memory and other cognitive skills: donepezil, approved in 1996; rivastigmine, approved in 2000; and galantamine, approved in 2001.

Memantine was approved by the FDA in 2003 for the treatment of moderate to severe AD. It is classified as an uncompetitive low-to-moderate affinity N-methyl-D-aspartate (NMDA) receptor antagonist, and it is the first Alzheimer drug of this type to be approved in the United States. According to the Alzheimer's Association, memantine acts by regulating the activity of glutamate, one of the brain's specialized messenger chemicals that are involved in information processing, storage, and retrieval.

The National Institutes of Health (http://www.clinical trials.gov/ct2/results?term=Alzheimer%27s) notes that in 2012 there were more than 1,000 clinical trials of new treatments for AD under way. Some research involved the use of drugs and vaccines to block the production of beta amyloid, which is thought to be the source of the problem, or to help rid the body of it quickly. Researchers are also looking at antiamyloid antibodies, proteins made by the immune system that counter the effects of beta amyloid, as a way to halt the progress of the disease early in its course. All the drugs being tested were intended to decrease the frequency or severity of the symptoms of AD and slow its progression, but none were expected to cure AD. The investigational drugs aim to address three aspects of AD: improve cognitive function in people with early AD; slow or postpone the progression of the disease; and control behavioral problems such as wandering, aggression, and agitation of patients with AD.

Investigational drug research targeting two enzymes—beta-secretase and gamma-secretase—that are involved in plaque formation may also benefit people suffering from AD. In "Modeling an Anti-amyloid Combination Therapy for Alzheimer's Disease" (*Science Translational Research*, vol. 2, no. 13, January 6, 2010), Vivian W. Chow et al. of Johns Hopkins University School of Medicine report that reduction of these two enzymes reduces the formation of amyloid beta protein or amyloid plaque in the brain.

It also appears that a combination of vitamin E and anti-inflammatory drugs play a role in slowing the progress of AD. According to Valory N. Pavlik et al. of Baylor College of Medicine, in "Vitamin E Use Is Associated with Improved Survival in an Alzheimer's Disease Cohort" (*Dementia and Geriatric Cognitive Disorders*, vol. 28, no. 6, December 2009), vitamin E at a dose of 2,000 international units

per day has been shown to delay AD progression. Even though some researchers question the safety of this high dose, Pavlik et al. find that the dose posed no safety risk and that vitamin E use actually improved the survival rates among AD patients. In "Combination Therapy of Acetylcholinesterase Inhibitor and Vitamin E in Alzheimer Disease" (*Journal of Clinical Psychopharmacology*, vol. 29, no. 5, October 2009), Daniel M. Bittner of Otto von Guericke University reports that a small study revealed that the combination of vitamin E and a cholinesterase inhibitor appear to act synergistically (the combined action is greater than the sum total of each acting separately) to address symptoms of AD.

Fang Cheng et al. note in "Suppression of Amyloid Beta A11 Antibody Immunoreactivity by Vitamin C: Possible Role of Heparan Sulfate Oligosaccharides Derived from Glypican-1 by Ascorbate-Induced, Nitric Oxide (NO) Catalyzed Degradation" (*Journal of Biological Chemistry*, vol. 286, no. 31, August 5, 2011) that vitamin C can dissolve the amyloid plaques in the brains of people with AD. Even though these preliminary research results are from animal studies, they may help identify another direction for researchers in developing treatment for people with AD.

THE IMPACT OF AD ON CAREGIVERS' HEALTH AND WELL-BEING. The suffering of a patient with AD is only part of the devastating emotional, physical, and financial trauma of AD. According to the Alzheimer's Association, in *2011 Alzheimer's Disease Facts and Figures*, 14.9 million Americans served as unpaid caregivers in 2011. People who care for loved ones with AD are considered to be the "second patients" of the disease. Caregivers often neglect their own needs, including their health and social lives, and the needs of other family members. As a result, they may develop more stress-related illnesses and are at a greater risk for depression.

The Alzheimer's Association 2010 Women and Alzheimer's Poll, which was conducted between August and September 2010, finds that three-quarters of caregivers said they are "somewhat" or "very concerned" about maintaining their own physical health. Nearly two-thirds (61%) said the emotional stress of caregiving is "high to very high" and one-third (33%) said they have symptoms of depression. More than half of caregivers also reported financial strain that was associated with caregiving (56%) and strained family relationships (52%).

Research also demonstrates that caregivers are more likely than their peers who do not provide care for people suffering from AD or other forms of dementia to suffer from mood and sleep disorders such as insomnia at least in part because they are awakened by their care-recipients at night. In "Insomnia in Caregivers of Persons with Dementia: Who Is at Risk and What Can Be Done about It?" (*Sleep Medicine Clinics*, vol. 4, no. 4, December 1, 2009), Susan M. McCurry et al. of the University of

Washington, Seattle, describe sleep as the "new vital sign" because of mounting evidence of its crucial role in maintaining health. AD caregivers, who may also be considered patients because of their increased risk for physical and mental health problems, are at greater risk of suffering negative consequences from chronic sleep loss in combination with the stress that is involved in caregiving. Health professionals assert that in view of caregivers' risks of developing health problems, there is an urgent need to exhort family caregivers to engage in activities such as regular exercise and preventive medical care that will benefit their own health, well-being, and longevity.

CHAPTER 7
INFECTIOUS DISEASES

Pursue him to his house, and pluck him thence;

Lest his infection, being of a catching nature,

Spread further.

—William Shakespeare, *Coriolanus* (1607–1608)

Infectious (contagious) diseases are caused by micro-organisms—viruses, bacteria, parasites, or fungi—that are transmitted from one person to another through casual contact, such as influenza; through bodily fluids, such as the human immunodeficiency virus (HIV; the virus that produces the acquired immunodeficiency syndrome [AIDS]); or via contaminated air, food, or water supplies. Infectious diseases may also spread by vectors of disease such as insects or arthropods that carry the infectious agent.

According to the World Health Organization (WHO), infectious diseases are a leading cause of death world-wide. Not long ago, the U.S. government and medical experts believed that the widespread use of vaccines, antibiotics, and public health measures had effectively eliminated the public health threat of infectious diseases. Throughout the world, however, new and rare diseases were emerging, and old diseases were resurfacing. Some of these infections reflected changes that were associated with increasing population, growing poverty, urban migration, drug-resistant microbes, and expanding international travel.

The mistaken belief that infectious diseases were problems of the past prompted the governments of many countries, including the United States, to neglect public health programs that were aimed at preventing and treating infectious disease. By the close of the 20th century, however, enough troubling new diseases had arisen and old ones recurred that the United States resurrected and intensified efforts to respond to and contain infections.

The National Electronic Telecommunications System for Surveillance (NETSS) is a computerized public health surveillance information system that provides the Centers

for Disease Control and Prevention (CDC) with weekly data to track certain infectious diseases (notifiable diseases). The CDC (November 17, 2011, http://www.cdc.gov/osels/ph_surveillance/nndss/netss.htm) defines a notifiable disease as "one for which regular, frequent, timely information on individual cases is considered necessary to prevent and control that disease." The list of nationally notifiable diseases is revised periodically. For example, a disease might be added to the list as a new pathogen (an organism that causes disease) emerges, or a disease might be deleted as its incidence declines. Physicians, clinics, and hospitals must report any occurrences of these diseases to the CDC each week. Table 7.1 shows the nationally notifiable infectious diseases that were tracked in 2012.

MOST FREQUENTLY REPORTED DISEASES

Among the CDC's notifiable diseases, the three most frequently reported infectious diseases in the United States in 2009 were chlamydia (1,244,180 cases—the highest it has been since voluntary reporting began during the mid-1980s), gonorrhea (301,174 cases), and HIV diagnoses (36,870 cases)—all sexually transmitted diseases (STDs). (See Table 7.2.) The remaining notifiable infectious diseases in the top 10 were:

- Salmonellosis (49,192 cases)—a food-borne disease that causes fever and intestinal disorders

- Syphilis, all stages (44,828 cases)—an STD that occurs in three stages; it can also be congenital (an infant can be born with the disease)

- Lyme disease (38,468 cases)—a disease that is spread by ticks

- Varicella (chicken pox; 20,482 cases)—a disease (usually of childhood) that is marked by a vesicular (small, blister-like elevations on the skin with fluid in them) rash on the face and body caused by the herpes varicella zoster virus

TABLE 7.1

Nationally notifiable infectious diseases, 2012

Infectious conditions

Anthrax
Arboviral neuroinvasive and non-neuroinvasive diseases
• California serogroup virus disease
• Eastern equine encephalitis virus disease
• Powassan virus disease
• St. Louis encephalitis virus disease
• West Nile virus disease
• Western equine encephalitis virus disease
Babesiosis
Botulism
• Botulism, foodborne
• Botulism, infant
• Botulism, other (wound & unspecified)
Brucellosis
Campylobacteriosis
Chancroid
Chlamydia trachomatis infection
Cholera
Coccidioidomycosis
Cryptosporidiosis
Cyclosporiasis
Dengue
• Dengue fever
• Dengue hemorrhagic fever
• Dengue shock syndrome
Diphtheria
Ehrlichiosis/anaplasmosis
• *Ehrlichia chaffeensis*
• *Ehrlichia ewingii*
• *Anaplasma phagocytophilum*
• Undetermined
Free-living amebae, infections caused by
Giardiasis
Gonorrhea
Haemophilus influenzae, invasive disease
Hansen disease (leprosy)
Hantavirus pulmonary syndrome
Hemolytic uremic syndrome, post-diarrheal
Hepatitis
• Hepatitis A, acute
• Hepatitis B, acute
• Hepatitis B, chronic
• Hepatitis B virus, perinatal infection
• Hepatitis C, acute
• Hepatitis C, past or present
HIV infection (*AIDS has been reclassified as HIV stage III*)
• HIV infection, adult/adolescent (age >= 13 years)
• HIV infection, child (age >= 18 months and < 13 years)
• HIV infection, pediatric (age < 18 months)
Influenza-associated hospitalizations
Influenza-associated pediatric mortality
Legionellosis
Listeriosis
Lyme disease
Malaria
Measles
Melioidosis
Meningococcal disease
Mumps
Novel influenza A virus infections
Pertussis
Plague
Poliomyelitis, paralytic
Poliovirus infection, nonparalytic
Psittacosis

Q Fever
• Acute
• Chronic
Rabies
• Rabies, animal
• Rabies, human
Rubella (German measles)
Rubella, congenital syndrome
Salmonellosis
Severe acute respiratory syndrome-associated coronavirus (SARS-CoV) disease
Shiga toxin-producing *escherichia coli* (STEC)
Shigellosis
Smallpox
Spotted fever rickettsiosis
Streptococcal toxic-shock syndrome
Streptococcus pneumoniae, invasive disease
Syphilis
• Primary
• Secondary
• Latent
• Early latent
• Late latent
• Latent, unknown duration
• Neurosyphilis
• Late, non-neurological
• Stillbirth
• Congenital
Tetanus
Toxic-shock syndrome (other than streptococcal)
Trichinellosis (trichinosis)
Tuberculosis
Tularemia
Typhoid fever
Vancomycin—intermediate *staphylococcus aureus* (VISA)
Vancomycin—resistant *staphylococcus aureus* (VRSA)
Varicella (morbidity)
Varicella (deaths only)
Vibriosis
Viral Hemorrhagic fevers, due to:
• Ebola virus
• Marburg virus
• Crimean-Congo Hemorrhagic Fever virus
• Lassa virus
• Lujo virus
• New world arenaviruses (Gunarito, Machupo, Junin, and Sabia viruses)
  Yellow fever

SOURCE: "2012 Nationally Notifiable Diseases and Conditions and Current Case Definitions," in *National Notifiable Diseases Surveillance System*, U.S. Department of Health and Human Services, Centers for Disease Control and Prevention, December 2011, http://www.cdc.gov/osels/ph_surveillance/nndss/nndsshis.htm (accessed January 2, 2012)

TABLE 7.2

Reported cases of notifiable diseases, by month, 2009

Disease	Jan	Feb	Mar	Apr	May	Jun	Jul	Aug	Sept	Oct	Nov	Dec	Month not stated	Total
Anthrax	—	—	—	—	—	—	—	—	—	—	—	1	—	1
Arboviral diseases[a]														
California serogroup virus														
Neuroinvasive	—	—	—	—	1	3	12	21	6	3	—	—	—	46
Nonneuroinvasive	—	2	—	—	—	—	1	3	2	—	1	—	—	9
Eastern equine encephalitis virus														
Neuroinvasive	—	—	—	—	—	—	2	—	1	—	—	—	—	3
Nonneuroinvasive	—	—	—	—	—	—	—	—	1	—	—	—	—	1
Powassan virus, neuroinvasive	1	—	—	1	—	2	—	1	1	—	—	—	—	6
St. Louis encephalitis virus														
Neuroinvasive	—	—	—	1	—	3	4	1	1	1	—	—	—	11
Nonneuroinvasive	—	—	—	—	—	—	—	—	—	—	1	—	—	1
West Nile virus														
Neuroinvasive	—	—	—	—	3	11	59	182	111	18	—	1	1	386
Nonneuroinvasive	—	—	—	1	4	8	57	174	74	16	14	18	—	334
Botulism, total	5	13	10	13	7	7	7	9	8	7	14	18	—	118
Foodborne	1	3	—	1	2	7	1	1	—	—	—	—	—	10
Infant	2	8	8	8	5	6	5	5	7	6	10	13	—	83
Other (wound and unspecified)	2	2	2	4	—	1	1	3	1	1	4	4	—	25
Brucellosis	1	4	9	12	12	10	7	13	11	8	7	21	—	115
Chancroid[b]	—	2	6	4	—	2	—	—	1	1	4	8	—	28
Chlamydia trachomatis genital infection[b]	93,356	100,303	98,845	98,846	114,944	98,941	94,182	125,258	94,924	120,816	85,399	118,366	—	1,244,180
Cholera	1	—	—	1	—	1	4	1	1	1	—	—	—	10
Coccidioidomycosis	654	496	628	527	726	1,448	1,204	1,571	1,174	1,476	1,304	1,718	—	12,926
Cryptosporidiosis, total	328	311	353	442	602	551	791	1,320	982	883	484	607	—	7,654
Confirmed	325	306	349	429	594	541	759	1,245	942	849	468	586	—	7,393
Probable	3	5	4	13	8	10	32	75	40	34	16	21	—	261
Cyclosporiasis	31	9	1	5	9	23	18	20	9	3	8	5	—	141
Ehrlichiosis/Anaplasmosis														
Ehrlichia chaffeensis	7	6	8	20	65	136	181	144	83	66	24	204	—	944
Ehrlichia ewingii	—	—	—	—	—	—	3	3	1	—	—	—	—	7
Anaplasma phagocytophilum	—	2	7	14	102	160	177	127	52	101	44	375	—	1,161
Undetermined	1	1	5	2	17	22	23	23	9	6	4	42	—	155
Giardiasis	1,078	1,215	1,256	1,328	1,468	1,273	1,754	2,294	1,970	2,117	1,505	2,141	—	19,399
Gonorrhea[b]	23,914	23,822	23,003	23,218	27,248	24,251	23,411	31,147	24,368	29,252	20,053	27,487	—	301,174
Haemophilus influenzae, invasive disease, all ages, serotypes	238	247	259	244	309	259	227	223	166	189	190	471	—	3,022
Age <5 yrs														
Serotype b	3	3	9	2	2	2	3	2	4	4	—	4	—	38
Nonserotype b	21	29	26	20	26	19	24	11	14	8	17	30	—	245
Unknown serotype	15	14	15	7	22	12	7	10	5	11	11	37	—	166
Hansen disease (Leprosy)	5	12	9	6	8	12	7	12	3	11	14	4	—	103
Hantavirus pulmonary syndrome	—	—	2	—	4	2	3	1	2	1	—	5	—	20
Hemolytic uremic syndrome, post-diarrheal	6	6	15	12	24	24	22	25	23	28	17	40	—	242
Hepatitis, viral, acute														
A	135	165	139	161	174	143	187	205	179	176	123	200	—	1,987
B	260	271	283	259	297	246	252	312	261	292	197	475	—	3,405
C	54	50	61	63	61	76	61	67	53	72	60	104	—	782
HIV diagnoses[c]	3,746	3,810	4,136	3,996	3,354	3,764	3,543	3,191	2,969	2,583	1,493	279	6	36,870

TABLE 7.2

Reported cases of notifiable diseases, by month, 2009 (CONTINUED)

Disease	Jan	Feb	Mar	Apr	May	Jun	Jul	Aug	Sept	Oct	Nov	Dec	Month not stated	Total
Influenza-associated pediatric mortality[d]	3	18	22	13	11	17	13	14	17	80	108	42	—	358
Legionellosis	135	118	132	115	192	352	439	583	426	445	264	321	—	3,522
Listeriosis	67	40	41	41	61	47	93	113	93	90	58	107	—	851
Lyme disease, total	686	756	914	1,118	2,407	5,826	8,818	7,038	2,980	2,637	1,591	3,697	—	38,468
Confirmed	488	555	650	744	1,772	4,917	7,421	5,579	2,194	1,985	1,104	2,550	—	29,959
Probable	198	201	264	374	635	909	1,397	1,459	786	652	487	1,147	—	8,509
Malaria	89	80	72	77	124	101	147	228	126	131	87	189	—	1,451
Measles, total	2	2	7	11	16	12	9	5	1	3	—	3	—	71
Indigenous	—	1	3	8	11	11	8	4	1	3	—	1	—	51
Imported	2	1	4	3	5	1	1	1	—	—	—	2	—	20
Meningococcal disease, all serogroups	59	102	118	87	103	59	66	59	49	76	81	121	—	980
Serogroup A, C, Y, and W-135	15	34	34	32	30	16	18	14	12	21	32	43	—	301
Serogroup B	9	18	28	11	21	12	12	8	7	13	11	24	—	174
Other serogroup	1	4	2	2	4	1	3	2	2	2	—	—	—	23
Serogroup unknown	34	46	54	42	48	30	33	35	28	40	38	54	—	482
Mumps	27	24	37	40	42	24	32	45	75	137	282	1,226	—	1,991
Pertussis	956	856	912	1,177	1,425	1,342	1,627	1,981	1,333	1,316	1,021	2,912	—	16,858
Plague	—	—	—	—	2	2	2	1	1	—	—	—	—	8
Poliomyelitis, paralytic	—	—	—	—	—	—	—	—	—	—	—	—	—	1
Psittacosis	—	1	3	—	1	—	1	1	1	—	—	1	—	9
Q Fever, total	6	5	9	10	14	8	10	8	9	12	4	18	—	113
Acute	5	3	7	10	13	6	9	8	6	11	3	12	—	93
Chronic	1	2	2	—	1	2	1	—	3	1	1	6	—	20
Rabies, animal	210	416	406	501	634	442	416	644	546	526	285	317	—	5,343
Human	—	—	—	—	—	1	—	—	—	1	1	1	—	4
Rocky Mountain spotted fever, total	39	34	34	72	190	259	278	233	122	70	26	458	—	1,815
Confirmed	2	1	5	6	17	33	23	29	7	15	3	10	—	151
Probable	37	33	29	65	173	226	254	204	115	55	23	448	—	1,662
Rubella	—	—	—	1	—	1	1	—	—	—	—	—	—	3
Rubella, congenital syndrome	—	1	—	—	—	—	—	—	—	—	1	—	—	2
Salmonellosis	2,798	2,194	2,356	2,658	3,855	4,068	4,976	7,030	5,301	5,567	3,624	4,765	—	49,192
Shiga toxin-producing E. coli (STEC)	253	201	168	258	429	426	506	705	475	505	303	414	—	4,643
Shigellosis	1,219	1,161	1,132	1,036	1,808	1,366	1,392	1,723	1,105	1,224	968	1,797	—	15,931
Streptococcal disease, invasive, group A	462	565	658	647	588	422	328	337	201	263	258	550	—	5,279
Streptococcal, toxic-shock syndrome	8	21	24	20	17	7	6	10	8	8	6	26	—	161
Streptococcus pneumoniae, invasive disease														
Drug resistant														
All ages	291	394	360	326	308	160	117	104	138	241	218	713	—	3,370
Age <5 yrs	36	69	63	55	57	31	19	24	28	53	53	95	—	583
Non-drug resistant, age <5 yrs	143	204	183	208	192	118	81	86	104	178	171	320	—	1,988
Syphilis, total, all stages[b,c]	3,263	3,590	3,672	3,569	4,315	3,499	3,351	4,503	3,546	4,254	2,988	4,278	—	44,828
Congenital (age <1 yr)[b]	45	39	42	33	34	23	38	40	35	32	25	41	—	427
Primary and secondary[b]	1,070	1,032	1,099	1,080	1,323	1,029	1,101	1,556	1,123	1,271	985	1,328	—	13,997
Tetanus	1	2	2	—	—	—	—	5	3	—	—	5	—	18
Toxic-shock syndrome	5	7	5	10	6	7	9	5	5	6	4	5	—	74
Trichinellosis	2	4	1	2	1	—	1	—	1	—	1	—	—	13
Tuberculosis[f]	531	710	850	942	947	1,114	1,001	949	931	988	891	1,691	—	11,545
Tularemia	2	1	3	3	4	14	14	17	9	12	5	9	—	93
Typhoid fever	33	35	32	23	33	28	17	62	53	30	16	35	—	397

TABLE 7.2

Reported cases of notifiable diseases, by month, 2009 [CONTINUED]

Disease	Jan	Feb	Mar	Apr	May	Jun	Jul	Aug	Sept	Oct	Nov	Dec	Month not stated	Total
Vancomycin-intermediate *Staphylococcus aureus* (VISA)	5	4	3	11	12	9	7	6	6	5	4	6	—	78
Vancomycin-resistant *Staphylococcus aureus* (VRSA)	—	—	—	—	—	—	—	—	—	—	—	1	—	1
Varicella (Chickenpox)														
Morbidity	1,961	2,304	2,275	2,277	3,062	1,255	787	777	1,205	1,730	1,240	1,607	—	20,480
Mortality[a]	—	—	—	1	—	—	—	—	—	—	1	—	—	2
Vibriosis	42	11	27	20	51	61	81	171	114	101	55	55	—	789

[a]Totals reported to the Division of Vector-Borne Infectious Diseases, National Center for Zoonotic, Vector-Borne, and Enteric Diseases (ArboNET Surveillance), as of May 28, 2010.
[b]Totals reported to the Division of STD Prevention, National Center for HIV/AIDS, Viral Hepatitis, STD, and TB Prevention (NCHHSTP), as of May 7, 2010.
[c]Total number of HIV cases reported to the Division of HIV/AIDS Prevention, NCHHSTP through December 31, 2009.
[d]Totals reported to the Influenza Division, National Center for Immunization and Respiratory Diseases (NCIRD), as of December 31, 2009.
[e]Includes the following categories: primary, secondary, latent (including early latent, late latent, and latent syphilis of unknown duration), neurosyphilis, late (including late syphilis with clinical manifestations other than neurosyphilis), and congenital syphilis.
[f]Totals reported to the Division of TB Elimination, NCHHSTP, as of May 14, 2010.
[g]Totals reported to the Division of Viral Diseases, NCIRD, as of June 30, 2010.
Note: No cases of diphtheria; poliovirus infection, nonparalytic; Powassan virus disease, neuroinvasive and non-neuroinvasive; and yellow fever were reported in 2009. Data on chronic hepatitis B and hepatitis C virus infection (past or present) are not included because they are undergoing data quality review. Data on human immunodeficiency virus (HIV) infections are not included because HIV infection reporting has been implemented on different dates and using different methods than for AIDS case reporting.

SOURCE: Patsy A. Hall-Baker et al., "Table 1. Reported Cases of Notifiable Diseases, by Month—United States, 2009," in "Summary of Notifiable Diseases—United States, 2009," *Morbidity and Mortality Weekly Report*, vol. 58, no. 53, May 13, 2011, http://www.cdc.gov/mmwr/pdf/wk/mm5853.pdf (accessed January 2, 2012)

- Giardiasis (19,399 cases)—a common protozoal infection of the small intestine that is spread via contaminated food and water and direct person-to-person contact

- Shigellosis (15,931 cases)—food-borne and water-borne dysentery

- Tuberculosis (11,545 cases)—an infection caused by the bacterium *Mycobacterium tuberculosis* that usually involves the lungs, but other organs also may be involved

RESISTANT STRAINS OF BACTERIA

Antibiotics have generally been considered "miracle drugs" that control or cure many bacterial infectious diseases. However, since 2000 nearly all the major bacterial infections in the world have become increasingly resistant to the most commonly prescribed antibiotic treatments, primarily because of repeated and improper uses of antibiotics. Decreasing inappropriate antibiotic use is the best way to control this resistance.

Bacteria such as pneumococcus, which causes pneumonia and children's ear infections—diseases long considered common and treatable—are evolving into strains that are proving to be untreatable with commonly used antibiotics. Pneumococcal bacteria cause many hundreds of thousands of cases of pneumonia and bacterial meningitis (inflammation of the tissue covering the brain and spinal cord). It also causes otitis media (middle-ear infection), which, according to Peter S. Morris and Amanda J. Leach in "Acute and Chronic Otitis Media" (*Pediatric Clinics of North America*, vol. 56, no. 6, December 2009), remains the most common indication for antibiotic prescribing in young children despite the fact that it is usually a mild condition that resolves spontaneously without any treatment.

Joseph P. Lynch and George G. Zhanel indicate in "Streptococcus Pneumoniae: Does Antimicrobial Resistance Matter?" (*Seminars in Respiratory and Critical Care Medicine*, vol. 30, no. 2, April 2009) that during the past three decades antimicrobial resistance among *Streptococcus pneumoniae*, the most common cause of community-acquired pneumonia, escalated significantly, with 15% to 30% of infections being multidrug-resistant (MDR), meaning they were resistant to three or more classes of antibiotics. The researchers point to a 2006 survey revealing that the national rate of MDR was 15.2%, with the highest MDR rate in the Southeast and lowest in the Northeast. Lynch and Zhanel explain that previous antibiotic use is the most common risk factor that is associated with antibiotic drug-resistance.

To treat patients with penicillin-resistant pneumococcus infections, physicians use a combination of other antibiotics, such as vancomycin, imipenem, and rifampin for resistant pneumonia and clindamycin or cefuroxime for ear infections. Another strategy to combat the illness is the pneumococcal vaccine. One of the reasons that public health professionals advocate widespread use of the pneumococcal vaccine is the hope that it will produce "herd immunity"—when a large proportion of the population is immune, the likelihood of person-to-person spread is so small that the disease does not proliferate and even nonimmune individuals are protected from disease. However, Lynch and Zhanel observe that some of the reduction in the occurrence of illness anticipated from the introduction of the pneumococcal vaccine has been offset by the increased prevalence of resistant infections that are not prevented by the current vaccine.

Methicillin-Resistant *Staphylococcus Aureus*

Methicillin-resistant *Staphylococcus aureus* (MRSA) are bacterial infections that resist treatment with customary antibiotics. According to the CDC, they are most common in hospitalized patients with weakened immune systems as well as in nursing home residents; however, they can also appear in people living in the community at large. MRSA infections vary from life-threatening illnesses to minor skin infections.

The CDC reports in "Protect Yourself from MRSA" (May 3, 2011, http://www.cdc.gov/Features/MRSAinHealth care/) that suspected staph and MRSA infections, which skyrocketed from just 2% of the total number of staph infections in 1974 to 63% in 2004, have declined in recent years. Furthermore, life-threatening MRSA infections that begin in hospitals declined by 28% between 2005 and 2008 and community-acquired infections fell by 17%. The CDC's National Healthcare Safety Network reports that MRSA bloodstream infections in hospitalized patients declined by about 50% between 1997 and 2007.

In "Trends in Antimicrobial Resistance in Intensive Care Units in the United States" (*Current Opinions in Critical Care*, vol. 17, no. 5, October 2011), Kavitha Prabaker and Robert A. Weinstein observe that antimicrobial resistance and a lack of new antimicrobial agents continue to threaten public health. The researchers note that MRSA bloodstream infection rates have declined, primarily due to interventions that have been aimed at decreasing infections related to vascular catheters. Even so, the rates of community-acquired MRSA infections continue to increase.

MRSA infections can be prevented by following infection control guidelines. Jane D. Siegel et al. of the Healthcare Infection Control Practices Advisory Committee describe in *Management of Multidrug-Resistant Organisms in Healthcare Settings, 2006* (2006, http://www.cdc.gov/hicpac/pdf/guidelines/MDROGuideline2006.pdf) the prevention and management of multidrug-resistant organisms (MDROs) such as MSRA. Table 7.3 describes the education, monitoring, prudent use of antimicrobial drugs, surveillance, and precautions to prevent the transmission of infection that can control MDROs in health care settings.

TABLE 7.3

Recommendations for prevention and control of multidrug-resistant organisms (MDROs) in health care settings

Administrative measures/ adherence monitoring	MDRO education	Judicious antimicrobial use	Surveillance	Infection control precautions to prevent transmission	Environmental measures	Decolonization
Make MDRO prevention/control an organizational priority. Provide administrative support and both fiscal and human resources to prevent and control MDRO transmission. *(IB)* Identify experts who can provide consultation and expertise for analyzing epidemiologic data, recognizing MDRO problems, or devising effective control strategies, as needed. *(II)* Implement systems to communicate information about reportable MDROs to administrative personnel and state/local health departments. *(II)* Implement a multi-disciplinary process to monitor and improve HCP adherence to recommended practices for standard and contact precautions. *(IB)* Implement systems to designate patients known to be colonized or infected with a targeted MDRO and to notify receiving healthcare facilities or personnel prior to transfer of such patients within or between facilities. *(IB)* Support participation in local, regional and/or national coalitions to combat emerging or growing MDRO problems. *(IB)* Provide updated feedback at least annually to healthcare providers and administrators on facility and patient-care unit MDRO infections. Include information on changes in prevalence and incidence, problem assessment and performance improvement plans. *(IB)*	Provide education and training on risks and prevention of MDRO transmission during orientation and periodic educational updates for HCP; include information on organizational experience with MDROs and prevention strategies. *(IB)*	In hospitals and LTCFs, ensure that a multi-disciplinary process is in place to review local susceptibility patterns (antibiograms), and antimicrobial agents included in the formulary, to foster appropriate antimicrobial use. *(IB)* Implement systems (e.g., CPOE, susceptibility report comment, pharmacy or unit director notification) to prompt clinicians to use the appropriate agent and regimen for the given clinical situation. *(IB)* Provide clinicians with antimicrobial susceptibility reports and analysis of current trends, updated at least annually, to guide antimicrobial prescribing practices. *(IB)* In settings with limited electronic communication system infrastructures to implement physician prompts, etc., at a minimum implement a process to review antibiotic use. Prepare and distribute reports to providers. *(II)*	Use standardized laboratory methods and follow published guidelines for determining antimicrobial susceptibilities of targeted and emerging MDROs. Establish systems to ensure that clinical micro labs (in-house and outsourced) promptly notify infection control or a medical director/designee when a novel resistance pattern for that facility is detected. *(IB)* In hospitals and LTCFs: ... develop and implement laboratory protocols for storing isolates of selected MDROs for molecular typing when needed to confirm transmission or delineate epidemiology of MDRO in facility. *(IB)* ... establish laboratory-based systems to detect and communicate evidence of MDROs in clinical isolates *(IB)* ... prepare facility-specific antimicrobial susceptibility reports as recommended by CLSI; monitor reports for evidence of changing resistance that may indicate emergence or transmission of MDROs *(IA/IC)* ... develop and monitor special-care unit-specific antimicrobial susceptibility reports (e.g., ventilator-dependent units, ICUs, oncology units). *(IB)* ... monitor trends in incidence of target MDROs in the facility over time to determine if MDRO rates are decreasing or if additional interventions are needed. *(IA)*	Follow standard precautions in all healthcare settings. *(IB)* Use of contact precautions (CP): —In *acute care settings*: Implement CP for all patients known to be colonized/infected with target MDROs. (IB) —In *LTCFs: Consider the individual patient's clinical situation and facility resources in deciding whether to implement CP (II)* —In *ambulatory and home care settings, follow standard precautions (II)* —In *hemodialysis units:* Follow dialysis specific guidelines *(IC)* No recommendation can be made regarding when to discontinue CP. *(unresolved issue)* Masks are not recommended for routine use to prevent transmission of MDROs from patients to HCWs. Use masks according to standard precautions when performing splash-generating procedures, caring for patients with open tracheostomies with potential for projectile secretions, and when there is evidence for transmission from heavily colonized sources (e.g., burn wounds). Patient placement in hospitals and LTCFs: When single-patient rooms are available, assign priority for these rooms to patients with known or suspected MDRO colonization or infection. Give highest priority to those patients who have conditions that may facilitate transmission, e.g., uncontained secretions or excretions. When single-patient rooms are not available, cohort patients with the same MDRO in the same room or patient-care area. *(IB)*	Follow recommended cleaning, disinfection and sterilization guidelines for maintaining patient care areas and equipment. Dedicate non-critical medical items to use on individual patients known to be infected or colonized with an MDRO. Prioritize room cleaning of patients on contact precautions. Focus on cleaning and disinfecting frequently touched surfaces (e.g., bedrails, bedside commodes, bathroom fixtures in patient room, doorknobs) and equipment in immediate vicinity of patient.	Not recommended routinely

TABLE 7.3

Recommendations for prevention and control of multidrug-resistant organisms (MDROs) in health care settings [CONTINUED]

Administrative measures/ adherence monitoring	MDRO education	Judicious antimicrobial use	Surveillance	Infection control precautions to prevent transmission	Environmental measures	Decolonization
				When cohorting patients with the same MDRO is not possible, place MDRO patients in rooms with patients who are at low risk for acquisition of MDROs and associated adverse outcomes from infection and are likely to have short lengths of stay. *(II)*		

Notes: MDRO=multidrug-resistant organism. HCP=health care provider. LTCF=long term care facility. CPOE=computerized provider order entry. CLSI=Clinical and Laboratory Standards Institute. ICU=intensive care unit. HCW=health care worker.

SOURCE: Jane D. Siegel et al., "Table 3. Tier 1. General Recommendations for Routine Prevention and Control of MDROs in Healthcare Settings," in *Management of Multidrug-Resistant Organisms in Healthcare Settings, 2006*, Centers for Disease Control and Prevention, Healthcare Infection Control Practices Advisory Committee, 2006, http://www.cdc.gov/hicpac/pdf/guidelines/MDROGuideline2006.pdf (accessed January 2, 2012)

Educating Physicians and Patients about the Appropriate Use of Antibiotics

According to the CDC, antibiotic resistance is among the most urgent public health problems in the world. In 1995 the CDC Division of Foodborne Bacterial and Mycotic Diseases began a national campaign to reduce antimicrobial resistance by encouraging the appropriate use of antibiotics.

Christopher A. Ohl and Elizabeth S. Dodds Ashley explain in "Antimicrobial Stewardship Programs in Community Hospitals: The Evidence Base and Case Studies" (*Clinical Infectious Diseases*, vol. 53, suppl. 1, August 2011) that reducing antibiotic use lowers the rates of drug-resistant bacteria. By changing and managing how physicians choose and administer antimicrobial drugs, hospitals are able to "prevent or slow the emergence of antimicrobial resistance; optimize the selection, dosing, and duration of antimicrobial therapy; reduce the incidence of drug-related adverse events; and lower rates of morbidity and mortality, length of hospitalization, and costs."

These findings highlight the need for professional and public awareness and understanding of the need to assume active roles in preventing antibiotic resistance. The consequences of the failure of antibiotics to treat formerly treatable illnesses could be dire: longer-lasting illnesses, more physician office visits or longer hospital stays, the need for more expensive and toxic medications, and even death.

In "Can a Nationwide Media Campaign Affect Antibiotic Use?" (*American Journal of Managed Care*, vol. 15, no. 8, August 2009), Beatriz Hemo et al. evaluate the effectiveness of a media campaign to decrease antibiotic overuse among children in Israel by reducing the parents' demands for antibiotics. During the winter of 2006 Israel's second-largest health maintenance organization, which provides health care services for 1.7 million people, launched a nationwide media campaign that was intended to heighten awareness of the misuse of antibiotics among the general public. The campaign focused on the inappropriate use of antibiotics in the treatment of influenza and upper respiratory infections caused by viruses. Hemo et al. find "a significant decrease in antibiotic purchases for the treatment of the conditions studied subsequent to the campaign and greater knowledge regarding appropriate antibiotic use among parents exposed to the campaign." Their findings suggest that the media campaign had a favorable impact on parents' attitudes and the actual use of antibiotics.

PREVENTION THROUGH IMMUNIZATION

Many infectious diseases can be prevented by immunizations. According to the CDC's National Immunization Program, in "List of Vaccine-Preventable Diseases" (May 8, 2009, http://www.cdc.gov/vaccines/vpd-vac/vpd-list.htm), there are 27 diseases that can be prevented by vaccination. However, immunization against only a portion of these diseases is recommended for the general public. Even though the other portion is preventable by vaccination, widespread administration of the vaccines is not recommended because the risk of contracting these diseases—such as anthrax, meningococcal infection, rotavirus, and smallpox—is not great enough to warrant it. (See Figure 2.1, Figure 2.2, and Figure 2.3 in Chapter 2 for the 2011 schedule of childhood, adolescent, and adult immunizations. Figure 7.1 lists vaccines that may be administered to adults based on their medical histories, lifestyles, occupational exposures, or other indications.) The vaccine-preventable diseases that the majority of adults should receive are:

- Diphtheria—this bacterial infection causes potentially fatal respiratory infections that are treated with antibiotics. People diagnosed with diphtheria are isolated until cultures are negative, to prevent the spread of the disease.

- Haemophilus influenza type b—this bacterial infection causes respiratory infections and other diseases, such as meningitis.

- Hepatitis A—this virus is spread through fecal (stool) or oral routes, although it may also be transmitted via blood or sexual contact. Outbreaks usually occur from contaminated food and water; military workers, children in day care centers, and their care providers are considered at high risk.

- Hepatitis B—this virus is transmitted by blood or sexual contact or from mother to unborn child; injection drug users, gay men, and health care workers are at high risk.

- Human papillomavirus (HPV)—HPV is transmitted by sexual contact, and ideally the vaccine is administered before potential exposure to HPV.

- Influenza—this viral infection produces sudden fever, muscle aches, and respiratory infection symptoms.

- Measles—this highly contagious viral disease produces red circular spots on the skin.

- Meningitis—the meningococcal vaccine was added to the 2005–06 schedule for select populations such as college students living in dormitories to prevent bacterial meningitis caused by infection with Neisseria meningitides. Meningitis means inflammation of the meninges (the covering of the brain and the spinal cord) and it is characterized by fever, vomiting, intense headache, and stiff neck.

- Mumps—this highly contagious viral disease produces swelling of the parotid glands (salivary glands that occur below and in front of the ear).

FIGURE 7.1

Vaccines recommended for some adults based on medical and other indications, 2009

| ☒ For all persons in this category who meet the age requirements and who lack evidence of immunity (e.g., lack documentation of vaccination or have no evidence of prior infection) | ▨ Recommended if some other risk factor is present (e.g., on the basis of medical, occupational, lifestyle, or other indications) | ☐ No recommendation |

Vaccine ▼ / Indication ▶	Pregnancy	Immuno-compromising conditions (excluding human immuno-deficiency virus [HIV])	HIV infection CD4+ T lymphocyte count <200 cells/µL	HIV infection CD4+ T lymphocyte count ≥200 cells/µL	Diabetes, heart disease, chronic lung disease, chronic alcoholism	Asplenia (including elective splenectomy and terminal complement component deficiencies)	Chronic liver disease	Kidney failure, end-stage renal disease, receipt of hemodialysis	Health-care personnel
Tetanus, diphtheria, pertussis (Td/Tdap)*	Td	Substitute 1-time dose of Tdap for Td booster; then boost with Td every 10 yrs							
Human papillomavirus (HPV)*		3 doses for females through age 26 yrs							
Varicella*	Contraindicated			2 doses					
Zoster	Contraindicated			1 dose					
Measles, mumps, rubella (MMR)*	Contraindicated			1 or 2 doses					
Influenza*		1 dose TIV annually							1 dose TIV or LAIV annually
Pneumococcal (polysaccharide)		1 or 2 doses							
Hepatitis A*		2 doses							
Hepatitis B*		3 doses							
Meningococcal*		1 or more doses							

TIV = Trivalent influenza vaccine. LAIV = Live attenuated influenza vaccine.

*Covered by the Vaccine Injury Compensation Program.

SOURCE: "Figure 2. Vaccines That Might Be Indicated for Adults Based on Medical and Other Indications—United States, 2009," in "Recommended Adult Immunization Schedule—United States, 2009," *MMWR*, vol. 57, no. 53, January 9, 2009, http://www.cdc.gov/mmwr/preview/mmwrhtml/mm5753a6 .htm?s_cid=mm5753a6_e (accessed January 2, 2012)

- Pertussis (whooping cough)—this bacterial infection causes illness that is marked by spasms of coughing.

- Pneumococcal—this bacteria causes pneumonia, an inflammation of the lungs.

- Poliomyelitis (polio)—a viral disease that causes fever, atrophy (wasting) of skeletal muscles, and paralysis.

- Rubella (German measles)—this viral infection is usually mild in children but can seriously harm an unborn child when contracted by a woman early during her pregnancy.

- Tetanus—the bacteria from this disease produce a toxin that causes victims to have painful muscle spasms.

- Varicella (chickenpox)—this is a highly contagious viral disease that is marked by skin eruptions of fluid-filled lesions that itch.

INFLUENZA

Influenza (the flu) is a contagious respiratory disease that is caused by a virus. When a person infected with the flu sneezes, coughs, or even talks, the virus is expelled into the air via droplets and may be inhaled by anyone nearby. It can also be transmitted by direct hand contact. The flu primarily affects the lungs, but the whole body experiences symptoms. The infected person usually becomes acutely ill, with fever, chills, weakness, loss of appetite, and aching muscles in the head, back, arms, and legs. The person with an influenza infection may also have a sore throat, a dry cough, nausea, and burning eyes. The accompanying fever increases quickly—sometimes reaching 104 degrees Fahrenheit (40 degrees Celsius)—but usually subsides after two or three days. Influenza leaves the patient exhausted.

For healthy individuals, the flu is typically a moderately severe illness, with most adults and children back to work or school within a week. However, for the very young, the very old, and people who are not in good general health, the flu can be extremely severe and even fatal. Complications such as secondary bacterial infections may develop, taking advantage of the body's weakened condition and lowered resistance. The most common bacterial complication is pneumonia, but sinuses, bronchi (lung tubes), or inner ears can also become secondarily infected with bacteria. Less common but very serious complications include viral pneumonia, encephalitis (inflammation of the brain), acute renal (kidney) failure, and nervous system disorders. These complications can be fatal.

Who Gets the Flu?

Anyone can get the flu, especially if there is an epidemic in the community. (An epidemic is a period when the number of cases of a disease exceeds the number that is expected based on past experience.) During an epidemic year, 20% to 30% of the population may contract influenza. Not surprisingly, people who are not healthy are considered to be at high risk for most strains of influenza and their complications. The high-risk population includes people who have chronic lung conditions, such as asthma, emphysema, chronic bronchitis, tuberculosis, or cystic fibrosis (an inherited disease that is characterized by chronic respiratory and digestive problems); people with heart disease, chronic kidney disease, diabetes, or severe anemia; people who are residing in nursing homes; people over the age of 65 years; and some health care workers.

Vaccines

Influenza can be prevented by inoculation with a current influenza vaccine, which is formulated annually so that it contains the influenza viruses that are expected to cause the flu the following year. The viruses are killed or inactivated to prevent those who are vaccinated from getting influenza from the vaccine. After being immunized, the person develops antibodies to the influenza viruses. The antibodies are most effective after one or two months. High-risk people should be vaccinated early during the fall because peak flu activity usually occurs around the beginning of the new calendar year. The flu season usually runs from October to May and peaks in December and January.

Each year's flu vaccine protects against only the viruses that were included in its formulation. If another strain of flu appears, people can still catch the new strain even though they were vaccinated for the primary expected strains.

Most people have little or no noticeable reaction to the vaccine; about a quarter may have a swollen, red, tender area where the vaccination was injected. Children may suffer a slight fever for 24 hours or have chills or a headache. Those who already suffer from a respiratory disease may experience worsened symptoms. Usually, these reactions are temporary. Because the egg in which the virus is grown cannot be completely extracted, people with egg protein allergies should consult their physician before receiving the vaccine and, if vaccinated, should be closely observed for any indications of an allergic reaction.

Older Adults Benefit from Flu Vaccinations

Influenza is a major cause of illness and death among people aged 65 years and older. According to Janet E. McElhaney of the University of British Columbia, Vancouver, in "Influenza Vaccination in the Elderly: Seeking New Correlates of Protection and Improved Vaccines" (*Aging Health*, vol. 4, no. 6, December 1, 2008), every year influenza and its complications are responsible for an estimated 60% of the nearly 300,000 excess hospitalizations for respiratory and circulatory problems and 85% to 90% or more of the 31,000 to 51,000 unexpected deaths in this population. McElhaney asserts, "Given their high risk for these serious, influenza-associated complications, the elderly are included among the high-priority groups for annual influenza vaccination in many countries." She also observes that influenza vaccination is a cost-saving intervention in older adults, at least in part because it prevents costly hospitalizations.

Recent research questions whether adults aged 65 years and older who obtain influenza vaccinations significantly reduce their risk of contracting influenza. In "Efficacy and Effectiveness of Influenza Vaccines: A Systematic Review and Meta-analysis" (*Lancet Infectious Diseases*, vol. 12, no. 1, January 2012), Michael T. Osterholm et al. examine 31 studies published between 1967 and 2011 that assessed the reduction in influenza risk of all circulating flu viruses after vaccination. The researchers find that "influenza vaccines can provide moderate protection against virologically confirmed influenza, but such protection is greatly reduced or absent in some seasons." Osterholm et al. also observe that "evidence for protection in adults aged 65 years or older is lacking" and call for "new vaccines with improved clinical efficacy and effectiveness" to further reduce influenza-related illness and deaths.

Pandemic Influenza

In "Pandemic Flu: Key Facts" (October 17, 2005, ftp://ftp.cdc.gov/pub/avian_influenza1/Appendix%20section%20of%20notebook/CDC%20Pandemic%20Influenza

%20Fact%20Sheet.pdf), the CDC defines pandemic flu as "a global outbreak of disease that occurs when a new influenza A virus appears or 'emerges' in the human population, causes serious illness, and then spreads easily from person to person worldwide." Pandemics are different from seasonal outbreaks or even epidemics of influenza. Seasonal outbreaks are caused by influenza viruses that already move from person to person, whereas pandemics are caused by new viruses, subtypes of viruses that have never passed between people, or subtypes that have not circulated among people for a very long time.

In the past, influenza pandemics produced high levels of illness, death, social disruption, and economic loss. The 20th century saw three pandemics. The CDC reports that the 1918–19 "Spanish flu" claimed half a million lives in the United States and as many as 50 million people throughout the world. Nearly half of the deaths were young, healthy adults. In 1957–58 the "Asian flu" was responsible for 70,000 deaths in the United States. The 1968–69 "Hong Kong flu" proved fatal for 34,000 people in the United States. All three pandemics involved avian influenza, or bird flu. The 1957–58 and 1968–69 pandemics were caused by viruses that contained a combination of genes from a human influenza virus and an avian influenza virus; the 1918–19 pandemic virus also appears to have been an avian flu.

AVIAN INFLUENZA. Avian influenza is an infectious disease of birds that is caused by type A strains of the influenza virus. The disease, which was first identified in Italy more than 100 years ago, occurs worldwide. Because these viruses usually do not infect humans, there is little or no immune protection against them. If an avian influenza virus infects people and gains the ability to spread easily from person to person, an influenza pandemic can begin. The first cases in humans probably resulted from contact with infected birds or surfaces that were contaminated with excretions from infected birds. The disease usually only affects birds and pigs; the first documented infection of humans occurred in Hong Kong in 1997. Outbreaks of avian flu have affected bird populations in countries throughout Asia and Europe. Avian flu affects humans as well—according to the WHO (http://www.who.int/influenza/human_animal_interface/EN_GIP_20111215Cumulative NumberH5N1cases.pdf), as of December 2011 human cases of influenza A (H5N1) infection had been reported in 15 countries (Azerbaijan, Bangladesh, Cambodia, China, Djibouti, Egypt, Indonesia, Iraq, Laos, Burma [Myanmar], Nigeria, Pakistan, Thailand, Turkey, and Vietnam).

The spread of H5N1 virus from person to person has been rare, but by late 2007 researchers were concerned that the virus had mutated to infect humans more easily. Maggie Fox reports in "H5N1 Bird Flu Virus Mutations Facilitate Human Infection" (Reuters Health Information,

October 5, 2007) that there remains considerable cause for concern and vigilance, because the recent avian flu outbreaks in Asia and Europe have killed more than half of those infected. Even more frightening, most cases have occurred in previously healthy children and young adults as opposed to the old and infirm, who generally succumb to influenza. Even though attention had turned in 2009 and 2010 to another influenza virus, H1N1, the WHO continued to monitor cases of H5N1 throughout the world. By December 2011 a total of 573 cases and 336 deaths had been reported worldwide.

In efforts to prepare for an avian flu pandemic, in April 2007 the U.S. Food and Drug Administration (FDA) approved the first human H5N1 vaccine, which could help protect people at the highest risk of exposure during the early critical months of a pandemic. Even though the vaccine is not available commercially, Michael O. Leavitt (1951–), the former secretary of the U.S. Department of Health and Human Services (HHS), notes in *Pandemic Planning Update VI* (January 8, 2009, http://www.flu.gov/pandemic/history/panflureport6.pdf) that at the end of 2008 the U.S. government had reached its "goal of stockpiling enough pandemic influenza antivirals to cover 44 million people, which will help slow the spread of an emerging pandemic."

According to the FDA, in "Influenza (Flu) Antiviral Drugs and Related Information" (http://www.fda.gov/drugs/drugsafety/informationbydrugclass/ucm100228.htm), as of January 2012 four different influenza antiviral medications—amantadine, rimantadine, oseltamivir phosphate, and zanamivir—had been approved for the treatment and/or prevention of influenza. All four usually work against influenza A viruses. However, the drugs are not always effective because influenza virus strains can become resistant to one or more of these medications.

The HHS supports pandemic influenza activities in the areas of surveillance, vaccine development and production, strategic stockpiling of antiviral medications, research, and risk communications. The HHS aims to have sufficient antiviral courses of drug treatment on hand in anticipation of a possible pandemic. There are also plans in place for pandemic preparedness for health care facilities, schools, local governments, businesses, and law enforcement agencies. Individuals and families can prepare for a pandemic flu by stockpiling nonperishable food and regular prescription medication.

SWINE FLU. In April 2009, H1N1, sometimes called swine flu because it has two genes from flu viruses that normally circulate in pigs as well as avian and human genes, was detected in people in the United States. On June 11, 2009, the WHO declared that the 2009 H1N1 influenza was a pandemic. In "2009 H1N1 Flu ('Swine Flu') and You" (February 10, 2010, http://www.cdc.gov/h1n1flu/qa.htm), the CDC describes the illness caused by

H1N1 as ranging from mild to severe, with typical influenza symptoms—fever, cough, sore throat, runny or stuffy nose, body aches, headache, chills, and fatigue. Severe illness, hospitalizations, and deaths from H1N1 were reported.

Because initial supplies of the H1N1 vaccine were limited as manufacturers shifted from seasonal flu vaccine production to H1N1 vaccine production, the CDC Advisory Committee on Immunization Practices (ACIP) recommended in "Vaccine against 2009 H1N1 Influenza Virus" (December 22, 2009, http://www.cdc.gov/h1n1flu/vaccination/public/vaccination_qa_pub.htm) that people at highest risk for complications from this virus, or those caring for high-risk individuals, receive the vaccine first. These target populations included pregnant women, people who live with or care for children younger than six months old, health care and emergency medical services workers, anyone six months through 24 years of age, and people aged 25 to 64 years at higher risk for H1N1 influenza because of certain chronic health conditions or compromised immune systems. The ACIP advised that once these target groups had been vaccinated, programs and providers should begin vaccinating everyone from age 25 to 64. Because research indicated that, unlike seasonal flu, the risk for H1N1 infection among people 65 years and older was less than the risk for younger age groups, older adults were not initially targeted to receive early doses of the vaccine. As the vaccine supply increased, the ACIP advised vaccination of people over the age of 65 years. By December 2009 many states were offering vaccination to people of all ages, and, even though older adults still appeared less likely to become ill with H1N1, severe infections and deaths had occurred in every age group, including older people.

Along with vaccination, the CDC encouraged other, general preventive measures including:

- Covering the nose and mouth with a tissue when coughing or sneezing and throwing the tissue in the trash after using it

- Washing hands often with soap and water and, when soap and water are unavailable, using an alcohol-based hand rub

- Avoiding touching the eyes, nose, and mouth to prevent the spread of virus

- Staying home from work or school when sick to limit contact with others and keep from infecting them

The CDC also advised the use of prescription antiviral drugs (oseltamivir and zanamivir), especially for people at high risk of developing serious flu-related complications. In a December 22, 2009, press briefing (http://www.cdc.gov/media/transcripts/2009/t091222.htm), Anne Schuchat, the CDC director of the National Center for Immunization and Respiratory Diseases, reported that hospitalizations for H1N1 influenza were largely among people with asthma or other chronic lung disease.

The CDC indicates that during the 2009–10 flu season the vast majority of influenza cases were attributable to H1N1, and H1N1 flu caused more illness in people aged 25 years and younger than in older people. According to Laura MacInnis and Stephanie Nebehay, in "Some Immunity Building Up against Pandemic Flu: WHO" (Reuters, January 8, 2010), the WHO noted that by January 2010 the H1N1 flu was responsible for 12,799 deaths, more than half of which occurred in Mexico, the United States, and Canada, where H1N1 disease activity appeared to have peaked in October 2009. The WHO also observed that Southern Hemisphere countries that experienced H1N1 in 2009 went on to display considerable population immunity, meaning that the virus spread much more slowly and less easily.

Figure 7.2 shows visits for influenza-like symptoms (fever of 100 degrees Fahrenheit [38.8 degrees Celsius] or higher and cough and/or sore throat) between September 2008 and December 2011. It clearly displays the spike in visits that were attributable to H1N1 flu and the below average visits during the 2011 flu season.

NEW FLU DEBUTS. In "CDC Confirms Detection of a Different Influenza A Variant Virus" (http://www.cdc.gov/media/haveyouheard/stories/Influenza_A_Variant.html), the CDC reports that in December 2011 an influenza A (H1N1) virus that had been found in swine in the United States but never before in humans was detected in a person from Wisconsin who had contact with swine. The new variant was a triple reassortant virus because it contained genes from avian, swine, and human influenza viruses; however, it was different from earlier triple reassortant influenza A H1N1 viruses in swine (tr-H1N1), because it had acquired the matrix gene from the 2009 influenza A (H1N1) pandemic virus. The virus was not transmitted to other humans. The CDC indicates that the virus is susceptible to the influenza antiviral medications oseltamivir and zanamivir.

TUBERCULOSIS

Tuberculosis (TB), a communicable disease that is caused by the bacterium *Mycobacterium tuberculosis*, is spread from person to person through the inhalation of airborne particles containing *M. tuberculosis*. The particles, called droplet nuclei, are produced when a person with infectious TB of the lungs or larynx forcefully exhales, such as when coughing, sneezing, speaking, or singing. These infectious particles can remain suspended in the air and may be inhaled by someone sharing the same air.

FIGURE 7.2

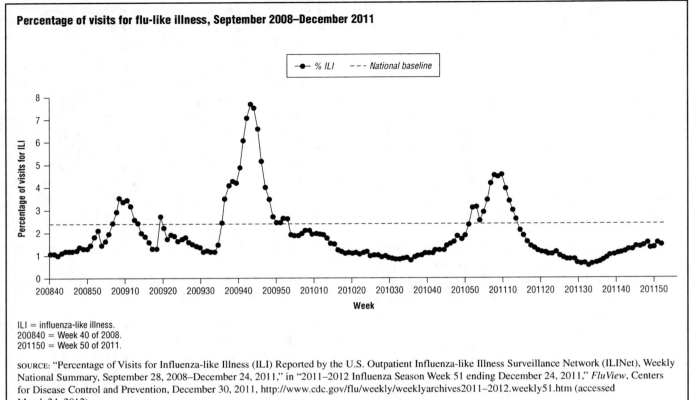

Percentage of visits for flu-like illness, September 2008–December 2011

Legend: ● % ILI - - - National baseline

Y-axis: Percentage of visits for ILI

X-axis: Week

ILI = influenza-like illness.
200840 = Week 40 of 2008.
201150 = Week 50 of 2011.

SOURCE: "Percentage of Visits for Influenza-like Illness (ILI) Reported by the U.S. Outpatient Influenza-like Illness Surveillance Network (ILINet), Weekly National Summary, September 28, 2008–December 24, 2011," in "2011–2012 Influenza Season Week 51 ending December 24, 2011," *FluView*, Centers for Disease Control and Prevention, December 30, 2011, http://www.cdc.gov/flu/weekly/weeklyarchives2011–2012.weekly51.htm (accessed March 24, 2012)

The CDC notes in the fact sheet "Questions and Answers about TB" (June 20, 2011, http://www.cdc .gov/tb/publications/faqs/qa_introduction.htm) that most TB occurs in the lungs (pulmonary TB). The risk of transmission is increased where ventilation is poor and when susceptible people share air for prolonged periods with a person who has untreated pulmonary TB. However, the disease may occur at any site of the body, such as the larynx, the lymph nodes, the brain, the kidneys, or the bones. This type of TB infection, which occurs outside the lungs, is referred to as extrapulmonary. Except for laryngeal TB, people with extrapulmonary TB are usually not considered infectious to others.

In the fact sheet "The Difference between Latent TB Infection and TB Disease" (June 20, 2011, http:// www.cdc.gov/tb/publications/factsheets/general/LTBIand ActiveTB.htm), the CDC explains that TB does not develop in everyone who is infected with the bacteria. In the United States about 90% of infected people never show symptoms of TB, but they are considered to have latent TB infections. The only indication of a latent TB infection is a positive reaction to the tuberculin skin test or special TB blood test. Between 5% and 10% of those infected develop active disease later in life, and about half of those who develop active TB do so within the first two years of infection. Table 7.4 shows the differences between latent TB infection and TB disease. People with compromised immune systems are at greater risk of developing TB than those with healthy immune systems. For example, the WHO notes in the fact sheet "Tuberculosis" (November 2010, http://www.who.int/mediacentre/factsheets/fs104/en/) that an individual who is HIV-positive and infected with TB bacilli is many times more likely to become sick with TB than someone infected with TB bacilli who is HIV-negative.

Ancient Enemy and Continuing Threat

According to the CDC, in the fact sheet "Data and Statistics" (December 13, 2011, http://www.cdc.gov/tb/ statistics/default.htm), TB is among the world's deadliest diseases. Overall, one-third of the world's population is infected with the TB bacillus. In 2010 about 9 million people worldwide became sick with TB and approximately 1.4 million people died from it. The numbers of people who become infected with and die from TB have increased dramatically since the HIV/AIDS epidemic swept through many countries. TB is a leading cause of death among people who are infected with HIV.

After several decades of decline, TB made a comeback in the United States during the late 1980s and early 1990s. (See Figure 7.3.) In 1992 the CDC reported 26,673 cases of TB, up from 22,201 in 1985. Since 1992 the number of cases has declined steadily, and by 2010 it had decreased by 58.1% to 11,182.

In "Reported Tuberculosis in the United States, 2010" (October 7, 2011, http://www.cdc.gov/tb/statistics/surv/surv2010/default.htm), the CDC reports that the proportion of TB cases in foreign-born people has increased steadily since 1993 and that in 2010 it accounted for 60% of all TB cases in the United States. (See Figure 7.4.) People born outside the United States have accounted for the majority of TB cases in the United States every year since 2002. (See Figure 7.5.)

TABLE 7.4

Distinguishing latent TB infection from TB disease

A person with latent TB infection	A person with TB disease
• Has no symptoms	• Has symptoms that may include: - a bad cough that lasts 3 weeks or longer - pain in the chest - coughing up blood or sputum - weakness or fatigue - weight loss - no appetite - chills - fever - sweating at night
• Does not feel sick	• Usually feels sick
• Cannot spread TB bacteria to others	• May spread TB bacteria to others
• Usually has a skin test or blood test result indicating TB infection	• Usually has a skin test or blood test result indicating TB infection
• Has a normal chest x-ray and a negative sputum smear	• May have an abnormal chest x-ray, or positive sputum smear or culture
• Needs treatment for latent TB infection to prevent active TB disease	• Needs treatment to treat active TB disease

TB = Tuberculosis

SOURCE: "The Difference between Latent TB Infection and TB Disease," in *Basic TB Facts*, Centers for Disease Control and Prevention, Division of Tuberculosis Elimination, July 1, 2010, http://www.cdc.gov/tb/topic/basics/default.htm (accessed January 3, 2012)

Treatment has become increasingly difficult because new strains of MDR TB have developed. If the disease is not properly treated or if treatment is not completed, some TB can become resistant to drugs, making it much harder to cure. According to the CDC, the proportion of patients with MDR TB decreased from 2.5% in 1993 to 1.2% in 2010. However, the proportion of MDR TB in foreign-born people increased from 25% in 1993 to 82% in 2010. Figure 7.6 shows the rates of MDR TB, termed "resistance to at least isoniazid and rifampin," among U.S.-born and foreign-born people.

March 24 of each year has been designated World TB Day by the CDC to recognize and increase awareness of the global threat to health posed by the disease. This annual event, first sponsored by the WHO, honors the date in 1882 when Robert Koch (1843–1910) announced his discovery of *M. tuberculosis*.

HIV/AIDS

AIDS is the late stage of an infection caused by HIV, a retrovirus that attacks and destroys certain white blood cells, which weakens the body's immune system and makes it susceptible to infections and diseases that ordinarily would not be life threatening. AIDS is considered to be a blood-borne STD because HIV is spread through contact with blood, semen, or vaginal fluids from an infected person.

Around the World

AIDS and HIV were virtually unknown before 1981, when testing and reporting of the disease became mandatory, but awareness grew as the annual number of

FIGURE 7.3

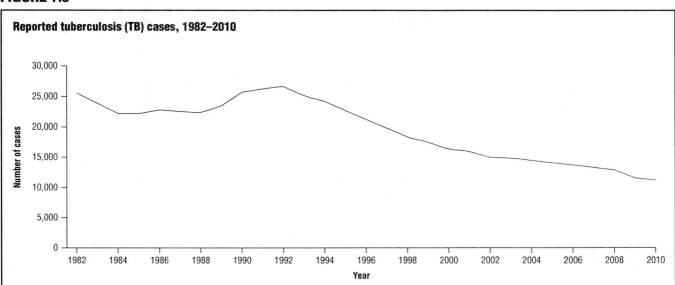

Reported tuberculosis (TB) cases, 1982–2010

SOURCE: "Slide 2. Reported TB Cases United States, 1982–2008," in *Reported Tuberculosis in the United States, 2010*, Centers for Disease Control and Prevention, October 7, 2011, http://www.cdc.gov/tb/statistics/surv/surv2010/default.htm (accessed January 3, 2012)

FIGURE 7.4

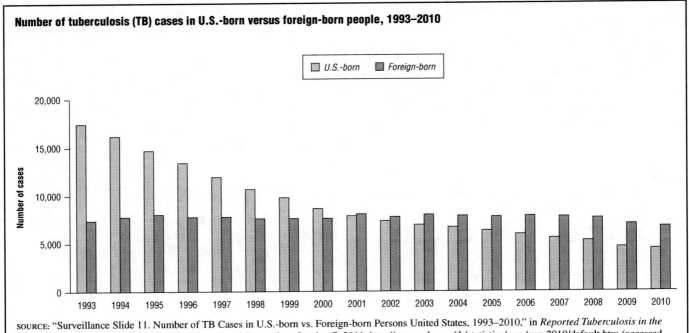

Number of tuberculosis (TB) cases in U.S.-born versus foreign-born people, 1993–2010

Legend: U.S.-born | Foreign-born

SOURCE: "Surveillance Slide 11. Number of TB Cases in U.S.-born vs. Foreign-born Persons United States, 1993–2010," in *Reported Tuberculosis in the United States, 2010*, Centers for Disease Control and Prevention, October 7, 2011, http://www.cdc.gov/tb/statistics/surv/surv2010/default.htm (accessed January 3, 2012)

FIGURE 7.5

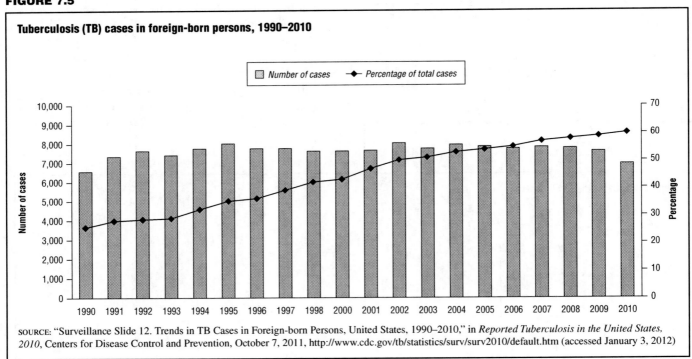

Tuberculosis (TB) cases in foreign-born persons, 1990–2010

Legend: Number of cases | Percentage of total cases

SOURCE: "Surveillance Slide 12. Trends in TB Cases in Foreign-born Persons, United States, 1990–2010," in *Reported Tuberculosis in the United States, 2010*, Centers for Disease Control and Prevention, October 7, 2011, http://www.cdc.gov/tb/statistics/surv/surv2010/default.htm (accessed January 3, 2012)

diagnosed cases and deaths steadily increased. In *UNAIDS Data Tables 2011* (2011, http://www.unaids .org/en/media/unaids/contentassets/documents/unaidspublication/2011/JC2225_UNAIDS_datatables_en.pdf), the Joint United Nations Programme on HIV/AIDS and the WHO note that there were about 2.7 million new HIV infections in 2010, down 21% from the height of the epidemic in 1997. Another 34 million people worldwide were estimated to be living with HIV/AIDS. About 1.8 million deaths were attributable to AIDS-related causes in 2010, down from 2.2 million deaths during the middle part of the first decade of the 21st century.

FIGURE 7.6

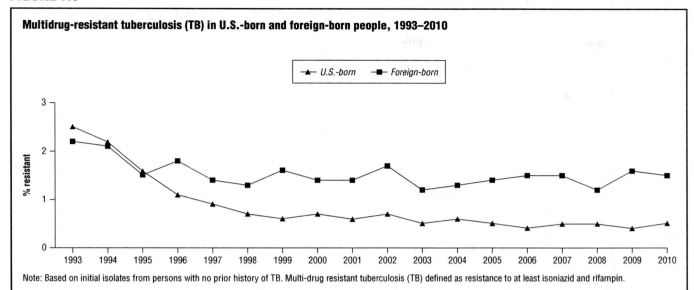

Multidrug-resistant tuberculosis (TB) in U.S.-born and foreign-born people, 1993–2010

Note: Based on initial isolates from persons with no prior history of TB. Multi-drug resistant tuberculosis (TB) defined as resistance to at least isoniazid and rifampin.

SOURCE: "Surveillance Slide 22. Primary MDR TB in U.S.-born vs. Foreign-born Persons United States, 1993–2010," in *Reported Tuberculosis in the United States, 2010*, Centers for Disease Control and Prevention, October 7, 2011, http://www.cdc.gov/tb/statistics/surv/surv2010/default.htm (accessed January 3, 2012)

In the United States

The CDC reports in *HIV Surveillance Report: Diagnoses of HIV Infection and AIDS in the United States and Dependent Areas, 2009* (February 2011, http://www.cdc.gov/hiv/surveillance/resources/reports/2009report/pdf/2009SurveillanceReport.pdf) that at the end of 2008 there were an estimated 479,868 people living with AIDS. In 2009 an estimated 42,011 diagnoses of HIV infection were made. Of these diagnosed cases, 9,973 were females and 31,872 were males. (See Table 7.5.) An estimated 166 HIV diagnoses were in children under the age of 13 years.

The CDC indicates that the rate of HIV diagnoses in the 40 states with name-based reporting was 17.4 per 100,000 population in 2009. Between 2006 and 2009 the rate of HIV diagnoses among males was unchanged, but in females it decreased. Three-quarters (76%) of HIV diagnoses were made in males of all ages. (See Table 7.5.)

Between 2006 and 2009 the annual number of HIV infections attributed to male-to-male sexual contact increased, while infections attributed to heterosexual contact were relatively unchanged. (See Table 7.5.) In contrast, infections attributed to injection drug use and infections attributed to male-to-male sexual contact and injection drug use decreased. In 2009, nearly one-third (31%) of diagnosed HIV infections were attributed to heterosexual contact.

The CDC's analysis of the groups most affected by HIV/AIDS confirms that the majority (57%) of infections continues to be diagnosed in men who have sex with men. The analysis also identifies the racial and ethnic distribution of new HIV infections. For example, African-Americans are the most affected by HIV/AIDS. In 2009 African-Americans accounted for 52% of all diagnoses of HIV infection. The rates per 100,000 population were 66.6 in the African-American population, 22.8 in the Hispanic population, 21 in the Native Hawaiian or Pacific Islander population, 16.7 in people reporting multiple races, 9.8 in the Native American or Alaskan Native population, 7.2 in the white population, and 6.4 in the Asian-American population.

The CDC reports that in 2009 the overall rate of AIDS diagnoses was 11.2 per 100,000 population. Between 2006 and 2009 AIDS diagnoses among people aged 15 to 19 years increased, whereas the rates remained stable for children aged 13 years and younger. The vast majority of AIDS diagnoses in children under the age of 13 years occurred in the African-American and Hispanic populations. (See Table 7.6.)

From the beginning of the AIDS epidemic through 2009, a total of 1,142,714 people in the United States and dependent areas had been reported as having AIDS. Since its recognition in 1981, the disease has killed 594,496 people in the United States.

How Is AIDS Spread?

HIV/AIDS is not transmitted through casual contact with an infected person. The CDC has identified several behavioral risk factors that greatly increase the likelihood of a person's chances of being infected. Table 7.7 shows the estimated numbers of those diagnosed with AIDS by year of diagnosis and the selected characteristics of

TABLE 7.5

HIV infections, by selected characteristics, 2006–09

	2006			2007			2008			2009		
		Estimated[a]			Estimated[a]			Estimated[a]			Estimated[a]	
	No.	No.	Rate	No.	No.	Rate	No.	No.	Rate	No.	No.	Rate
Age at diagnosis (yr)												
<13	204	215	0.5	190	204	0.5	194	215	0.5	141	166	0.4
13–14	55	57	0.9	37	40	0.6	34	37	0.6	19	21	0.3
15–19	1,530	1,605	9.6	1,742	1,861	11.0	1,817	1,996	11.8	1,752	2,036	12.0
20–24	4,481	4,695	28.2	4,700	5,020	30.1	5,156	5,662	33.8	5,327	6,237	36.9
25–29	5,117	5,370	33.7	5,351	5,723	34.9	5,239	5,743	34.4	5,078	5,951	35.2
30–34	4,917	5,155	34.1	4,732	5,056	33.6	4,685	5,160	34.0	4,294	5,020	32.5
35–39	5,995	6,287	38.5	5,562	5,944	36.3	4,961	5,450	33.5	4,448	5,232	32.6
40–44	6,281	6,590	37.7	5,833	6,238	36.4	5,244	5,752	34.3	4,704	5,519	33.6
45–49	4,677	4,899	27.4	4,734	5,059	28.2	4,630	5,093	28.4	4,141	4,865	27.1
50–54	3,029	3,176	19.7	3,185	3,412	20.6	2,977	3,271	19.3	2,834	3,323	19.3
55–59	1,629	1,705	11.9	1,715	1,827	12.7	1,761	1,926	13.1	1,691	2,004	13.4
60–64	749	786	7.4	829	884	7.7	872	953	7.9	772	900	7.2
≥65	665	696	2.3	731	780	2.6	679	747	2.4	624	736	2.3
Race/ethnicity												
American Indian/Alaska Native	156	163	8.8	175	185	9.9	175	193	10.2	163	189	9.8
Asian	345	366	5.5	434	473	6.9	418	466	6.6	395	470	6.4
Black/African American	19,701	20,672	65.7	19,542	20,922	65.7	19,667	21,709	67.4	18,320	21,652	66.6
Hispanic/Latino[b]	6,931	7,285	25.1	6,977	7,463	24.8	6,568	7,177	23.0	6,318	7,347	22.8
Native Hawaiian/other Pacific Islander	44	46	31.4	39	41	27.1	29	31	20.0	29	34	21.0
White	11,576	12,099	7.4	11,592	12,332	7.5	10,873	11,860	7.2	10,160	11,803	7.2
Multiple races	576	606	21.8	582	631	21.9	519	567	19.0	440	516	16.7
Transmission category												
Male adult or adolescent												
Male-to-male sexual contact	15,979	20,877	—	16,292	22,177	—	16,030	22,849	—	15,488	23,846	—
Injection drug use	2,040	3,245	—	1,676	2,907	—	1,269	2,540	—	1,018	2,449	—
Male-to-male sexual contact and injection drug use	1,040	1,407	—	904	1,318	—	744	1,188	—	632	1,131	—
Heterosexual contact[c]	2,971	4,541	—	2,893	4,680	—	2,705	4,634	—	2,266	4,399	—
Other[d]	6,745	101	—	7,342	55	—	7,729	72	—	7,749	47	—
Subtotal	**28,775**	**30,171**	**31.9**	**29,107**	**31,137**	**32.6**	**28,477**	**31,283**	**32.4**	**27,153**	**31,872**	**32.7**
Female adult or adolescent												
Injection drug use	1,067	1,954	—	887	1,756	—	791	1,654	—	591	1,483	—
Heterosexual contact[c]	4,896	8,826	—	4,674	8,894	—	4,268	8,813	—	3,453	8,461	—
Other[d]	4,387	71	—	4,482	55	—	4,519	40	—	4,487	29	—
Subtotal	**10,350**	**10,851**	**10.9**	**10,043**	**10,705**	**10.7**	**9,578**	**10,506**	**10.4**	**8,531**	**9,973**	**9.8**

TABLE 7.5

HIV infections, by selected characteristics, 2006–09 [CONTINUED]

	2006			2007			2008			2009		
		Estimated[a]			Estimated[a]			Estimated[a]			Estimated[a]	
	No.	No.	Rate	No.	No.	Rate	No.	No.	Rate	No.	No.	Rate
Child (<13 yrs at diagnosis)												
Perinatal	173	182	—	161	173	—	156	171	—	112	131	—
Other[e]	31	34	—	29	32	—	38	44	—	29	35	—
Subtotal	**204**	**215**	**0.5**	**190**	**204**	**0.5**	**194**	**215**	**0.5**	**141**	**166**	**0.4**
Total[f]	**39,329**	**41,237**	**17.5**	**39,341**	**42,047**	**17.7**	**38,249**	**42,005**	**17.5**	**35,825**	**42,011**	**17.4**

Note: Data include persons with a diagnosis of HIV infection regardless of stage of disease at diagnosis.
[a]Estimated numbers resulted from statistical adjustment that accounted for reporting delays and missing risk-factor information, but not for incomplete reporting. Rates are per 100,000 population. Rates are not calculated by transmission category because of the lack of denominator data.
[b]Hispanics/Latinos can be of any race.
[c]Heterosexual contact with a person known to have, or to be at high risk for, HIV infection.
[d]Includes hemophilia, blood transfusion, perinatal exposure, and risk factor not reported or not identified.
[e]Includes hemophilia, blood transfusion, and risk factor not reported or not identified.
[f]Because column totals for estimated numbers were calculated independently of the values for the subpopulations, the values in each column may not sum to the column total.

SOURCE: "Table 1a. Diagnoses of HIV infection, by Year of Diagnosis and Selected Characteristics, 2006–2009—40 States with Confidential Name-Based HIV Infection Reporting," in "Diagnoses of HIV Infection and AIDS in the United States and Dependent Areas, 2009," *HIV/AIDS Surveillance Report*, vol. 21, February 2011, http://www.cdc.gov/hiv/surveillance/resources/reports/2009report/pdf/2009SurveillanceReport.pdf (accessed January 3, 2012)

TABLE 7.6

AIDS diagnoses among children <13 years of age, by race/ethnicity, 2006–09 and cumulative

Race/ethnicity	2006		2007		2008		2009		Cumulative[a]	
	No.	Est. no.[b]	No.	Est. no.[b]	No.	Est. no.[b]	No.	Est. no.[b]	No.	Est. no.[b]
American Indian/Alaska Native	0	0	0	0	0	0	0	0	31	31
Asian[c]	1	1	0	0	2	2	0	0	47	48
Black/African American	28	30	21	22	20	23	6	8	5,748	5,799
Hispanic/Latino[d]	7	8	4	4	4	4	3	3	2,261	2,279
Native Hawaiian/other Pacific Islander	0	0	0	0	0	0	0	0	7	7
White	3	3	4	4	6	7	1	1	1,592	1,602
Multiple races	1	1	0	0	4	4	0	0	109	110
Total[e]	**40**	**42**	**29**	**31**	**36**	**41**	**10**	**13**	**9,796[f]**	**9,878**

[a]From the beginning of the epidemic through 2009.
[b]Estimated numbers resulted from statistical adjustment that accounted for reporting delays, but not for incomplete reporting.
[c]Includes Asian/Pacific Islander legacy cases.
[d]Hispanics/Latinos can be of any race.
[e]Because column totals for estimated numbers were calculated independently of the values for the subpopulations, the values in each column may not sum to the column total.
[f]Includes children of unknown race/ethnicity.

SOURCE: "Table 6b. AIDS Diagnoses among Children <13 Years of Age, by Race/Ethnicity, 2006–2009 and Cumulative—United States and 5 U.S. Dependent Areas," in "Diagnoses of HIV Infection and AIDS in the United States and Dependent Areas, 2009," *HIV/AIDS Surveillance Report*, vol. 21, February 2011, http://www.cdc.gov/hiv/surveillance/resources/reports/2009report/pdf/2009SurveillanceReport.pdf (accessed January 3, 2012)

people with AIDS, including the transmission category—ways in which they contracted the disease.

More than 25 years of research and observation have definitively concluded that the HIV infection can only be transmitted by the following methods:

- By oral, anal, or vaginal sex with an infected person; worldwide, heterosexual sex is the most common mode of transmission

- By sharing drug needles or syringes with an infected person

- From an infected mother to her baby at the time of birth and possibly through breast milk

- By receiving a transplanted organ or bodily fluids, such as blood transfusions or blood products, from an infected person

Because avoiding these methods of transmission virtually eliminates the possibility of becoming infected with HIV, unlike some other infectious diseases, AIDS is considered to be almost entirely preventable.

High concentrations of HIV have been found in blood, semen, and cerebrospinal fluid. Concentrations 1,000 times less have been found in saliva, tears, vaginal secretions, breast milk, and feces. There have been no reports, however, of HIV transmission from saliva, tears, or human bites. Research, such as that done by Julián Campo et al., in "Oral Transmission of HIV, Reality or Fiction? An Update" (*Oral Diseases*, vol. 12, no. 3, May 2006), confirms that the risk of transmission from these other body fluids is very low.

Opportunistic Infections

Once HIV has destroyed the immune system, the body can no longer protect itself against bacterial, fungal, parasitic, or viral agents that take advantage of the compromised condition, causing opportunistic infections (OIs). OIs are illnesses caused by organisms that would not normally harm a healthy person. Because the patient is considered to have AIDS if at least one OI appears, OIs are considered to be AIDS-defining events. OIs are not the only AIDS-defining events; the diagnosis of malignancies such as Kaposi's sarcoma (a rare skin carcinoma that is capable of spreading to internal organs), Burkitt's lymphoma, invasive cervical cancer, and primary brain lymphoma are also considered to be AIDS-defining events.

One of the most common OIs is *Pneumocystis carinii* pneumonia, a lung infection that is caused by a fungus. Other infections that AIDS patients are susceptible to are toxoplasmosis (a contagious disease that is caused by a one-cell parasite), oral candidiasis (thrush), esophageal candidiasis (an infection of the esophagus), extrapulmonary cryptococcosis (a systemic fungus that enters the body through the lungs and may invade any organ of the body), pulmonary TB, extrapulmonary TB, *Mycobacterium avium* complex (a serious bacterial infection that can occur in one part of the body, such as the liver, bone marrow, and spleen, or can spread throughout the body), and cytomegalovirus disease (a member of the herpes virus group).

Treatment of AIDS

The first drug thought to delay symptoms was azidothymidine (now called zidovudine [ZDV]), but its effects were found to be temporary at best. Several other drugs work on the same principle as ZDV, but until the advent of protease inhibitors (PIs; a class of drugs that became available during the mid-1990s) it seemed that there was no way of stopping HIV. PIs appear to keep HIV from

TABLE 7.7

AIDS diagnoses, by year of diagnosis and selected characteristics, 2006–09 and cumulative

	2006			2007			2008			2009			Cumulative[b]	
	No.	Estimated[a] No.	Rate	No.	Estimated[a] No.	Rate	No.	Estimated[a] No.	Rate	No.	Estimated[a] No.	Rate	No.	Est. No.[a]
Age at diagnosis (yr)														
<13	40	42	0.1	29	31	0.1	36	41	0.1	10	13	0.0	9,796	9,878
13–14	75	80	0.9	75	81	1.0	52	59	0.7	40	60	0.7	1,319	1,380
15–19	387	410	1.9	424	458	2.1	438	490	2.2	379	488	2.2	7,125	7,436
20–24	1,569	1,659	7.7	1,775	1,908	8.9	1,695	1,892	8.7	1,679	2,110	9.7	42,948	44,264
25–29	3,231	3,412	16.4	3,193	3,442	16.1	3,112	3,485	16.0	2,795	3,531	16.1	131,010	133,765
30–34	4,140	4,378	22.2	3,880	4,179	21.3	3,803	4,248	21.4	3,287	4,120	20.4	216,911	220,905
35–39	6,043	6,397	30.1	5,433	5,869	27.6	4,872	5,479	25.9	3,966	4,996	24.0	236,470	241,608
40–44	6,915	7,326	32.4	6,328	6,844	30.9	5,654	6,355	29.3	4,615	5,840	27.4	193,538	198,832
45–49	5,362	5,679	24.7	5,427	5,863	25.4	5,014	5,669	24.6	4,402	5,602	24.2	125,725	130,009
50–54	3,511	3,722	18.0	3,422	3,690	17.4	3,363	3,763	17.3	3,212	4,080	18.5	71,709	74,430
55–59	1,953	2,069	11.2	1,898	2,045	11.1	1,916	2,136	11.4	1,762	2,244	11.7	38,817	40,286
60–64	925	981	7.2	942	1,016	6.9	987	1,100	7.2	827	1,039	6.5	20,620	21,331
≥65	823	873	2.3	756	818	2.1	752	836	2.1	688	872	2.2	17,983	18,589
Race/ethnicity														
American Indian/Alaska Native	138	145	—	132	141	—	161	177	—	127	155	—	3,601	3,702
Asian[c]	395	422	—	416	454	—	436	492	—	329	429	—	8,038	8,369
Black/African American	16,377	17,321	—	15,947	17,194	—	15,236	17,077	—	13,206	16,759	—	453,443	466,829
Hispanic/Latino[d]	7,445	7,920	—	7,098	7,696	—	6,630	7,476	—	5,833	7,442	—	217,309	223,671
Native Hawaiian/other Pacific Islander	47	49	—	51	55	—	40	44	—	41	52	—	821	851
White	9,926	10,487	—	9,331	10,050	—	8,643	9,672	—	7,598	9,471	—	418,198	426,230
Multiple races	646	686	—	607	656	—	548	616	—	528	686	—	12,251	12,749
Transmission category														
Male adult or adolescent														
Male-to-male sexual contact	13,139	16,665	—	12,755	16,680	—	12,004	16,637	—	10,891	17,171	—	479,147	535,570
Injection drug use	2,986	4,126	—	2,561	3,744	—	2,260	3,554	—	1,661	3,207	—	173,351	199,565
Male-to-male sexual contact and injection drug use	1,628	1,994	—	1,431	1,841	—	1,281	1,729	—	1,020	1,608	—	73,006	79,693
Heterosexual contact[e]	2,941	4,080	—	2,706	4,004	—	2,643	4,066	—	2,237	3,956	—	59,593	75,901
Other[f]	4,857	202	—	5,003	167	—	5,115	190	—	4,761	159	—	96,977	12,931
Subtotal	**25,551**	**27,067**	**22.2**	**24,456**	**26,435**	**21.5**	**23,303**	**26,175**	**21.0**	**20,570**	**26,102**	**20.8**	**882,074**	**903,661**
Female adult or adolescent														
Injection drug use	1,673	2,553	—	1,545	2,453	—	1,260	2,192	—	936	1,982	—	73,712	90,102
Heterosexual contact[e]	4,745	7,172	—	4,513	7,139	—	4,109	7,007	—	3,367	6,740	—	101,068	131,886
Other[f]	2,965	195	—	3,038	185	—	2,986	137	—	2,779	157	—	47,319	7,185
Subtotal	**9,383**	**9,920**	**7.8**	**9,096**	**9,777**	**7.6**	**8,355**	**9,337**	**7.2**	**7,082**	**8,879**	**6.8**	**222,099**	**229,173**
Child (<13 yrs at diagnosis)														
Perinatal	37	39	—	28	30	—	32	36	—	9	12	—	8,971	9,046
Other[g]	3	3	—	1	1	—	4	5	—	1	1	—	825	832
Subtotal	**40**	**42**	**0.1**	**29**	**31**	**0.1**	**36**	**41**	**0.1**	**10**	**13**	**0.0**	**9,796**	**9,878**

TABLE 7.7

AIDS diagnoses, by year of diagnosis and selected characteristics, 2006–09 and cumulative [CONTINUED]

	2006			2007			2008			2009				
		Estimated[a]			Estimated[a]			Estimated[a]			Estimated[a]		Cumulative[b]	
	No.	No.	Rate	No.	No.	Rate	No.	No.	Rate	No.	No.	Rate	No.	Est. No.[a]
Region of residence														
Northeast	8,742	9,369	17.1	8,298	9,082	16.5	6,986	8,064	14.6	5,807	8,171	14.8	330,979	340,357
Midwest	3,903	4,154	6.3	3,675	4,006	6.0	3,687	4,218	6.3	3,435	4,394	6.6	112,560	116,029
South	15,718	16,453	15.1	15,371	16,383	14.8	15,003	16,506	14.7	13,188	15,806	13.9	419,910	430,141
West	5,796	6,174	9.0	5,506	5,964	8.5	5,332	5,967	8.4	4,670	5,875	8.2	217,265	222,083
U.S. dependent areas	815	878	20.3	732	810	18.6	686	798	18.3	562	747	17.1	33,257	34,103
Total[h]	**34,974**	**37,029**	**12.2**	**33,582**	**36,244**	**11.8**	**31,694**	**35,553**	**11.5**	**27,662**	**34,993**	**11.2**	**1,113,971[i]**	**1,142,714**

[a]Estimated numbers resulted from statistical adjustment that accounted for reporting delays and missing risk-factor information, but not for incomplete reporting. Rates are per 100,000 population. Rates by race/ethnicity are not provided because U.S. census information is limited for U.S. dependent areas. Rates are not calculated by transmission category because of the lack of denominator data.
[b]From the beginning of the epidemic through 2009.
[c]Includes Asian/Pacific Islander legacy cases.
[d]Hispanics/Latinos can be of any race.
[e]Heterosexual contact with a person known to have, or to be at high risk for, HIV infection.
[f]Includes hemophilia, blood transfusion, perinatal exposure, and risk factor not reported or not identified.
[g]Includes hemophilia, blood transfusion, and risk factor not reported or not identified.
[h]Because column totals for estimated numbers were calculated independently of the values for the subpopulations, the values in each column may not sum to the column total.
[i]Includes persons of unknown race/ethnicity.

SOURCE: "Table 2b. AIDS Diagnoses, by Year of Diagnosis and Selected Characteristics, 2006–2009 and Cumulative—United States and 5 U.S. Dependent Areas," in "Diagnoses of HIV Infection and AIDS in the United States and Dependent Areas, 2009," *HIV/AIDS Surveillance Report*, vol. 21, February 2011, http://www.cdc.gov/hiv/surveillance/resources/reports/2009report/pdf/2009SurveillanceReport.pdf (accessed January 3, 2011)

reproducing, unlike ZDV and similar drugs, which helps keep HIV out of the cell's chromosomes. Even if the PIs are not entirely effective long term in reducing patients' viral "loads," they have improved patients' prospects simply by creating more roadblocks for HIV. However, HIV mutates so rapidly that it eventually becomes resistant to most drugs when they are used alone.

Treatment recommendations change rapidly in response to the development of new drugs and clinical trials indicating the effectiveness of different combinations of antiretroviral drugs. Researchers are acting quickly to develop new mixtures of the recently approved and older drugs. Because HIV mutates to resist any drug it faces, including all PIs, researchers have found that varying the combination of drugs that are prescribed can "fool" the virus before it has time to mutate.

Still, there are reasons for optimism in the battle against HIV/AIDS. In "HIV Surveillance—United States, 1981–2008" (*Morbidity and Mortality Weekly Report*, vol. 60, no. 21, July 3, 2011), Lucia Torian et al. report that because of the use of combinations of drugs that target different proteins involved in HIV pathogenesis (a treatment strategy known as highly active antiretroviral therapy), the rates of diagnosis and death in the United States and other industrialized countries have been dramatically reduced. By 2008 AIDS diagnoses and deaths had stabilized at an average of 38,279 diagnoses and 17,489 deaths per year.

According to the FDA, in "Antiretroviral Drugs Used in the Treatment of HIV Infection" (http://www.fda.gov/forconsumers/byaudience/forpatientadvocates/hivandaids activities/ucm118915.htm), as of August 2011, 35 antiretroviral medications were approved by the FDA that target HIV, and researchers were pursuing novel strategies for prevention and vaccine development. Even if a cure for the disease is not imminent, new and better drugs that are being used in various combinations have made HIV infection a chronic but manageable disease, much like diabetes.

COMPLICATIONS AND SIDE EFFECTS OF TREATMENT. Patients undergoing therapy with new drugs or drug combinations must be highly disciplined. For example, indinavir must be taken on an empty stomach, every eight hours, not less than two hours before or after a meal, and with large amounts of water to prevent the development of kidney stones. Patients must also be careful to never skip doses of indinavir, otherwise HIV will quickly grow immune to its effect. (Indinavir has been found to generate cross-resistance, meaning that it can make patients resistant to other PIs.) Saquinavir mesylate must be taken in large doses. Ritonavir must be carefully prescribed and administered because it interacts negatively with some antifungals and antibiotics that are used by AIDS patients. Because there are many minor and serious risks

that are associated with use of these drugs, patients must be closely monitored.

The drug regimens are complicated, and many produce severe side effects in a substantial number of patients. The difficulty of dealing with a complicated regimen of daily medication and maintaining the personal resolve to continue the regimen are ongoing issues for many HIV/AIDS patients. When effective AIDS drugs were introduced, patients sometimes had to wake up in the middle of the night to take pills, and some treatment regimens consisted of as many as 50 or 60 pills administered several times a day. Even with intense pressure to simplify treatment regimens, pharmaceutical companies remained skeptical about an effective once-a-day pill despite the consensus opinion that it would help more people start, and stick with, treatment. As recently as 2005, many combined HIV/AIDS medication regimens were administered two to three times per day. Once-a-day regimens were sought after but were not available until 2006.

In "Epidemiology of Treatment Failure: A Focus on Recent Trends" (*Current Opinion in HIV and AIDS*, vol. 4, no. 6, November 2009), Mark W. Hull et al. observe that the development of more potent antiretroviral drugs that are better tolerated (with fewer side effects) and have simpler treatment regimens result in fewer instances of treatment failure. Hull et al. assert, "Improved tolerability has aided adherence, which remains a key determinant of treatment success."

LYME DISEASE

Spread by the bites of infected deer ticks, Lyme disease is the most commonly reported vector-borne disease in the United States. (Vector-borne means the indirect transmission of an infectious agent that occurs when any animal that transmits human disease touches or bites an individual.) Lyme disease is caused by the *Borrelia burgdorferi* organism and produces early symptoms such as skin rashes, headache, fever, and general illness; if untreated, the disease can cause arthritis and heart damage.

The CDC began tracking Lyme disease in 1982, and the disease was added to the list of nationally notifiable diseases in 1990. In 2010 the CDC received reports of 22,572 confirmed cases of Lyme disease and 7,597 probable cases, with most cases occurring in northeastern and north-central states. (See Figure 7.7 and Table 7.8.) Even though there is some variability from year to year, there was a considerable increase in the number of reported cases between 1997 and 2010.

The FDA and the CDC warn that people must take precautions against ticks. Wearing long-sleeved shirts and long pants, tucking pant legs into socks, and spraying the skin and/or clothing with tick repellents can keep

FIGURE 7.7

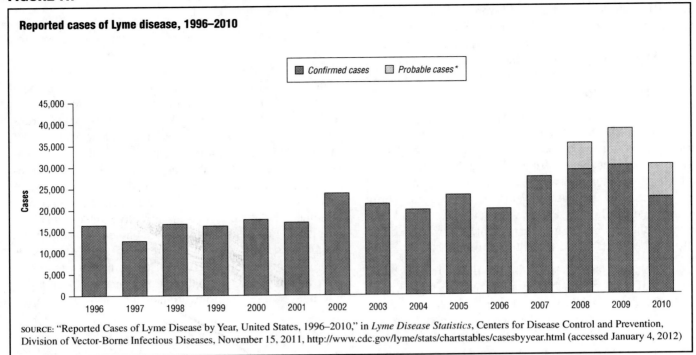

Reported cases of Lyme disease, 1996–2010

SOURCE: "Reported Cases of Lyme Disease by Year, United States, 1996–2010," in *Lyme Disease Statistics*, Centers for Disease Control and Prevention, Division of Vector-Borne Infectious Diseases, November 15, 2011, http://www.cdc.gov/lyme/stats/chartstables/casesbyyear.html (accessed January 4, 2012)

ticks away from the skin. If a tick is found on the body, it should be removed promptly, and the affected individual should be alert for early symptoms of the disease. Immediate medical care, which consists of antibiotic treatment, is imperative to prevent long-term health damage from Lyme disease.

WEST NILE VIRUS

The West Nile virus (WNV) is common in Africa, West Asia, and the Middle East, and it can infect birds, mosquitoes, horses, humans, and other mammals. It is spread by bites from infected mosquitoes, and even though most people who become infected have few or no symptoms, some develop serious and even fatal illnesses. The virus was first reported in the United States in 1999, and the CDC has tracked its westward spread across the United States. In "West Nile Virus: Statistics, Surveillance, and Control" (January 10, 2012, http://www.cdc.gov/ncidod/dvbid/westnile/surv&controlCaseCount11_detailed.htm), the CDC indicates that in 2011 WNV caused 690 cases of human illness and 43 deaths in the United States.

According to the CDC, the presence of WNV in either humans or infected mosquitoes is permanently established in the United States. Even though human illness from the virus is relatively rare, the disease is more likely to be fatal in older adults and young children. Figure 7.8 shows the distribution of human WNV cases by state as well as by infection of birds, animals, or mosquitoes.

The CDC advises taking precautions against mosquito bites, such as using insect repellent; wearing long pants and long-sleeved shirts that are treated with insect repellent; remaining indoors during dawn, dusk, and early evening, the hours when mosquitoes are the most likely to bite; and removing standing water to prevent mosquitoes from laying eggs and breeding near homes and other populated areas.

SEVERE ACUTE RESPIRATORY SYNDROME

In "Frequently Asked Questions about SARS" (May 3, 2005, http://www.cdc.gov/sars/about/faq.html), the CDC explains that severe acute respiratory syndrome (SARS) is a viral respiratory illness caused by a coronavirus that was first reported in southern China in November 2002. The illness spread to more than 24 countries in North America, South America, Europe, and Asia before the global outbreak was contained in July 2003. SARS seems to be transmitted primarily by person-to-person contact through respiratory droplets, which travel via coughs or sneezes to the mucous membranes of other people or to surfaces that others touch. Symptoms of the disease may include high fever, body aches, malaise (overall discomfort), diarrhea, and mild respiratory symptoms; after two to seven days the infected person may develop a dry cough. The disease then progresses to pneumonia in most people.

According to the CDC, 8,098 people worldwide became sick with SARS during the outbreak, and 774 died. In the United States eight people—all of whom had

TABLE 7.8

Reported Lyme disease cases by state, 2000–10

State	2000	2001	2002	2003	2004	2005	2006	2007	2008	2009†	2010 Confirmed	2010 Probable	2010 Incidence*
Alabama	6	10	11	8	6	3	11	13	6	3	1	1	0.0
Alaska	2	2	3	3	3	4	3	10	6	7	7	0	1.0
Arizona	2	3	4	4	13	10	10	2	2	3	2	0	0.0
Arkansas	7	4	3	0	0	0	0	1	0	0	0	0	0.0
California	96	95	97	86	48	95	85	75	74	117	137	3	0.4
Colorado	0	0	1	0	0	0	0	0	2	0	1	2	0.0
Connecticut	3,773	3,597	4,631	1,403	1,348	1,810	1,788	3,058	2,738	2,751	1,964	1,104	55.0
Delaware	167	152	194	212	339	646	482	715	772	984	656	0	73.1
DC	11	17	25	14	16	10	62	116	71	53	34	8	5.7
Florida	54	43	79	43	46	47	34	30	72	77	56	28	0.3
Georgia	0	0	2	10	12	6	8	11	35	40	10	0	0.1
Hawaii	0	0	0	0	0	0	0	0	0	0	0	0	0.0
Idaho	4	5	4	3	6	2	7	9	5	4	6	3	0.4
Illinois	35	32	47	71	87	127	110	149	108	136	135	0	1.1
Indiana	23	26	21	25	32	33	26	55	42	61	62	16	1.0
Iowa	34	36	42	58	49	89	97	123	85	77	68	17	2.2
Kansas	17	2	7	4	3	3	4	8	16	18	7	3	0.2
Kentucky	13	23	25	17	15	5	7	6	5	1	5	0	0.1
Louisiana	8	8	5	7	2	3	1	2	3	0	2	1	0.0
Maine	71	108	219	175	225	247	338	529	780	791	559	192	42.1
Maryland	688	608	738	691	891	1,235	1,248	2,576	1,746	1,466	1,163	454	20.1
Massachusetts	1,158	1,164	1,807	1,532	1,532	2,336	1,432	2,988	3,960	4,019	2,380	883	36.3
Michigan	23	21	26	12	27	62	55	51	76	81	76	19	0.8
Minnesota	465	461	867	474	1,023	917	914	1,238	1,046	1,063	1,293	667	24.4
Mississippi	3	8	12	21	0	0	3	1	1	0	0	0	0.0
Missouri	47	37	41	70	25	15	5	10	6	3	4	0	0.1
Montana	0	0	0	0	0	0	1	4	6	3	3	1	0.3
Nebraska	5	4	6	2	2	2	11	7	8	4	7	1	0.4
Nevada	4	4	2	3	1	3	4	15	9	10	2	0	0.1
New Hampshire	84	129	261	190	226	265	617	896	1,211	996	830	509	63.0
New Jersey	2,459	2,020	2,349	2,887	2,698	3,363	2,432	3,134	3,214	4,598	3,320	392	37.8
New Mexico	0	1	1	1	1	3	3	5	4	1	3	2	0.1
New York	4,329	4,083	5,535	5,399	5,100	5,565	4,460	4,165	5,741	4,134	2,385	1,040	12.3
North Carolina	47	41	137	156	122	49	31	53	16	21	21	61	0.2
North Dakota	2	0	1	0	0	3	7	12	8	10	21	12	3.1
Ohio	61	44	82	66	50	58	43	33	40	51	21	23	0.2
Oklahoma	1	0	0	0	3	0	0	1	1	2	0	0	0.0
Oregon	13	15	12	16	11	3	7	6	18	12	7	32	0.2
Pennsylvania	2,343	2,806	3,989	5,730	3,985	4,287	3,242	3,994	3,818	4,950	3,298	507	26.0
Rhode Island	675	510	852	736	249	39	308	177	186	150	115	66	10.9
South Carolina	25	6	26	18	22	15	20	31	14	25	19	10	0.4
South Dakota	0	0	2	1	1	2	1	0	3	1	1	0	0.1
Tennessee	28	31	28	20	20	8	15	31	7	10	6	30	0.1
Texas	77	75	139	85	98	69	29	87	105	88	55	87	0.2
Utah	3	1	5	2	1	2	5	7	3	6	3	0	0.1
Vermont	40	18	37	43	50	54	105	138	330	323	271	85	43.3
Virginia	149	156	259	195	216	274	357	959	886	698	911	334	11.4
Washington	9	9	11	7	14	13	8	12	22	15	12	4	0.2
West Virginia	35	16	26	31	38	61	28	84	120	143	128	17	6.9
Wisconsin	631	597	1,090	740	1,144	1,459	1,466	1,814	1,493	1,952	2,505	983	44.0
Wyoming	3	1	2	2	4	3	1	3	1	1	0	0	0.0
U.S. total	**17,730**	**17,029**	**23,763**	**21,273**	**19,804**	**23,305**	**19,931**	**27,444**	**28,921**	**29,959**	**22,572**	**7,597**	**7.3**

†Confirmed cases presented for all years except most recent.
*Confirmed cases per 100,000 population.

SOURCE: "Reported Lyme Disease Cases by State, 2000–2010," in *Lyme Disease Statistics*, Centers for Disease Control and Prevention, Division of Vector-Borne Infectious Diseases, November 15, 2011, http://www.cdc.gov/lyme/stats/chartstables/reportedcases_statelocality.html (accessed January 4, 2012)

traveled to parts of the world where the virus was present—contracted the disease.

In 2005 the National Institute of Allergy and Infectious Diseases (NIAID) began applying its resources to establishing diagnostics, developing vaccines, and identifying antiviral compounds to combat SARS-associated coronavirus (SARS-CoV). Among the many projects that have received NIAID support are the development of a SARS chip, a deoxyribonucleic acid (DNA) microarray to rapidly identify SARS sequence variants, and a SARS diagnostic test based on polymerase chain reaction (PCR) technology. (PCR is a technique for amplifying DNA sequences by as many as 1 billion times, and it is important in biotechnology, medicine, and genetic research.)

FIGURE 7.8

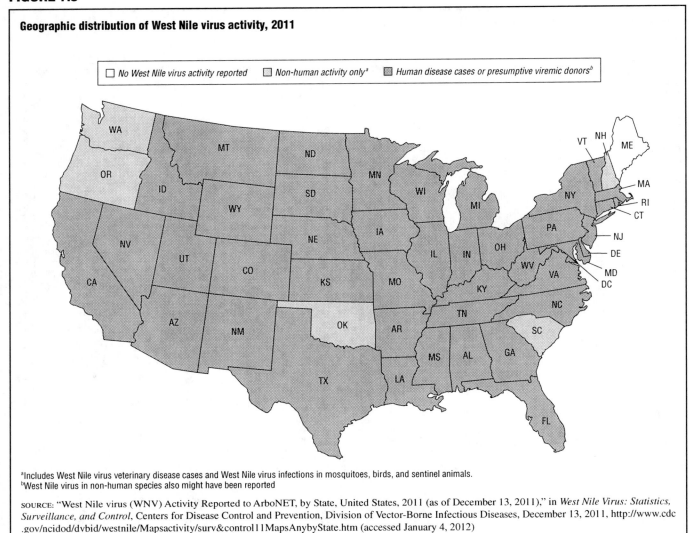

Geographic distribution of West Nile virus activity, 2011

☐ No West Nile virus activity reported ☐ Non-human activity only[a] ▨ Human disease cases or presumptive viremic donors[b]

[a]Includes West Nile virus veterinary disease cases and West Nile virus infections in mosquitoes, birds, and sentinel animals.
[b]West Nile virus in non-human species also might have been reported

SOURCE: "West Nile virus (WNV) Activity Reported to ArboNET, by State, United States, 2011 (as of December 13, 2011)," in *West Nile Virus: Statistics, Surveillance, and Control*, Centers for Disease Control and Prevention, Division of Vector-Borne Infectious Diseases, December 13, 2011, http://www.cdc .gov/ncidod/dvbid/westnile/Mapsactivity/surv&control11MapsAnybyState.htm (accessed January 4, 2012)

The CDC reports in "SARS News and Alerts Archive" (December 15, 2011, http://www.cdc.gov/sars/ media/index.html) that there has been no known SARS transmission anywhere in the world since April 2004; as of February 2012, this situation remained unchanged. The 2002 outbreak of human cases of SARS-CoV infection occurred in China, and the cases were considered to be laboratory-acquired infections. The WHO notes in "Cumulative Number of Reported Probable Cases of Severe Acute Respiratory Syndrome (SARS)" (2012, http://www .who.int/csr/sars/country/en/index.html) that by the time SARS had run its course, just 27 cases were reported in the United States, and there were no U.S. SARS-related deaths.

RESPONDING TO BIOLOGIC TERRORISM: INTENTIONAL EPIDEMICS

In September and October 2001, in an unprecedented event, 22 letters containing *Bacillus anthracis* spores that were sent through the U.S. Postal Service caused anthrax outbreaks in seven states: Connecticut, one case; Pennsylvania, one case; Florida, two cases; Virginia, two cases; Maryland, three cases; New Jersey, five cases; and New York City, eight cases (includes the case of a New Jersey resident who was exposed in New York City). Five of the letters resulted in fatal cases of anthrax.

Anthony S. Fauci (1940–), the director of the NIAID, states in "The Power of Biomedical Research" (*Washington Times*, July 8, 2003) that these anthrax attacks "starkly exposed the vulnerability of the United States—and, indeed, the rest of the world—to bioterrorism." Accordingly, the NIAID devotes considerable attention to accelerated programs to prevent, diagnose, and treat possible intentional epidemics. The NIAID explains in "Biodefense and Emerging Infectious Diseases" (October 28, 2011, http://www.niaid.nih.gov/TOPICS/BIODEFENSERELATED/ BIODEFENSE/Pages/qanda.aspx) that since 2001 its research mission has shifted "from the 'one bug-one drug' approach toward a more flexible and broad strategy" that is aimed at developing broad-spectrum antibiotics and antivirals.

The NIAID asserts that "overall, the United States is much better prepared to respond to an infectious disease threat today than it was 10 years ago in part because of the strong investment in basic and applied research, product development, and technology development for biodefense and emerging infectious diseases." However, some experts question whether the United States is adequately prepared for a biological attack. In "How Ready Are We for Bioterrorism?" (*New York Times*, October 26, 2011), Wil S. Hylton quotes retired U.S. Air Force colonel Randall Larsen, who successfully smuggled a biological weapon into Vice President Dick Cheney's (1941–) office shortly after the September 11, 2001, terrorist attacks against the United States. White House guards had searched Larsen's belongings, but Larsen explained, "They were looking for the wrong things. They still are."

Hylton also notes that after evaluating the U.S. biodefense program, the Congressional Commission on the Prevention of Weapons of Mass Destruction Proliferation and Terrorism observed in January 2010, "Especially troubling is the lack of priority given to the development of medical countermeasures—the vaccines and medicines that would be required to mitigate the consequences of an attack." In early 2011 Kathleen Sebelius (1948–), the U.S. secretary of the HHS, characterized the countermeasure program as "full of leaks, choke points and dead ends," and many high ranking past and current military and government officials concurred. The congressional commission concluded, "To date, the U.S. government has invested most of its nonproliferation efforts and diplomatic capital in preventing nuclear terrorism. The commission believes that it should make the more likely threat—bioterrorism—a higher priority."

CHAPTER 8
MENTAL HEALTH AND ILLNESS

Mental health may be measured in terms of an individual's ability to think and communicate clearly, to learn and grow emotionally, to deal productively and realistically with change and stress, and to form and maintain fulfilling relationships with others. Mental health is a principal component of wellness—self-esteem, resilience, and the ability to cope with adversity influence how people feel about themselves and whether they choose lifestyles and behaviors that promote or jeopardize their health.

Mental illness refers to all identifiable mental health disorders and mental health problems. In the landmark study *Mental Health: A Report of the Surgeon General* (1999, http://profiles.nlm.nih.gov/ps/access/NNBBHS.pdf), the Office of the Surgeon General defines mental disorders as "health conditions that are characterized by alterations in thinking, mood, or behavior (or some combination thereof) associated with distress and/or impaired functioning." The surgeon general distinguishes mental disorders from mental problems, describing the signs and symptoms of mental health problems as less intense and of shorter duration than those of mental health disorders. However, it acknowledges that both mental health disorders and problems may be distressing and disabling.

The symptoms of mental disorders differentiate one type of problem from another; however, the symptoms of mental illness vary far more widely in both type and intensity than do the symptoms of most physical illnesses. In general, people are usually considered mentally healthy if they are able to maintain their mental and emotional balance in times of crisis and stress and to cope effectively with the problems of daily life. When their coping ability is lost, then there is some degree of mental dysfunction. The goals of diagnosis and treatment of mental disorders are to recognize and understand the conditions, to reduce their underlying causes, and to work toward regaining mental and emotional equilibrium.

HOW MANY PEOPLE ARE MENTALLY ILL?

It is complicated to determine how many people suffer from mental illness due to changing definitions of mental illness and the difficulties in classifying, diagnosing, and reporting mental disorders. There are social stigmas that are attached to mental illness, such as being labeled "crazy," being treated as a danger to others, and being denied a job or health insurance coverage, that keep some sufferers from seeking help, and many of those in treatment do not reveal it on surveys. Some patients do not realize that their symptoms are caused by mental disorders. Because knowledge about the way the brain works is relatively narrow, mental health professionals must continually reassess how mental illnesses are defined and diagnosed. In addition, what might be considered, for example, delusional thinking in one culture may well be widely accepted in another; the symptoms of mental illness are notoriously fluid, and diagnosis may be skewed by cultural differences or other bias on the part of both patient and practitioner.

In "The Numbers Count: Mental Disorders in America" (August 10, 2009, http://wwwapps.nimh.nih.gov/health/publications/the-numbers-count-mental-disorders-in-america.shtml), the National Institute of Mental Health (NIMH) estimates that 26.2% of Americans aged 18 years and older are affected by mental disorders and that 6% suffer from serious mental illness. Community surveys estimate that as many as 30% of the adult population in the United States suffer from mental disorders. The National Center for Chronic Disease Prevention and Health Promotion reports that between 2003 and 2009 more than 10% of American adults said they experience frequent mental distress, as defined by "14 or more mentally unhealthy days." (See Figure 8.1.) The Harvard School of Medicine in its National Comorbidity Survey (July 2007, http://www.hcp.med.harvard.edu/ncs/) uses a national sample of 10,000 respondents to assess the prevalence of mental

FIGURE 8.1

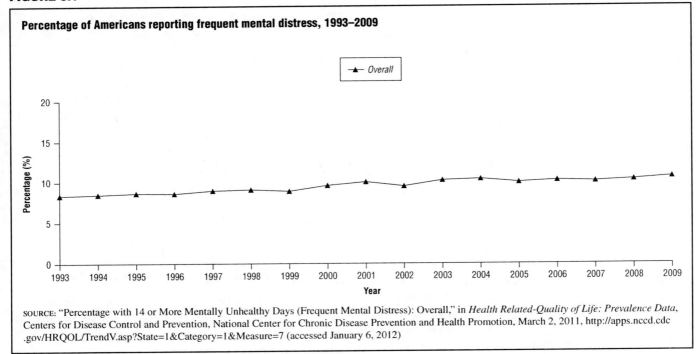

Percentage of Americans reporting frequent mental distress, 1993–2009

SOURCE: "Percentage with 14 or More Mentally Unhealthy Days (Frequent Mental Distress): Overall," in *Health Related-Quality of Life: Prevalence Data*, Centers for Disease Control and Prevention, National Center for Chronic Disease Prevention and Health Promotion, March 2, 2011, http://apps.nccd.cdc .gov/HRQOL/TrendV.asp?State=1&Category=1&Measure=7 (accessed January 6, 2012)

disorders in the United States. The survey indicates that in any given year 32.4% of all Americans meet the criteria for having a mental illness and that the lifetime prevalence of any diagnosable mental disorder is 57.4%.

How Many Children Suffer from Mental Illness?

Data describing the prevalence of mental disorders in children vary. Christian Kieling et al. estimate in "Child and Adolescent Mental Health Worldwide: Evidence for Action" (*Lancet*, vol. 378, no. 9801, October 22, 2011) that between 10% and 20% of children and adolescents worldwide have mental health problems. The National Health and Nutrition Examination Survey (NHANES), which was conducted by the NIMH and the National Center for Health Statistics, surveyed 3,042 children aged eight to 15 years between 2001 and 2004 to determine the prevalence of mental health problems in this population. The NHANES found that 13% of children had at least one mental disorder in the year prior to the survey and close to 2% of respondents had more than one disorder. In "Prevalence and Treatment of Mental Disorders among US Children in the 2001–2004 NHANES" (*Pediatrics*, vol. 125, no. 1, January 1, 2010), an analysis of the NHANES data, Kathleen Ries Merikangas et al. find that boys were more than twice as likely as girls to have attention deficit/hyperactivity disorder (ADHD; problems concentrating, focusing, and paying attention, coupled with excessive restlessness and movement), whereas girls were twice as likely to suffer from mood disorders (primarily depression). There were no differences between boys and girls in the rates of anxiety disorders or conduct

disorders. Merikangas et al. observe that even though these prevalence rates are lower than many of those previously reported, just half of children with mental health disorders sought treatment from a mental health professional.

The National Health Interview Study (NHIS), a continuing, nationwide survey that is conducted by the National Center for Health Statistics, reports lower rates—between 2001 and 2009 the percentage of children with serious emotional or behavioral difficulties was stable at about 5%. During this same period the percentage of children with serious emotional or behavioral difficulties differed by gender and age. Parents reported that in 2009 more boys (7%) than girls (4%) had difficulties. (See Figure 8.2.)

Many mental disorders that begin during childhood and adolescence recur or continue into adulthood. Children and teens with mood and anxiety disorders suffer from unfounded fears, prolonged sadness or tearfulness, withdrawal, low self-esteem, and feelings of worthlessness and hopelessness. These children and adolescents often suffer from more than one mental health problem (e.g., symptoms of depression and anxiety together). In 2009 the percentage of adolescents aged 12 to 17 years that had a major depressive episode (MDE; defined as a period of at least two weeks of depressed mood or loss of interest or pleasure in daily activities plus at least four additional symptoms of depression such as problems with sleeping, eating, energy, concentration, and feelings of self-worth) was 8%. (See Figure 8.3.) The prevalence of MDE was more than twice as high among girls and higher in older teens than in younger ones.

FIGURE 8.2

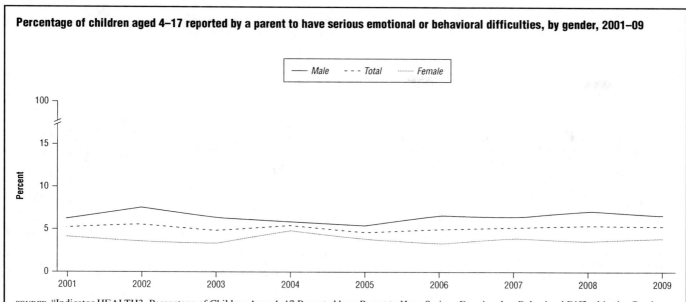

Percentage of children aged 4–17 reported by a parent to have serious emotional or behavioral difficulties, by gender, 2001–09

SOURCE: "Indicator HEALTH3. Percentage of Children Ages 4–17 Reported by a Parent to Have Serious Emotional or Behavioral Difficulties by Gender, 2001–2009," in *America's Children: Key National Indicators of Well-Being, 2011*, Federal Interagency Forum on Child and Family Statistics, 2011, http://childstats.gov/americaschildren/health3.asp (accessed January 6, 2012)

FIGURE 8.3

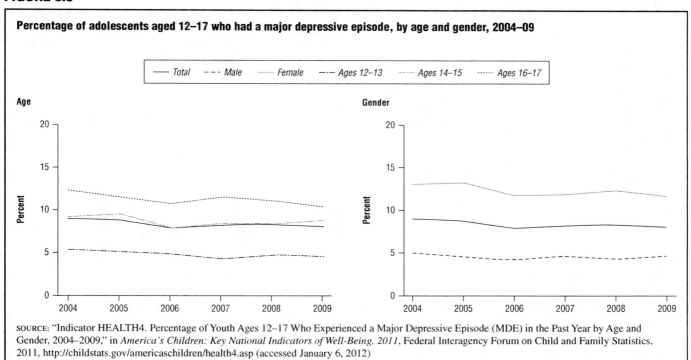

Percentage of adolescents aged 12–17 who had a major depressive episode, by age and gender, 2004–09

SOURCE: "Indicator HEALTH4. Percentage of Youth Ages 12–17 Who Experienced a Major Depressive Episode (MDE) in the Past Year by Age and Gender, 2004–2009," in *America's Children: Key National Indicators of Well-Being, 2011*, Federal Interagency Forum on Child and Family Statistics, 2011, http://childstats.gov/americaschildren/health4.asp (accessed January 6, 2012)

Some Americans Experience Serious Mental Distress

The NHIS poses questions about psychological distress. These questions ask how often a respondent experienced certain symptoms of psychological distress during the 30 days preceding the survey. In the first half of 2011 about 3.5% of adults aged 18 years and older said they had experienced serious psychological distress during the past 30 days. Figure 8.4 shows that the percentage of adults reporting serious psychological distress during the past 30 days was lowest in 1999 (2.4%) and highest in January–June 2011 (3.5%).

The NHIS reveals that people aged 45 to 65 years (4.7%) were more likely to have experienced serious psychological distress during the 30 days preceding the

FIGURE 8.4

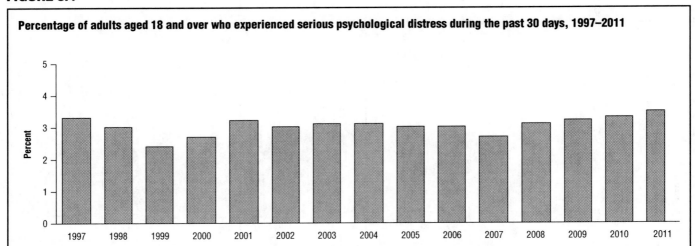

Percentage of adults aged 18 and over who experienced serious psychological distress during the past 30 days, 1997–2011

Notes: Data are based on household interviews of a sample of the civilian noninstitutionalized population. Six psychological distress questions are included in the National Health Interview Survey's Sample Adult Core component. These questions ask how often a respondent experienced certain symptoms of psychological distress during the past 30 days. The response codes (0–4) of the six items for each person are summed to yield a scale with a 0–24 range. A value of 13 or more for this scale is used here to define serious psychological distress (9).

SOURCE: "Figure 13.1. Percentage of Adults Aged 18 Years and over Who Experienced Serious Psychological Distress during the Past 30 Days: United States, 1997–June 2011," in *Early Release of Selected Estimates Based on Data from the January–June 2011 National Health Interview Survey*, Centers for Disease Control and Prevention, National Center for Health Statistics, December 2011, http://www.cdc.gov/nchs/data/nhis/earlyrelease/201112_13.pdf (accessed January 6, 2012)

survey than people aged 18 to 44 years (2.9%) and 65 years and older (2.9%). (See Figure 8.5.) Among people in all age groups, women were more likely than men to report serious psychological distress during the 30 days preceding the survey.

The percentage of adults in the first half of 2011 that experienced serious psychological distress during the 30 days preceding the survey varied by ethnicity—Hispanics were more likely to report such distress than were non-Hispanic whites or non-Hispanic African-Americans. The age-sex-adjusted prevalence of serious psychological distress was 4.6% for Hispanics, 3.4% for non-Hispanic whites, and 3.3% for non-Hispanic African-Americans. (See Figure 8.6.)

Not All People Need or Seek Treatment

The NIMH observes that not all mental disorders require treatment, because many people with mental disorders have relatively brief, self-limiting illnesses that are not disabling enough to warrant treatment. However, William C. Reeves et al. report in "Mental Illness Surveillance among Adults in the United States" (*Morbidity and Mortality Weekly Report*, vol. 60, no. 3, September 2, 2011) that even though one-quarter of adults in the United States said they had suffered a mental illness during the past year, just 5% of outpatient visits were attributable to a diagnosis of a mental health disorder. It is likely that more than 5% of adults receive some sort of treatment, but clearly there are many more people in need of mental health treatment than receive it. Reeves et al. assert that "many mental illnesses can be managed successfully, and increasing access to and

FIGURE 8.5

Percentage of adults aged 18 and over who experienced serious psychological distress during the past 30 days, by age group and sex, January–June 2011

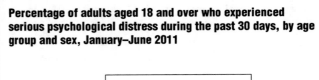

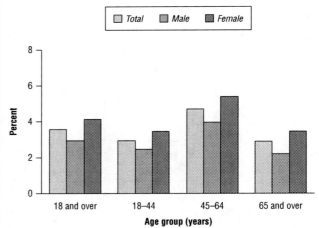

Notes: Data are based on household interviews of a sample of the civilian noninstitutionalized population. Six psychological distress questions are included in the National Health Interview Survey's Sample Adult Core component. These questions ask how often a respondent experienced certain symptoms of psychological distress during the past 30 days. The response codes (0–4) of the six items for each person are summed to yield a scale with a 0–24 range. A value of 13 or more for this scale is used here to define serious psychological distress (9).

SOURCE: "Figure 13.2. Percentage of Adults Aged 18 Years and over Who Experienced Serious Psychological Distress during the Past 30 Days, by Age Group and Sex: United States, January–June 2011," in *Early Release of Selected Estimates Based on Data from the January–June 2011 National Health Interview Survey*, Centers for Disease Control and Prevention, National Center for Health Statistics, December 2011, http://www.cdc.gov/nchs/data/nhis/earlyrelease/201112_13.pdf (accessed January 6, 2012)

FIGURE 8.6

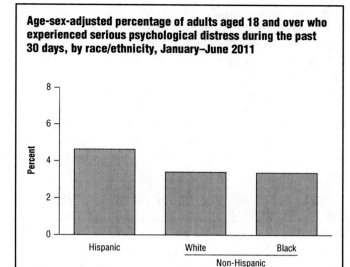

Age-sex-adjusted percentage of adults aged 18 and over who experienced serious psychological distress during the past 30 days, by race/ethnicity, January–June 2011

Notes: Data are based on household interviews of a sample of the civilian noninstitutionalized population. Six psychological distress questions are included in the National Health Interview Survey's Sample Adult Core component. These questions ask how often a respondent experienced certain symptoms of psychological distress during the past 30 days. The response codes (0–4) of the six items for each person are summed to yield a scale with a 0–24 range. A value of 13 or more for this scale is used here to define serious psychological distress (9). Estimates are age-sex-adjusted using the projected 2000 U.S. population as the standard population and using three age groups: 18–44, 45–64, and 65 and over.

SOURCE: "Figure 13.3. Age-Sex-Adjusted Percentage of Adults Aged 18 Years and over Who Experienced Serious Psychological Distress during the Past 30 Days, by Race/Ethnicity: United States, January–June 2011," in *Early Release of Selected Estimates Based on Data from the January–June 2011 National Health Interview Survey*, Centers for Disease Control and Prevention, National Center for Health Statistics, December 2011, http://www.cdc.gov/nchs/data/nhis/earlyrelease/201112_13.pdf (accessed January 6, 2012)

use of mental health treatment services could substantially reduce the associated morbidity."

In "Service Utilization for Lifetime Mental Disorders in U.S. Adolescents: Results of the National Comorbidity Survey-Adolescent Supplement (NCS-A)" (*Journal of the American Academy of Child and Adolescent Psychiatry*, vol. 50, no.1, January 2011), Kathleen Ries Merikangas et al. report that between 2002 and 2004 just one-third (36.2%) of adolescents with mental disorders received treatment. Even though the likelihood of receiving treatment rose with increasing severity of the disorder, 50% of adolescents with "severely impairing mental disorders had never received mental health treatment for their symptoms." Adolescents with ADHD (59.8%) and behavior disorders (45.4%; inappropriate behaviors that sharply deviate from accepted norms) were the most likely to receive treatment. African-American and Hispanic youth were less likely to receive treatment for mood and anxiety disorders than were white youth.

TYPES OF DISORDERS

Psychiatrists have identified a wide range of mental disorders, from phobias (intense, irrational, and persistent fears) to depression to schizophrenia. Psychiatric diagnoses are made based on criteria that are described in the fourth edition of the *Diagnostic and Statistical Manual of Mental Disorders* (*DSM-IV*) by the American Psychiatric Association. (In May 2013 the fifth edition of the *DSM*, *DSM-V*, is scheduled to replace the *DSM-IV*. See Chapter 3 for a discussion of the new diagnostic manual.) Some disorders are relatively mild and affect an individual's life in only a minor way. Others can be overwhelming, completely debilitating, and life-threatening.

Anxiety disorders, which include phobias, and depression are the two most common mental disorders. In "Any Anxiety Disorder among Adults" (2012, http://www.nimh.nih.gov/statistics/1ANYANX_ADULT.shtml), the National Institutes of Health indicates that in a given year 18.1% of the adults in the United States have an anxiety disorder and 4.1% of these are considered "severe." On average, anxiety disorders begin at age 11, and women are more likely to be affected than men. The types of anxiety disorders and the lifetime prevalence in adults aged 18 years and older in the United States include post-traumatic stress disorder (3.5%), generalized anxiety disorder (3.1%), panic disorder (2.7%), obsessive-compulsive disorder (1%), and phobias—specific phobia (8.7%), social phobia (6.8%), and agoraphobia (0.8%). Many people suffer from more than one mental disorder at a time (comorbidity). For example, millions of Americans suffer from substance (drug or alcohol) abuse combined with one or more other mental disorders.

Children suffer from many of the same mental disorders that afflict adults. The lifetime prevalence of anxiety disorder in adolescents aged 13 to 18 years is 25.1%. The types of anxiety disorders and the lifetime prevalence in adolescents aged 13 to 18 years in the United States include post-traumatic stress disorder (4%), panic disorder (2.3%), generalized anxiety disorder (1%), and phobias—specific phobia (15.1%), social phobia (5.5%), and agoraphobia (2.4%). Children may also be affected by developmental disorders. Children with disorganized thinking and difficulty communicating verbally, and those who have trouble understanding and navigating the world around them, may be diagnosed with autism or another pervasive developmental disorder. These disorders may be among the most disabling because they are associated with serious learning difficulties and impaired intelligence. Examples of pervasive developmental disorders include autism, Asperger's disorder, and Rett's disorder.

AUTISM SPECTRUM DISORDERS (PERVASIVE DEVELOPMENTAL DISORDERS)

Autism is a spectrum of disorders affecting a person's ability to communicate and interact with others. Autism spectrum disorders (ASDs), also known as pervasive developmental disorders, are conditions that result from a neurological disorder that typically appears during the first three years of childhood and continues throughout life. These disorders were first described in 1943 by Leo Kanner (1894–1981), who reported on 11 children who displayed an unusual lack of interest in other people but were extremely interested in unusual aspects of the inanimate environment. Autistic children appear unattached to parents or caregivers, assume rigid or limp body postures when held, suffer impaired language, and exhibit behavior such as head banging, violent tantrums, and screaming. They are often self-destructive and uncooperative and experience delayed mental and social skills. Autism is associated with a variety of neurological symptoms such as seizures and persistence of reflexes—involuntary muscle reactions and responses (e.g., the sucking reflex when the area around the mouth is stimulated) that are normal in infancy but usually disappear during normal child development. Autism is the most common of the pervasive developmental disorders. The NIMH reports in "Autism" (2012, http://www.nimh .nih.gov/statistics/1AUT_CHILD.shtml) that one out of every 110 eight-year-old children may be diagnosed with an ASD. In "Autism Spectrum Disorders (ASDs)" (May 13, 2010, http://www.cdc.gov/ncbddd/autism/data.html), the Centers for Disease Control and Prevention notes that the prevalence of autism is four to five times more frequent in boys than in girls.

Even though ASDs were once thought to have psychological origins or occur as the result of bad parenting, both of these hypotheses have been discarded in favor of biological and genetic explanations of causality. The cause of autism remains unknown, but the disorder has been associated with maternal rubella infection, phenylketonuria (an inherited disorder of metabolism), tuberous sclerosis (an inherited disease of the nervous system and skin), lack of oxygen at birth, and encephalitis (inflammation of the brain). There is considerable evidence of the heritability of autism.

Several genes and mutations that are associated with autism have been identified. In "Association of Autism with Polymorphisms in the Paired-Like Homeodomain Transcription Factor 1 (PITX1) on Chromosome 5q31: A Candidate Gene Analysis" (BMC Medical Genetics, vol. 8, December 6, 2007), Anne Philippi et al. suggest that at least three genes may be implicated in the development of autism. One is a regulator of the pituitary-hypothalamic axis (the pituitary is a small gland in the brain that produces hormones, and the hypothalamus is a part of the brain that controls body temperature, hunger, sleep, and thirst). Another is involved in the development of nerves, and a third is involved in X-chromosome inactivation in females, which may explain the disproportionate (four-to-one) number of males who are affected by autism.

Simon G. Gregory et al. report in "Genomic and Epigenetic Evidence for Oxytocin Receptor Deficiency in Autism" (BMC Medicine, vol. 7, October 22, 2009) the identification of an inherited disruption of gene expression in a part of the brain system that mediates the disturbed social behavior that is observed in autism. Gregory et al. find the same disruption in the oxytocin receptor gene in both a person with autism and his mother; the mother had obsessive-compulsive disorder, which, like autism, often involves repetitive behaviors. This genetic variant may prove to be a biomarker for autism that would enable the diagnosis to be made with a blood test. This finding also supports other research suggesting that treatment with oxytocin, a hormone produced by the pituitary gland that is involved in reproduction and social behavior, may help people with autism.

In "Genetic Basis of Autism: Is There a Way Forward?" (Current Opinion in Psychiatry, vol. 24, no. 3, May 2011), Valsamma Eapen of the University of New South Wales, Sydney, explains that about 103 genes have been implicated in autism. These genes overlap with other disorders such as intellectual deficiency, epilepsy, schizophrenia, and ADHD. This suggests that autism is not a single-gene disorder; rather, it is a complex disorder that results from simultaneous genetic variations in multiple genes as well as interactions between genetic, epigenetic (heritable changes in gene function that do not involve a change in deoxyribonucleic acid sequence), and environmental factors.

Autism varies from mild to quite severe, and the prognosis depends on the extent of the individual's disabilities and whether he or she receives the early, intensive interventions that are associated with improved outcomes. A diagnosis of atypical autism or "pervasive developmental disorder not otherwise specified" is generally used to refer to mild cases of autism or children with impaired social interaction and verbal and nonverbal communication who are not asocial enough to be considered autistic. Treatment of autism is individualized and may include applied behavior analysis, medications, dietary management and supplements, music therapy, occupational therapy, physical therapy, speech and language therapy, and vision therapy.

Asperger's disorder is a milder form of autism, and sufferers are sometimes called "high-functioning children with autism." The disorder is named for the Austrian pediatrician Hans Asperger (1906–1980), who first described it in 1944. The DSM-IV states that Asperger's disorder appears to be more common in boys. Affected children tend to be socially isolated and behave oddly. They have impaired social interactions, are unable to express pleasure in others' happiness, and lack social and emotional reciprocity. They are below average in nonverbal communication, and their speech is marked by peculiar abnormalities of inflection and a repetitive pattern. Unlike autism, however, cognitive and communicative development is normal or near normal during the first years of life, and verbal skills are usually relatively strong. Sufferers also have impaired gross motor skills, tend to be clumsy, and may engage in repetitive finger flapping, twisting, or awkward whole-body movements. They usually have very narrow areas of interest that are highly specific, idiosyncratic, and so consuming that they do not pursue age-appropriate activities. Examples of such interests include train schedules, spiders, or telegraph pole insulators.

Rett's disorder (also known as Rett's syndrome) is sometimes mistaken for autism when diagnosed in very young children (and is linked to autism, Asperger's disorder, ADHD, and schizophrenia), but it is much less prevalent and has a distinctive onset and course. The condition occurs primarily in girls who, after early normal development, experience slower-than-expected head growth during the first months of life and a loss of purposeful hand motions between ages five and 30 months. Affected children are usually profoundly mentally retarded and exhibit stereotypical repetitive behaviors such as hand wringing or hand washing. Interest in socialization diminishes during the first few years of the disorder but may resume later in life, despite severe impairment in expressive and receptive language development. Affected individuals experience problems in the coordination of gait or trunk movements, and walking may become difficult.

DEPRESSION

According to Reeves et al., in "Mental Illness Surveillance among Adults in the United States," depression affects about 8.7% of the U.S. population. Women are affected more often than men. The prevalence of depression is higher among women and non-Hispanic African-Americans, compared with other populations. The NIMH reports in "Major Depressive Disorder among Adults" (2012, http://www.nimh.nih.gov/statistics/1MDD_ADULT .shtml) that 6.7% of the U.S. adult population suffers from depression in a given year and that 30.4% of cases are severe. Even though depression can occur at any age, the average age when it begins is 32 and younger adults aged 18 to 59 years are more likely to have experienced depression than people aged 60 years and older.

Defining Depression

Depression is a "whole body" illness, involving physical, mental, and emotional problems. A depressive disorder is not a temporary sad mood, and it is not a sign of personal weakness or a condition that can be willed away. People with depressive illness cannot just "pull themselves together" and hope that they will become well. Without treatment, the symptoms can persist for months or even years. Table 8.1 lists the symptoms that characterize depression. Not everyone who is depressed experiences all the symptoms. Some people have few symptoms, and some have many. Like other mental illnesses, the severity and duration of the symptoms of depression vary.

TABLE 8.1

Symptoms of depression

Persistent sad, anxious, or "empty" feelings
Feelings of hopelessness or pessimism
Feelings of guilt, worthlessness, or helplessness
Irritability, restlessness
Loss of interest in activities or hobbies once pleasurable, including sex
Fatigue and decreased energy
Difficulty concentrating, remembering details, and making decisions
Insomnia, early-morning wakefulness, or excessive sleeping
Overeating, or appetite loss
Thoughts of suicide, suicide attempts
Aches or pains, headaches, cramps, or digestive problems that do not ease even with treatment.

SOURCE: "What Are the Signs and Symptoms of Depression?" in *Depression*, National Institute of Mental Health, 2011, http://www.nimh.nih.gov/health/publications/depression/depression-booklet.pdf (accessed January 9, 2012)

There are several types of depressive disorders. The most common form is dysthymic disorder (dysthymia), a less severe but chronic form of depression that by definition lasts at least two years in adults or at least one year in children. Dysthymic disorders commonly appear for the first time in children, teens, and young adults, and even though they may not disable people as severely as other forms of depression, these disorders can ruin lives by robbing them of joy, energy, and productivity. According to the NIMH, in "Dysthymic Disorder among Adults" (2012, http://www.nimh.nih.gov/statistics/1DD_ADULT.shtml), 1.5% of American adults suffer from dysthymic disorder.

Major depression is a more severe and disabling form. In fact, it is a leading cause of disability among Americans aged 15 to 44 years.

Causes of Depression

Combinations of genetic, psychological, and environmental factors are involved in the development of depressive disorders. Some types of depression run in families, and research studies of twins demonstrate that genetic factors determine susceptibility to depression. Major depression seems to recur in generation after generation of some families, but it also occurs in people with no family history of depression.

Studies of the brain support the premise that depression may have a biological and chemical basis. Even though brain imaging studies clearly indicate that there are differences in the brain between those who suffer from depression and those who do not, it is not yet known if these differences cause the depression or result from it. Researchers speculate that the problem may be caused by the complex neurotransmission (chemical messaging) system of the brain and that people suffering from depression have either too much or too little of certain neurochemicals in the brain. Researchers also believe that depressed patients with normal levels of neurotransmitters may suffer from an inability to regulate them. Most antidepressant drugs that are currently used to treat the disorder attempt to correct these chemical imbalances.

A person's psychological makeup is another factor in depressive disorders. People who are easily overwhelmed by stress or who suffer from low self-esteem or a pessimistic view of themselves, of life, and of the world tend to be prone to depression. Events outside the person's control can also trigger a depressive episode. A major change in the patterns of daily living—such as a serious loss, a chronic illness, a difficult relationship, or financial problems—can trigger the onset of depression.

Treatment of Depression

Antidepressant medications that alter brain chemistry have been used to treat depressive disorders effectively. Antidepressant medications—including selective serotonin reuptake inhibitors (SSRIs) such as fluoxetine hydrochloride, tricyclic antidepressants such as amitriptyline, and monoamine oxidase inhibitors—work by influencing the function of neurotransmitters such as dopamine or norepinephrine. SSRIs have fewer reported side effects (such as sedation, headache, weight gain or loss, and nausea) than tricyclic antidepressants.

Antidepressants do not offer immediate relief from symptoms; most take full effect in about four weeks, and some take up to eight weeks to achieve optimal therapeutic effect. Patients must be closely monitored by health professionals for side effects, dosage, and effectiveness. The most common side effects of antidepressants include headache, nausea, sleeplessness or drowsiness, agitation, sexual problems, dry mouth, constipation, bladder problems, and blurred vision. In cases of chronic depression, medication may be needed continuously and on a long-term basis to prevent the recurrence of the disease.

In 2004 the U.S. Food and Drug Administration (FDA) issued a warning that depression may worsen or suicidal thoughts may occur in people, particularly children and adolescents, who take any of the popular antidepressants. This is most likely to occur at the beginning of treatment or when the doses are increased or decreased. The FDA ordered manufacturers to revise the labeling of antidepressants to increase awareness of these side effects. The NIMH reports in *Depression* (2011, http://www.nimh.nih.gov/health/publications/depression/depression-booklet.pdf) that research conducted between 1988 and 2006 suggests that the benefits of antidepressant medications likely outweigh their risks to children and adolescents with major depression and anxiety disorders.

Psychotherapy has also been demonstrated as effective therapy for mild to moderate depression. Talking about problems with mental health professionals can help patients better understand their feelings. Two types of short-term therapy lasting 10 to 20 weeks appear to improve symptoms of depression. Interpersonal psychotherapy (IPT) concentrates on helping patients improve personal relationships with family and friends. Cognitive behavioral therapy (CBT) attempts to help patients replace negative thoughts and feelings with more positive, optimistic approaches and actions.

Some people respond well to psychotherapy, and others respond well to antidepressants. Many do best with a combination of treatment—drugs for relatively quick relief of symptoms and therapy to learn how to cope with life's problems more effectively. John S. March et al. find in "The Treatment for Adolescents with Depression Study (TADS): Long-Term Effectiveness and Safety Outcomes" (*Archives of General Psychiatry*, vol. 64, no. 10, October 2007) that depressed adolescents recovered more quickly when they received drug treatment (fluoxetine) alone or in combination with CBT than those who received CBT alone.

In "Antidepressant Drug Effects and Depression Severity" (*Journal of the American Medical Association*, vol. 303, no. 1, January 6, 2010), a meta-analysis that reviews the results of six studies spanning 30 years of antidepressant drug treatment, Jay C. Fournier et al. suggest that people with severe depression benefit most from antidepressant medications, while there is little or no benefit for people with the less-severe symptoms of mild depression. The researchers assert that the benefit of antidepressant medication is comparable to placebo for people with mild to moderate symptoms.

Electrical stimulation of the brain, known as electroconvulsive therapy (ECT; formerly called shock therapy), may also be used to treat people with severe depression that has not responded to medication. Electric shocks that are administered to one side of the patient's head while he or she is under general anesthesia cause brain seizures that somehow relieve depression. The mechanism by which ECT works is as yet unknown. The treatment requires multiple sessions to achieve results; patients usually receive one, sometimes two, treatments per week over the course of nine to 12 weeks. Because ECT has the potential for serious side effects (e.g., reactions to anesthesia and memory loss) and because of the history of abuses of the treatment, ECT is a controversial treatment of last resort for people with the most refractory (treatment-resistant) depression.

Children Also Suffer from Depression

The most frequently diagnosed mood disorders in children and adolescents are major depressive disorder, dysthymic disorder, and bipolar disorder. Children who are depressed are not unlike their adult counterparts. They may be teary and sad, lose interest in friends and activities, and become listless, self-critical, and hypersensitive to criticism from others. They feel unloved, helpless, and hopeless about the future, and they may think about suicide. Depressed children and adolescents may also be irritable, aggressive, and indecisive. They may have problems concentrating and sleeping and often become careless about their appearance and hygiene. Depressed children often display anxiety symptoms, such as clinging to parents or not wanting to go to school. They also experience more somatic symptoms, such as general aches and pains, stomachaches, and headaches, than adults with depression.

Dysthymic disorder usually begins in childhood or early adolescence and is a chronic but milder depressive disorder with fewer symptoms. The child or adolescent is depressed on a daily basis for at least one year. Because the average duration of the disorder is about four years, some children become so accustomed to feeling depressed that they may not identify themselves as being depressed or complain about symptoms. In "Dysthymic Disorder among Children" (2012, http://www.nimh.nih.gov/statistics/1DD_CHILD.shtml), the NIMH estimates a lifetime prevalence of 11.2% of adolescents aged 13 to 18 years. Of these, 3.3% suffer a "severe" depressive disorder.

Reactive depression is the most common mental health problem in children and adolescents. It is not considered a mental disorder, and many health professionals consider occasional bouts of reactive depression as entirely consistent with normal adolescent development. It is characterized by transient depressed feelings in response to some negative experience, such as a rejection from a boyfriend or girlfriend or a failing grade. Sadness or listlessness spontaneously resolves in a few hours or may last as long as two weeks. Generally, distraction, in the form of a change of activity or setting, helps improve the mood of affected individuals.

BIPOLAR DISORDER

Bipolar disorder, also known as manic depression, is characterized by alternating periods of persistently elevated, expansive, or irritable mood—called mania—and periods of depression. During a manic episode, a person may feel inflated self-esteem and decreased need for sleep and be unusually talkative and easily distracted. He or she may also have flights of ideas, racing thoughts, increased goal-directed activity such as shopping, and excessive involvement in high-risk activities. According to the NIMH, in "Bipolar Disorder among Adults" (2012, http://www.nimh.nih.gov/statistics/1BIPOLAR_ADULT.shtml), bipolar disorder affects about 2.6% of the U.S. adult population, and the median age of onset is 25.

During the early stages of the illness patients may experience few symptoms or even symptom-free periods between relatively mild episodes of mania and depression. As the illness progresses, however, manic and depressive episodes become more serious and more frequent. Patients are less likely to experience intermissions, manic euphoria is increasingly replaced by irritability, and depressions deepen. Some individuals suffer psychotic episodes during periods of mania or depression. Bipolar disorder is one of the most lethal illnesses. According to Frederick K. Good-

win and Kay Redfield Jamison, in *Manic-Depressive Illness* (2007), "Patients with depressive and manic-depressive illnesses are far more likely to commit suicide than individuals in any other psychiatric or medical risk group. The mortality rate for untreated manic-depressive patients is higher than it is for most types of heart disease and many types of cancer."

The onset of bipolar illness is usually a depressive episode during adolescence. Manic episodes may not appear for months or even years. During manic episodes adolescents are tireless, overly confident, and tend to have rapid-fire or pressured speech. They may perform tasks and schoolwork quickly and energetically but in a wildly disorganized manner. Manic adolescents may seriously overestimate their capabilities, and the combination of bravado and loosened inhibitions may prompt them to participate in high-risk behaviors, such as vandalism, drug abuse, or unsafe sex. The NIMH reports in "Bipolar Disorder among Children" (2012, http://www.nimh.nih.gov/statistics/1BIPOLAR_CHILD.shtml) that the lifetime prevalence of bipolar disorder may be as high as 3% of adolescents aged 13 to 18 years. The disorder can run in families, and treatment for children and adolescents is similar to the treatment that is given to adults.

In "Trends in Antipsychotic Drug Use by Very Young, Privately Insured Children" (*Journal of the American Academy of Child and Adolescent Psychiatry*, vol. 49, no. 1, January 2010), Mark Olfsen et al. confirm that the number of very young children (aged two to five years) who were diagnosed with bipolar disorder and other mental disorders and prescribed powerful antipsychotic drugs increased between 2001 and 2007. During this same period there was a slight decrease in the proportion of very young children who received psychotherapy. Olfsen et al. observe that "most very young children treated with antipsychotic medications did not receive a mental health assessment, a psychotherapy visit, or treatment from a psychiatrist during the year of antipsychotic use" and that one out of 70 privately insured children in 2007 received a prescription drug that was intended to treat a mental disorder.

Treatments for Bipolar Disorder

Lithium has been widely used to treat bipolar disorder since the 1960s, and it is still the mood-stabilizing drug of choice for controlling the illness. During the 1970s psychiatrists also began using anticonvulsant drugs, including carbamazepine, clonazepam, and valproate, to treat patients who could not tolerate lithium or for whom the drug did not work. Other anticonvulsants, such as gabapentin, lamotrigine, and oxcarbazepine, have also been evaluated to treat the mania that is associated with bipolar disorder. Chlorpromazine and haloperidol, both antipsychotics, are also helpful in some cases. Antimanic and other antipsychotic agents, such as olanzapine, risperidone, and zipraisidone, are often combined with antidepressants to relieve depressive symptoms and to promote better sleep patterns, an important factor in maintaining patients' mood stability. These medication strategies have proven highly effective in treating bipolar disorder; however, many patients still experience a residual pattern of ups and downs.

Medications may become less effective over time and have to be changed. Another major concern among practitioners and patients are medication side effects, especially of lithium. Because therapeutic blood levels of the drug are close to fatal levels, patients taking lithium must consume adequate amounts of water and salt to prevent dehydration, which would cause lithium blood levels to rise to toxic levels. People who take lithium must have their blood level of the drug checked frequently, and they must also be aware of the signs of lithium poisoning. Long-term usage of the drug has been shown to cause kidney damage; however, adequate consumption of water and careful dosage monitoring are believed to reduce the risk of kidney disease.

The NIMH also explains in "How Is Bipolar Disorder Treated?" (http://www.nimh.nih.gov/health/publications/bipolar-disorder/how-is-bipolar-disorder-treated.shtml) that a combination of psychotherapy and medication may help people with bipolar disorder to "live symptom-free for longer periods and to recover from episodes more quickly." Research is under way to find out whether psychotherapy may delay the start of bipolar disorder in children who are at high risk for the illness.

When medication and psychotherapy are not effective, ECT may prove beneficial. Even though ECT may cause short-term side effects such as confusion, disorientation, and memory loss, these side effects generally subside after treatment.

SCHIZOPHRENIA

A person who hears voices, becomes violent, and sometimes ends up being homeless, muttering and shouting incomprehensibly, frequently suffers from schizophrenia. This disease generally presents in adolescence, causing hallucinations, paranoia, delusions, and social isolation. The effects begin slowly and, initially, are often considered to be the normal behavioral changes of adolescence. Gradually, voices take over in the schizophrenic's mind, obliterating reality and directing the person to all kinds of erratic behaviors. Suicide attempts and violent attacks are not uncommon to schizophrenics. In an attempt to escape the torment that is inflicted by their brains, many schizophrenics turn to drugs. The NIMH observes in "Schizophrenia" (November 21, 2011, http://www.nimh.nih.gov/health/publications/schizophrenia/complete-index.shtml) that people who have schizophrenia abuse alcohol and/or drugs more often than the general population.

In "Numbers Count," the NIMH reports that 1.1% of the U.S. population suffers from schizophrenia and similar disorders. Even though the precise causes of schizophrenia are unknown, for years researchers have hypothesized that genetic susceptibility is a risk factor for schizophrenia and bipolar disorder. According to Undine E. Lang et al., in "Molecular Mechanisms of Schizophrenia" (*Cellular Physiology and Biochemistry*, vol. 20, no. 6, 2007), "family, twin and adoption studies [demonstrate] a high heritability of the disease."

Imaging studies of the brain reveal abnormal brain development in children who have schizophrenia, and imaging studies of adults with the disease find enlargement of the ventricles of the brain. Some studies suggest that the brain of a person with schizophrenia manufactures too much dopamine, a chemical that is vital to normal nerve activity. Conventional drug treatment focuses on blocking dopamine receptors in the brain, but not all people with schizophrenia respond to treatment. This type of treatment can produce serious side effects. Newer antipsychotic medications that are used to treat the disorder, such as risperidone, have fewer side effects than previously used medications. Regardless, patients who take these medications must be monitored closely for serious side effects such as the loss of the white blood cells that fight infection.

ANXIETY DISORDERS

Everyone experiences some degree of anxiety almost every day. In the 21st century, a certain amount of anxiety is unavoidable and, in some cases, may even be beneficial. For example, mild anxiety before an exam or a job interview may actually improve performance. Anxiety before a surgical operation, giving a speech, or driving in bad weather is normal.

Nevertheless, when anxiety becomes extreme or when an attack of anxiety strikes suddenly, without an apparent external cause, it can be both debilitating and destructive. Its symptoms may include nervousness, fear, a "knot" in the stomach, rapid heartbeat, or increased blood pressure. If the anxiety is severe and long lasting, more serious problems may develop. People suffering from anxiety over an extended period may have headaches, ulcers, irritable bowel syndrome, insomnia, and depression. Because anxiety tends to create various other emotional and physical symptoms, a "snowball" effect can occur in which these problems produce even more anxiety.

Chronic anxiety can interfere with an individual's ability to lead a normal life. Mental health professionals consider a person who has prolonged anxiety as having an anxiety disorder. In "Anxiety Disorders: Introduction" (July 7, 2009, http://www.nimh.nih.gov/health/publications/anxiety-disorders/introduction.shtml), the NIMH estimates that approximately 40 million Americans aged 18 years and older suffer from anxiety disorders.

Panic Disorder

Extremely high levels of anxiety may produce panic attacks that are both unanticipated and seemingly without cause. In one type of panic attack, called unexpected, the sufferer is unable to predict when an attack will occur. Other types of panic attacks are linked to a particular location, circumstance, or event and are called situationally bound or situationally predisposed panic attacks. These panic episodes can last as long as 30 minutes and are marked by an overwhelming sense of impending doom while the person's heart races and breathing quickens to the point of gasping for air. Sweating, weakness, dizziness, terror, and feelings of unreality are also typical. Individuals undergoing a panic attack fear they are going to lose control, "lose their mind," or even die. The NIMH estimates in "Panic Disorder" (July 15, 2011, http://www.nimh.nih.gov/health/publications/anxiety-disorders/panic-disorder.shtml) that about 6 million Americans suffer from panic disorders. It also notes that panic disorders are twice as common in women as in men and usually begin in early adulthood.

Repeated panic attacks may be called a panic disorder. Research reveals that people who experience panic attacks tend to suppress their emotions. Researchers hypothesize that this tendency leads to an emotional buildup for which a panic attack is a form of release. Interestingly, most people who suffer from panic attacks do not experience anxiety between attacks.

The usual treatment for panic disorder is CBT combined with antianxiety drugs to treat the fear of the attacks. Sometimes antidepressant medications are used, even though people suffering from anxiety disorders are usually not clinically depressed. Relaxation therapy has also proved beneficial.

Phobias

Phobias are defined as unreasonable fears that are associated with a particular situation or object. The most common of the many varieties of phobias are specific phobias. Fear of bees, snakes, rodents, heights, odors, blood, needles, and storms are examples of common specific phobias. Specific phobias, especially animal phobias, are common in children, but they can occur at any age. According to the NIMH, in "Specific Phobias" (July 7, 2009, http://www.nimh.nih.gov/health/publications/anxiety-disorders/specific-phobias.shtml), 19.2 million American adults suffer from specific phobias. Most people with a phobia understand that their fears are unreasonable, but this awareness does not make them feel any less anxious.

Some specific phobias, such as a fear of heights, usually do not interfere with daily life or cause as much distress as more severe forms, such as agoraphobia. People suffering from severe phobias may rearrange their lives drastically to avoid the situations they fear will trigger panic attacks.

SOCIAL PHOBIAS. Social phobias (also called social anxiety disorders) can be more serious than specific phobias. A person with social phobia is intensely afraid of being judged by others. At social gatherings the person with social phobia expects to be singled out, scrutinized, judged, and found lacking. People with social phobias are usually very anxious about feeling humiliated or embarrassed. They are often so crippled by their own fears that they may have a hard time thinking clearly, remembering facts, or carrying on normal conversations. The individual with social phobia may tremble, sweat, or blush and often fears fainting or losing bladder or bowel control in social settings. In response to these overwhelming fears, the person with social phobia tries to avoid public situations and gatherings of people. The NIMH estimates in "Anxiety Disorders: Social Phobia (Social Anxiety Disorder)" (July 7, 2009, http://www.nimh.nih.gov/health/publications/anxiety-disorders/social-phobia-social-anxiety-disorder.shtml) that about 15 million adults suffer from social phobias. Social phobias tend to start at around age 13 and, if not treated, can continue throughout life.

Because social phobics fear being the center of attention or the subject of criticism, public speaking, asking questions, eating in front of others, or even attending social events create anxiety. Social phobias should not be confused with shyness, which is considered to be a normal variation in personality. Social phobias can be disabling, preventing sufferers from attending school, working, and having friends.

AGORAPHOBIA. Many people who experience panic attacks go on to develop agoraphobia—the fear of crowds and open spaces. The term comes from the Greek word *agora*, which means "marketplace." This type of phobia is a severely disabling disorder that often traps its victims, rendering them virtual prisoners in their own home, unable to work, shop, or attend social activities.

Agoraphobia normally develops slowly, following an initial unexpected panic attack. For example, on an ordinary day, while shopping, driving to work, or doing errands, the individual is suddenly struck by a wave of terror that is characterized by symptoms such as trembling, a pounding heart, profuse sweating, and difficulty in breathing normally. The person desperately seeks safety and reassurance from friends or family. The panic subsides and all is well—until another panic attack occurs.

The person with agoraphobia begins to avoid all places and situations where an attack occurred and then begins to avoid places where an attack could possibly occur or where it might be difficult to escape and get help. Gradually, the victim becomes more and more limited in the choice of places that are "safe." Eventually, the person with agoraphobia cannot venture outside the immediate neighborhood or leave the house. The fear ultimately expands to touch every aspect of the victim's life.

In "Agoraphobia" (2012, http://www.nimh.nih.gov/statistics/pdf/NCS-R_Agoraphobia.pdf), the NIMH explains that agoraphobia usually begins during the late teens or 20s and that the average age-of-onset is 20.

PHOBIA TREATMENT PROGRAMS. Phobia treatment programs use a wide variety of CBT techniques to help patients face and overcome their fears. In addition, drugs may be used to ease the symptoms of anxiety, fear, and depression and to help the person return to a normal life more quickly. Antidepressants have been shown to help people who suffer from panic attacks and agoraphobia. In addition, antianxiety drugs are useful in treating the generalized anxiety that frequently accompanies phobias.

Deborah C. Beidel et al. indicate in "SET-C versus Fluoxetine in the Treatment of Childhood Social Phobia" (*Journal of the American Academy of Child and Adolescent Psychiatry*, vol. 46, no. 12, December 2007) that behavioral therapy was more effective than drug treatment in helping children overcome social phobias. Even though many children were helped by treatment with fluoxetine, the behavioral therapy appeared to offer more global benefits by also helping the children to improve their social skills and overall functioning.

In "Attention Training in Individuals with Generalized Social Phobia: A Randomized Controlled Trial" (*Journal of Consulting and Clinical Psychology*, vol. 77, no. 5, October 2009), Nader Amir et al. consider whether people suffering from social phobia can be conditioned to divert their attention from a perceived threat and thus reduce symptoms of social anxiety. In the study's Attention Modification Program (AMP), participants were shown pictures of faces with either threatening or neutral emotional expressions that were placed at different locations on a computer screen. Participants in this group were given a prompt on the screen that directed them to the neutral faces, thereby directing attention away from the threatening ones. In the control group, the prompt appeared with equal frequency in the position of the threatening and neutral faces. The results of the study, which measured clinician-observed and self-reported symptoms, show the AMP group had reduced symptoms of anxiety and suggest that such training may be helpful for treating social phobia.

Obsessive-Compulsive Disorder

Obsessive-compulsive disorder (OCD) is an anxiety disorder that is marked by unwanted, often unpleasant recurring thoughts (obsessions) and repetitive, often mechanical behaviors (compulsions). The repetitive behaviors, such as continually checking to be certain windows and doors are locked or repeated hand washing, are intended to dispel the obsessive thoughts that trigger them—that an intruder will enter the house through an unlocked door or window, or that disease will be prevented by hand washing. The vicious cycle of obsessions and compulsions only serves to heighten anxiety; OCD can debilitate those who have the disorder.

The symptoms of OCD generally appear during childhood or adolescence. Imaging studies using positron emission tomography (PET) reveal that people with OCD have different patterns of brain activity than those without the disorder. Furthermore, the PET scans show that the part of the brain that is most affected by OCD (the striatum) changes and responds to both medication and behavioral therapy.

Many of the medications that are used to treat other anxiety disorders appear effective for patients with OCD, as has a behavioral type of therapy called "exposure and response prevention," during which patients with OCD learn new ways to manage their obsessive thoughts without resorting to compulsive behaviors.

Anxiety among Children and Adolescents

Children and adolescents suffer from many of the same anxiety disorders as do adults. Taken together, the different types of anxiety disorders constitute the mental disorders that are most prevalent among children and adolescents. In "Service Utilization for Lifetime Mental Disorders in U.S. Adolescents," Merikangas et al. find that most adolescents with mental disorders do not receive treatment for their symptoms and that the "treatment gap is especially pronounced for anxiety."

Separation anxiety disorder is a type of anxiety disorder that is found specifically in children. It is normal for infants, toddlers, and very young children to experience anxiety when separated from their parents or caregivers. For example, nearly every child experiences at least a momentary pang of separation anxiety on the first day of preschool or kindergarten. When this condition occurs in older children or adolescents and it is severe enough to impair social, academic, or job functioning for at least one month, it is considered separation anxiety disorder. The risk factors that are associated with separation anxiety disorder include stress, the illness or death of a family member, geographic relocation, and physical or sexual assault.

Children with separation anxiety may be clingy, and often they harbor fears that accidents or natural disasters will forever separate them from their parents. Because they fear being apart from their parents, they may resist attending school or going anywhere without a parent. Separation anxiety can produce physical symptoms such as dizziness, nausea, or palpitations. It is often associated with symptoms of depression. Young children with separation anxiety may have difficulty falling asleep alone in their room and may have recurrent nightmares.

According to the U.S. Department of Health and Human Services (HHS), research suggests that some children develop OCD following an infection with a specific type of streptococcus. This condition is known as pediatric autoimmune neuropsychiatric disorders associated with streptococcal (PANDAS) infections. It is believed that antibodies intended to combat the strep infection mistakenly attack a region of the brain and trigger an inflammatory reaction, which in turn leads to the development of OCD. In "The PANDAS Subgroup of Tic Disorders and Childhood-Onset Obsessive-Compulsive Disorder" (*Journal of Psychosomatic Research*, vol. 67, no. 6, December 2009), Davide Martino, Giovanni Defazio, and Gavin Giovannoni suggest that in addition to childhood-onset OCD, the PANDAS spectrum may also include ADHD. SSRIs are effective in reducing or even eliminating the symptoms of OCD in many affected children and adolescents. However, side effects such as dry mouth, sleepiness, dizziness, fatigue, tremors, and constipation are common and may themselves impair functioning.

ATTENTION DEFICIT/ HYPERACTIVITY DISORDER

Attention deficit disorder (ADD) and attention deficit/hyperactivity disorder (ADHD) are relatively new names for psychiatric disorders that usually begin or become apparent in children going to preschool and elementary school. Children with ADHD cannot sit still, have difficulty controlling their impulsive actions, and are unable to focus on projects long enough to complete them; those who are diagnosed with ADD have the same symptoms but do not display hyperactivity. Even though teachers originally dubbed ADHD a "learning problem," the disorder affects more than just schoolwork. Children with ADHD have trouble socializing, are often unable to make friends, and suffer from low self-esteem. If left untreated, ADHD can leave children unable to cope academically or socially, possibly leading to depression.

According to the NIMH, in "What Conditions Can Coexist with ADHD?" (January 23, 2009, http://www.nimh .nih.gov/health/publications/attention-deficit-hyperactivity-disorder/what-conditions-can-coexist-with-adhd .shtml), the condition frequently coexists with other mental health problems, such as a learning disability, anxiety and depression, bipolar disorder, Tourette syndrome (a neurological disorder that is characterized by repeated, involuntary movements and uncontrollable vocal sounds), or antisocial behavior. According to Merikangas et al., in "Prevalence and Treatment of Mental Disorders among US Children in the 2001—2004 NHANES," the NHANES finds that higher rates of ADHD were reported in children of lower socioeconomic status. Children diagnosed with ADHD are usually affected into their teen years, but for most, symptoms subside in adulthood and adults become more adept at controlling their behavior. Regardless, vigilance is warranted because research reveals an increased incidence in juvenile delinquency and subsequent encounters with the criminal justice sys-

tem among adults who were diagnosed with ADHD during their youth.

The reported incidence of ADHD has increased over the past 25 years, possibly because of better diagnosis, changing expectations, or insufficient supportive social structures. In the absence of clear criteria for ADHD or guidelines by which to diagnose it, researchers fear that the disorder may be under- or overdiagnosed. The cause of ADHD is as yet unknown. According to the NIMH, in "What Causes ADHD?" (January 23, 2009, http://www.nimh.nih.gov/health/publications/attention-deficit-hyperactivity-disorder/what-causes-adhd.shtml), "many studies suggest that genes play a large role." The NIMH also notes that ADHD is likely caused by a combination of things and suggests that environmental factors, brain injuries, nutrition, and social environment may play a role. A biological explanation of ADHD arose because its symptoms respond to treatment with stimulants such as methylphenidate, which increase the availability of dopamine—the neurotransmitter that is vital for purposeful movement, motivation, and alertness. As a result, researchers theorize that ADHD may be caused by the unavailability of dopamine in the central nervous system.

Genes have been offered as a cause of ADHD, but the evidence of a genetic component has been inconclusive. There is an increased incidence of ADHD in children with a first-degree relative with ADHD, conduct disorders, antisocial personality, substance abuse, and other problems, but this observation does not resolve the question of whether nature (genetics) or nurture (family and environmental influences) contributes more strongly to the origins of ADHD. Twin studies find that when ADHD is present in one twin, it is significantly more likely to be present in an identical twin than in a fraternal twin. These findings support inheritance as an important risk in a proportion of children with ADHD.

Even though imaging studies reveal differences in the brains of children with ADHD, and scientists have found a link between the inability to pay attention and the diminished utilization of glucose in parts of the brain, some researchers question whether these changes cause the disorder. They argue that the observed changes may result from the disorder, or simply coexist with it. As a result, some mental health professionals and educators concede that some children are legitimately diagnosed with ADHD and that others are mislabeled. They speculate that the latter group may be simply high-spirited, undisciplined, or misbehaving.

Treatment for ADHD

Much controversy about ADHD has focused on its treatment. NIMH research indicates that there are two effective treatment methods for elementary-school children with ADHD: a closely monitored medication regimen and a combination of medication and behavioral interventions. Behavioral interventions include psychotherapy, CBT, social skills training, support groups, and parent-educator skills training.

Even though some researchers still question the wisdom of treatment with potentially addicting, powerful stimulants, prescription stimulants (such as methylphenidate, dextromethamphetamine, and amphetamine) have proved to be safe and effective for short-term treatment of ADHD. Another prescription medication that is used to treat ADHD, atomoxetine, is a nonstimulant drug, but it carries the risk of serious side effects, including cardiovascular symptoms, psychotic symptoms, and increased suicidal tendencies.

In "A One Year Trial of Methylphenidate in the Treatment of ADHD" (*Journal of Attention Disorders*, vol. 15, no. 1, January 2011), Paul H. Wender et al. find that adults with ADHD who responded well to short-term treatment with methylphenidate also benefited from long-term treatment. Wender et al. report that long-term drug treatment resulted in "marked improvements in ADHD symptoms and psychosocial functioning."

Janice Pellow, Elizabeth M. Solomon, and Candice N. Barnard report in "Complementary and Alternative Medical Therapies for Children with Attention-Deficit/Hyperactivity Disorder (ADHD)" (*Alternative Medicine Review*, vol. 16, no. 4, December 2011) that people are becoming increasingly concerned about drug side effects and the long-term use of stimulants and as a result are turning to complementary and alternative medicine (CAM) approaches to ADHD treatment. Examples of CAM treatments include dietary modifications, such as eliminating refined carbohydrates; nutritional supplementation, such as adding essential fatty acids, vitamin B6, magnesium, iron, calcium, and zinc; and use of herbal medicine, including rhodiola, chamomile, and St. John's wort, to relive restlessness and anxiety. Pellow, Solomon, and Barnard observe that "CAM appears to be most effective when prescribed holistically and according to each individual's characteristic symptoms."

DISRUPTIVE DISORDERS

Children and adolescents with disruptive disorders, which include oppositional defiant disorder and conduct disorder, display antisocial behaviors. Like separation anxiety, the diagnosis of a disruptive disorder largely depends on assessing whether behavior is age appropriate. For example, just as clinging may be considered normal for a toddler but abnormal behavior in an older child, toddlers and very young children often behave aggressively (e.g., grabbing toys and even biting one another). When, however, a child older than age five displays such aggressive behavior, it may indicate an emerging oppositional defiant or conduct disorder.

It is important to distinguish isolated acts of aggression or the normal childhood and adolescent phases of testing limits from the pattern of ongoing, persistent defiance, hostility, and disobedience that is the hallmark of oppositional defiant disorder (ODD). Children with ODD are argumentative, lose their temper, refuse to adhere to rules, blame others for their own mistakes, and are spiteful and vindictive. Their behaviors often alienate them from family and peers and cause problems at school.

Family strife, volatile marital relationships, frequently changing caregivers, and inconsistent child-rearing practices may increase the risk for the disorder. Some practitioners consider ODD a gateway condition to conduct disorder. According to the Office of the Surgeon General, in *Mental Health*, estimates of the prevalence of ODD range from 1% to 6%, depending on the population and the way the disorder is evaluated. Prepubescent boys are diagnosed more often with ODD than girls of the same age, but after puberty the rates in both genders are equal.

Children or adolescents with conduct disorder are aggressive. They may fight, sexually assault, or behave cruelly to people or animals. Because lying, stealing, vandalism, truancy, and substance abuse are common behaviors, adults, social service agencies, and the criminal justice system often view affected young people as "bad" rather than as mentally ill. The American Academy of Child and Adolescent Psychiatry describes in "Conduct Disorders" (July 2004, http://www.aacap.org/cs/root/facts _for_families/conduct_disorder) an array of generally antisocial behaviors that when exhibited by children or adolescents suggest a diagnosis of conduct disorder. These actions and behaviors include:

- Bullying, threatening, or intimidating others
- Initiating physical fights
- Using a weapon such as a bat, brick, knife, or gun that can cause serious physical harm
- Being physically cruel to people or animals
- Stealing from a victim while confronting him or her
- Engaging in coercive or forced sexual activity
- Deliberately setting fires with the intention of causing damage
- Deliberately destroying others' property
- Breaking into a building, house, or car
- Lying to obtain goods or favors or to avoid obligations
- Stealing items without confronting a victim
- Staying out at night despite parental objections
- Running away from home
- Being truant from school

Conduct disorder severely compromises the lives of affected children and adolescents. Their schoolwork suffers, as do their relationships with adults and peers. The HHS finds that youths with conduct disorders have higher rates of injury and sexually transmitted diseases and are likely to be expelled from school and have problems with the law. Rates of depression, suicidal thoughts, suicide attempts, and suicide are all higher in children and teens who are diagnosed with conduct disorder. Children in whom the disorder presents before the age of 10 years are predominantly male. Early onset places them at a greater risk for adult antisocial personality disorder. More than a quarter of severely antisocial children become antisocial adults.

As of February 2012, there were no medications that had proven effective in treating conduct disorder. Even though psychosocial interventions can reduce their antisocial behavior, children or adolescents with a conduct disorder still create high levels of stress for the entire family. Support programs train parents how to positively reinforce appropriate behaviors and how to strengthen the emotional bonds between parent and child. Identifying and intervening with high-risk children to enhance their social interaction and prevent academic failure can mitigate some of the potentially harmful long-term consequences of conduct disorder. In "Five- to Six-Year Outcome and Its Prediction for Children with ODD/CD Treated with Parent Training" (*Journal of Child Psychology and Psychiatry*, vol. 51, no. 5, May 2010), May B. Drugli et al. find that the combination of parent training, which educates parents about the strategies for managing their child's behavior, and child treatment is effective for young children with conduct disorders.

Research demonstrates that preventive measures may help reduce conduct problems in children who exhibit the most aggressive or disruptive behaviors. E. Michael Foster et al. find in "Can a Costly Intervention Be Cost-Effective?: An Analysis of Violence Prevention" (*Archives of General Psychiatry*, vol. 63, no. 11, November 2006) that the costs of providing targeted interventions were small when compared with the personal and societal costs of family strife and crime that can result from untreated conduct disorders.

EATING DISORDERS

American society is preoccupied with body image. Advertisers of many products suggest that to be thin and beautiful is to be happy. Many prominent weight-loss programs reinforce this suggestion. A well-balanced, low-fat food plan, combined with exercise, can help most overweight people achieve a healthier weight and lifestyle. Dieting to achieve a healthy weight is quite different from dieting obsessively to become "model" thin, which can have consequences ranging from mildly harmful to life threatening. In *Eating Disorders* (2011, http://www.nimh.nih.gov/health/publications/eating-disorders/eating-disorders.pdf), the NIMH observes that eating disorders frequently coexist with other mental disorders, including depression, substance abuse, and anxiety disorders.

Preteens, teens, and college-age women are at special risk for eating disorders. In fact, most of those who develop an eating disorder are young women. However, James I. Hudson et al. report in "The Prevalence and Correlates of Eating Disorders in the National Comorbidity Survey Replication" (*Biological Psychiatry*, vol. 61, no. 3, February 2007) the results of an analysis of national survey data and suggest that as many as 25% of people with eating disorders are male. Researchers do not know exactly how many teenage boys and men are afflicted. Until recently, there has been a lack of awareness that eating disorders can be a problem for males, perhaps because men are more likely to mask the symptoms of eating disorders with excuses and rationales such as preventing heart disease or diabetes or trying to build a more muscular physique.

Research reveals that many people believe certain foods are addictive and that some people can become addicted to behaviors, such as fasting, bingeing, purging, and using laxatives, that are associated with disordered eating. People with bulimia may talk of being "hooked" on certain foods and needing to feed their "habits." This addictive behavior can carry over into other areas of a person's life, resulting, for example, in substance abuse. Many people with eating disorders suffer from comorbidities (having more than one disease or disorder at the same time), such as severe depression, which increases their risk for suicide. In "Beliefs about Eating and Eating Disorders" (*Eating Behaviors*, vol. 10, no. 3, August 2009), G. Terence Wilson et al. note that because some researchers and clinicians view eating disorders as addictions, some of the types of treatments that are prescribed for eating disorders are comparable to substance (alcohol and drug) abuse and addiction treatment.

Anorexia Nervosa

Anorexia nervosa involves severe weight loss—a minimum of 15% below normal body weight. People with anorexia literally starve themselves, although they may be very hungry. For reasons that researchers do not yet fully understand, people with anorexia are irrationally fearful about gaining weight. They are often obsessed with food and weight, develop strange eating habits, refuse to eat with other people, and exercise strenuously to burn calories and prevent weight gain. Individuals with anorexia continue to believe they are overweight even when they are dangerously thin.

The medical complications of anorexia are similar to starvation. When the body attempts to protect its most vital organs—the heart and the brain—it goes into "slow gear." Monthly menstrual periods stop, and breathing, pulse, blood pressure, and thyroid function slow down. The nails and hair become brittle, and the skin dries. Water imbalance causes constipation, and the lack of body fat causes an inability to withstand cold temperatures. Depression, weakness, and a constant obsession with food are also symptoms of the disease. In addition, personality changes may occur. The person suffering from anorexia may have outbursts of anger and hostility or may withdraw socially. In the most serious cases, death can result.

Bulimia Nervosa

People who have bulimia nervosa eat compulsively and then purge (get rid of the food) through self-induced vomiting; use of laxatives, diuretics, strict diets, fasts, or exercise; or a combination of several of these compensatory behaviors. The NIMH reports in *Numbers Count* that an estimated 1.1% to 4.2% of females suffer from bulimia.

Many people with bulimia are at a normal body weight or higher because of their frequent binge-purge behavior, which can occur from once or twice per week to several times per day. Those people with bulimia who maintain normal weight may manage to keep their eating disorder secret for years. As with anorexia, bulimia usually begins during adolescence, but many people with bulimia do not seek help until they are in their 30s or 40s.

Both binge eating and purging are dangerous practices. Hudson et al. suggest that binge-eating disorder (bingeing that is not followed by purging, often resulting in obesity) is more prevalent than bulimia, with 3.5% of women and 2% of men suffering from it at some point during their lifetimes. In rare cases, bingeing can cause stomach ruptures. Purging can result in heart failure because the body loses vital minerals. The acid in vomit wears down tooth enamel and can cause scarring on the hands when fingers are pushed down the throat to induce vomiting. The esophagus may become inflamed, and glands in the neck may become swollen.

Causes of Eating Disorders

Mounting evidence suggests that there is a genetic component to susceptibility to eating disorders. For example, in "Understanding the Relation between Anorexia Nervosa and Bulimia Nervosa in a Swedish National Twin Sample" (*Biological Psychiatry*, vol. 67, no. 1, January 2010), Cynthia M. Bulik et al. examine the heritability of anorexia nervosa and bulimia nervosa and identify an overlap of genetic and environmental factors that influence the development of both eating disorders. The results of another twin study, "Shared and Unique Genetic and Environmental Influences on Binge Eating and Night Eating: A Swedish Twin Study" (*Eating Behaviors*, vol. 11, no. 2, April 2010) by Tammy L. Root et al., find that genetic factors make a strong contribution to risk for binge eating.

People with bulimia and anorexia seem to have different personalities. Those with bulimia are likely to be impulsive (acting without considering the consequences) and are more likely to abuse alcohol and drugs. People with anorexia tend to be perfectionists, good students, and competitive athletes. They usually keep their feelings to themselves and rarely disobey their parents. Regardless, people with bulimia and anorexia share certain traits: they lack self-esteem, they have feelings of helplessness, and they fear gaining weight. In both disorders the eating problems appear to develop as a way of handling stress and anxiety.

The person with bulimia consumes huge amounts of food in a search for comfort and stress relief. The bingeing, however, brings only guilt and depression. In contrast, people with anorexia restrict food to gain a sense of control and mastery over some aspect of their lives. Controlling their body weight seems to offer two advantages: they can take control of their body and can gain approval from others.

Treatment of Eating Disorders

Generally, a physician treats the medical complications of the disorder, while a nutritionist advises the affected individual about specific diet and eating plans. To help the person with an eating disorder face his or her underlying problems and emotional issues, psychotherapy is usually necessary. People with eating disorders, whether they are normal weight, overweight, or obese, should seek help from a mental health professional such as a psychiatrist, psychologist, or clinical social worker for their eating behavior. Sometimes the challenge is to convince people with eating disorders to seek and obtain treatment; other times it is difficult to gain their adherence to treatment. Many anorexics deny their illness, and getting and keeping anorexic patients in treatment can be difficult. Treating bulimia is similarly difficult. Many bulimics are easily frustrated and want to leave treatment if their symptoms are not quickly relieved.

Several approaches are used to treat eating disorders. CBT teaches people how to monitor their eating and change unhealthy eating habits. It also teaches them how to change the way they respond to stressful situations. CBT is based on the premise that thinking influences emotions and behavior—that feelings and actions originate with thoughts. CBT posits that it is possible to change the way people feel and act, even if their circumstances do not change. It teaches the advantages of feeling calm when faced with undesirable situations. CBT clients learn that they will confront undesirable events and circumstances whether they become troubled about them or not. When they are troubled about events or circumstances, they have two problems: the troubling event or circumstance, and the troubling feelings about the event or circumstance. Clients learn that when they do not become troubled about trying events and circumstances, they can reduce the number of problems that they face by half.

IPT helps people to look at their relationships with friends and family and make changes to resolve problems. IPT is short-term therapy that has demonstrated effectiveness for the treatment of depression. According to the International Society for Interpersonal Psychotherapy, IPT does not assume that mental illness arises exclusively from problematical interpersonal relationships. It does emphasize, however, that mental health and emotional problems occur within an interpersonal context. For this reason, the therapy aims to intervene specifically in social functioning to relieve symptoms.

Like other forms of psychotherapy, IPT may be used in conjunction with medications. Because eating disorders frequently recur, it is recommended that successful short-term treatment be combined with ongoing maintenance therapy, such as monthly sessions following completion of the short-term phase.

Group therapy has been found helpful for bulimics, who are relieved to find that they are not alone or unique in their binge-eating behaviors. A combination of behavioral therapy and family systems therapy is often the most effective with anorexics. Family systems therapy considers the family as the unit of treatment and focuses on relationships and communication patterns within the family rather than on the personality traits or symptoms that are displayed by individual family members. Family systems therapy also considers the family as an entity that is more than the sum of its individual members and uses systems theory to determine family members' roles within the system as a whole. Problems are addressed by modifying the system rather than by trying to change an individual family member. People with eating disorders who also suffer from depression may benefit from antidepressant and antianxiety medications to help relieve coexisting mental health problems.

Recovery from eating disorders is uneven. The Eating Disorders Coalition for Research, Policy, and Action characterizes recovery as a process that frequently entails multiple rehospitalizations, limited ability to work or attend school, and limited capacity for interpersonal relationships.

In "The Myths of Motivation: Time for a Fresh Look at Some Received Wisdom in the Eating Disorders?" (*International Journal of Eating Disorders*, vol. 45, no. 1, January 2012), Glenn Waller of the Vincent Square Eating Disorders Clinic in London, England, observes that the lack of motivation to change, arising from feelings of helplessness or hopelessness, may impede recovery from eating disorders. He opines that behavioral strategies to enhance motivation should be explored to improve the effectiveness of eating disorders treatment.

PRESCRIBING PSYCHOACTIVE MEDICATION TO CHILDREN

In "Treatment of Children with Mental Illness" (2009, http://www.nimh.nih.gov/health/publications/treatment-of-children-with-mental-illness-fact-sheet/nimh-treatment-children-mental-illness-faq.pdf), a publication aimed at the parents of children with a range of mental disorders, the NIMH acknowledges public concern that psychotropic medication is being prescribed to very young children and that the safety and efficacy of most psychotropic medications, especially for children under the age of six years, have not yet been established. Several widely used drugs have not received FDA approval for use in young children simply because there are not enough data to support their use.

The data are lacking because historically there were ethical concerns about involving children in clinical trials to determine not only the most effective treatments but also the proper dosage, the potential side effects, and the long-term effects of drug use on learning and development. Policies about research involving children affect the FDA approval process and recommendations for use. For example, methylphenidate is approved for use in children aged six years and older, but its use was not evaluated in children younger than age six. In contrast, dextromethamphetamine received approval for use in children as young as three years old because by the time approval was sought, study guidelines permitted participation of younger children. Highlighting the discrepancies in the approved starting ages of patients for certain drugs, Table 8.2 lists the brand and generic names of prescription

TABLE 8.2

Prescription drugs used to treat ADHD

Trade name	Generic name	FDA-approved age
ADHD medications		
(All of these ADHD medications are stimulants, except Strattera.)		
Adderall	amphetamine	3 and older
Adderall XR	amphetamine (extended release)	6 and older
Concerta	methylphenidate (long acting)	6 and older
Daytrana	methylphenidate patch	6 and older
Desoxyn	methamphetamine	6 and older
Dexedrine	dextroamphetamine	3 and older
Dextrostat	dextroamphetamine	3 and older
Focalin	dexmethylphenidate	6 and older
Focalin XR	dexmethylphenidate (extended release)	6 and older
Metadate ER	methylphenidate (extended release)	6 and older
Metadate CD	methylphenidate (extended release)	6 and older
Methylin	methylphenidate (oral solution and chewable tablets)	6 and older
Ritalin	methylphenidate	6 and older
Ritalin SR	methylphenidate (extended release)	6 and older
Ritalin LA	methylphenidate (long-acting)	6 and older
Strattera	atomoxetine	6 and older
Vyvanse	lisdexamfetamine dimesylate	

ADHD = Attention Deficit Hyperactivity Disorder
FDA = Food & Drug Administration

SOURCE: "ADHD Medications," in *Mental Health Medications: Alphabetical List of Medications*, National Institute of Mental Health, April 25, 2011, http://www.nimh.nih.gov/health/publications/mental-health-medications/alphabetical-list-of-medications.shtml (accessed January 9, 2012)

TABLE 8.3

Prescription drugs used to treat anxiety disorders

Trade name	Generic name	FDA-approved age
Antianxiety medications		
(All of these antianxiety medications are benzodiazepines, except BuSpar.)		
Ativan	lorazepam	18 and older
BuSpar	buspirone	18 and older
Klonopin	clonazepam	18 and older
Librium	chlordiazepoxide	18 and older
Oxazepam (generic only)	oxazepam	18 and older
Tranxene	clorazepate	18 and older
Valium	diazepam	18 and older
Xanax	alprazolam	18 and older

FDA = Food & Drug Administration

SOURCE: "Anti-Anxiety Medications," in *Mental Health Medications: Alphabetical List of Medications*, National Institute of Mental Health, April 25, 2011, http://www.nimh.nih.gov/health/publications/mental-health-medications/alphabetical-list-of-medications.shtml (accessed January 9, 2012)

medications that are used to treat ADHD in children and adolescents and indicates FDA approval of their use in children aged six years and older and aged three years and older. In contrast, none of the drugs that are prescribed to treat anxiety are FDA approved for use in people under the age of 18 years. (See Table 8.3.)

Because the FDA approval process often requires years of research to demonstrate safety and efficacy, and practitioners are eager to provide symptom relief for severely troubled children, many recommend off-label use of medications. Off-label treatment may involve the use of a medication that has not yet received official FDA approval for use in children or the use of a drug the FDA has approved for use in children for a different condition. As such, they are prescribed off-label when used in pediatric and adolescent medicine. The NIMH observes that some off-label use is supported by data from well-controlled studies but cautions that other off-label prescribing, particularly to very young children whose responses to these drugs have not been scrutinized, should be performed prudently.

In "Which Groups Have Special Needs When Taking Psychiatric Medications?" (January 9, 2012, http://www.nimh.nih.gov/), the NIMH notes that there is strong support for the safety and efficacy of several medications for a variety of conditions, specifically psychostimulants for ADHD. However, the NIMH also indicates that there is a lack of information about the safety and efficacy of other medications and warns that children may have different reactions to drugs than do adults. The NIMH also cautions that antidepressants and ADHD medications carry FDA warnings about potentially dangerous side effects for young people. The NIMH concludes, "In addition to medications, other treatments for young people with mental disorders should be considered. Psy-chotherapy, family therapy, educational courses, and behavior management techniques can help everyone involved cope with the disorder."

SUICIDE

Suicide may be the ultimate expression or consequence of depression or another serious mental disorder. Not all people who suffer from depression contemplate suicide, nor do all those who attempt suicide suffer from depressive or other mental illnesses. Regardless, except for certain desperate medical situations, suicide in the United States is generally considered to be an unacceptable act. It is often referred to as a "long-term solution to a short-term problem."

In *Health, United States, 2010* (2011, http://www.cdc.gov/nchs/data/hus/hus10.pdf), the National Center for Health Statistics observes that since 1970 the death rate for suicide has decreased from 13.1 suicides per 100,000 resident population to 11.3 deaths per 100,000 in 2007. According to the NIMH, in "Suicide in the U.S.: Statistics and Prevention" (September 27, 2010, http://www.nimh.nih.gov/health/publications/suicide-in-the-us-statistics-and-prevention.shtml), in 2007 suicide ranked as the 10th-leading cause of death in the United States. It was the seventh-leading cause of death for males and the 15th-leading cause of death for females. In 2008 suicidal behavior resulted in 323,342 emergency department visits, 197,838 hospitalizations, and 35,045 deaths. (See Figure 8.7.)

FIGURE 8.7

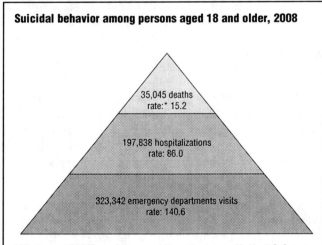

Suicidal behavior among persons aged 18 and older, 2008

35,045 deaths
rate:* 15.2

197,838 hospitalizations
rate: 86.0

323,342 emergency departments visits
rate: 140.6

*All rates per 100,000 population; population estimates provided by U.S. Census Bureau.

SOURCE: Alex E. Crosby et al., "Figure 1. Public Health Burden of Suicidal Behavior among Adults Aged ≥18 Years—United States, 2008," in "Suicidal Thoughts and Behaviors among Adults Aged ≥18 Years—United States, 2008–2009," *Morbidity and Mortality Weekly Report*, vol. 60, no. 3, October 21, 2011, http://www.cdc.gov/mmwr/pdf/ss/ss6013.pdf (accessed January 9, 2012)

Who Commits Suicide?

Suicide occurs among men and women of all racial, occupational, religious, and social groups, as well as all age groups, with the exception of the very young. Alex E. Crosby et al. explain in "Suicidal Thoughts and Behaviors among Adults Aged ≥18 Years—United States, 2008–2009" (*Morbidity and Mortality Weekly Report*, vol. 60, no. 13, October 21, 2011) that suicide is the fourth-leading cause of death among children aged 10 to 14 years, the third among people aged 15 to 24 years, the fourth among people aged 25 to 44 years, and the eighth among those aged 45 to 64 years.

The number of completed suicides does not give an accurate picture of the problem, because for every completed suicide there are many unsuccessful suicide attempts. Crosby et al. report that between 2007 and 2008 approximately 569,000 people visited the emergency department for "self-directed violence" and nearly three-quarters of these visits involved suicide attempts. Furthermore, research reveals that more than half of the people who engage in suicidal behavior are not counted because they do not seek medical care or treatment.

Crosby et al. find that suicidal thoughts are more prevalent in young adults aged 18 to 29 years and among females. Suicidal thoughts, plans, and suicide attempts were also more common among young adults—people aged 18 to 29 years had a significantly higher prevalence of suicide planning than those aged 30 years and older.

According to Crosby et al., only a small proportion of those who attempt suicide eventually die by suicide. Nonfatal suicidal behavior is different from fatal suicidal behavior. For example, the rates of fatal suicidal behavior are higher among males and middle-aged or older adults, whereas females, adolescents, and young adults have higher rates of nonfatal suicidal behavior. People with a history of suicide attempts are at greater risk for dying by suicide than those who have no history of suicidal behavior.

Interestingly, female suicide rates do not change as drastically as men's do as they age. One widely held theory about the high rates among white men older than the age of 65 years is that these men, who traditionally have been in positions of power, have great difficulty adjusting to a life they may consider useless or diminished.

Why Do People Commit Suicide?

People commit suicide for various reasons. Notes left by people who have killed themselves usually tell of life crises that they believed were unbearable. Many describe enduring chronic pain, losing loved ones, being unable to pay bills, or finding themselves incapable of living independently. Crosby et al. observe that depression, substance abuse, physical abuse, and sexual abuse are risk factors for suicide attempts by adolescents.

Some suicides are committed on an irrational, impulsive whim. Researchers observe that even among those who are most determined to commit suicide, the desire is not as much to die as it is to escape the life they are leading and to end the pain they are suffering. Whatever the cause of their despair, they are desperately crying out for help.

Follow-up studies on suicide survivors reveal their intense ambivalence about actually dying. Not all survivors are glad to be alive, but for most, the attempted suicide marked a definite turning point. It was an urgent and dramatic signal that their problems demanded serious and immediate attention. Most of the survivors said that what they really wanted was to change their lives.

Suicide among the Terminally Ill

Not all suicides are categorized as the acts of people who are mentally ill. Some people consider suicides committed by people who are terminally ill as rational choices. They argue that people who are terminally ill have the right to die—that is, the right to control the manner of their death. Patients with terminal diseases often worry that they will suffer long and painful deaths and that they stand a good chance of losing everything: health, independence, jobs, insurance, homes, and contact with loved ones and friends.

Researchers find that factors with significant impact on the quality of life include security, family, love, pleasurable activity, and freedom from pain and suffering. Sufferers of debilitating disease may lose all of these. For some, suicide is a last recourse to relieve pain, suffering, insecurity, dependence, or hopelessness.

The right to die and to choose the time and manner of death remains a hotly debated topic throughout the world. In the United States, just three states—Oregon, Washington, and Montana—have legalized physician-assisted suicide. Since 1994 Oregon's Death with Dignity Act has allowed a terminally ill adult to request a prescription for a lethal dose of drugs. The legislation contains many restrictions that are intended to protect both patients and the physicians who prescribe the drugs. In an analysis of the law's application, Ronald A. Lindsay of the Center for Inquiry in Amherst, New York, observes in "Oregon's Experience: Evaluating the Record" (*American Journal of Bioethics*, vol. 9, no. 3, March 2009) that none of the untoward consequences feared by the law's staunchest opponents—specifically that it would affect "vulnerable groups disproportionately, that legal assisted dying could not be confined to the competent terminally ill who voluntarily request assistance, and that the practice would result in frequent abuses"—have materialized. Lindsay asserts that Oregon's experience "argues in favor of legalization of assistance in dying."

In March 2008 Washington became the second state to permit physician-assisted suicide. Like the Oregon legislation, Washington's law aims to restrict the practice to minimize the potential for abuse. Patients must make two requests, more than two weeks apart, and one must be in writing. The patient must be of sound mind and not suffering from depression, and two physicians must approve the request for a lethal dose of drugs. In December 2009 Montana became the third state to legalize physician-assisted suicide.

Suicide's Warning Signs

Researchers believe that most suicidal people convey their intentions to someone among their friends and family, either openly or indirectly. The people they signal are those who know them well and are in the best position to recognize the signs and provide help. Comments such as "You'd be better off without me," "No one will have to worry about me much longer," or even a casual "I've had it" may be signals of upcoming attempts. Some people who are suicidal put their affairs in order. They draw up wills, give away prized possessions, or act as if they are preparing for a long trip. They may even talk about going away.

Often, the indicator is a distinct change in personality or behavior. A normally happy person may become increasingly depressed, a regular churchgoer may stop attending services, or an avid runner may quit exercising. These types of changes, if added to expressions of worthlessness or hopelessness, can indicate not only that the person is seriously depressed but also that he or she may have decided to commit suicide. Even though the vast majority of people who are depressed are not suicidal, most of the suicide-prone are depressed. Researchers and health care practitioners caution that suicide threats and attempts should not be discounted as harmless bids for attention. Anyone thinking, talking about, or planning suicide should receive immediate professional evaluation and treatment.

CHAPTER 9
COMPLEMENTARY AND ALTERNATIVE MEDICINE

The National Center for Complementary and Alternative Medicine (NCCAM; formerly the Office of Alternative Medicine, established in 1992) is one of the 27 institutes and centers of the National Institutes of Health (NIH). The center was created because consumers of complementary and alternative medicine (CAM) and health care practitioners wanted to know whether available alternative medical options were safe and effective. In "NCCAM Facts-at-a-Glance and Mission" (January 2, 2012, http://nccam.nih.gov/about/ataglance/), the NCCAM states that its mission is to "define, through rigorous scientific investigation, the usefulness and safety of complementary and alternative medicine interventions and their roles in improving health and health care." To determine a method's or product's effectiveness and safety, the organization uses a hierarchy of evidence. (See Figure 9.1.) Studies indicate that data on the efficacy and safety of CAM therapies span a continuum ranging from anecdotes and case studies to encouraging information that has been obtained from large, well-developed clinical trials.

In "What Is Complementary and Alternative Medicine?" (July 2011, http://nccam.nih.gov/health/whatiscam/), the NCCAM defines complementary and alternative medicine as "a group of diverse medical and health care systems, practices, and products that are not generally considered part of conventional medicine." Even though there is some overlap between them, the NCCAM further distinguishes between complementary, alternative, and integrative medicine in the following manner:

- Alternative medicine is therapy or treatment that is used instead of conventional medical treatment. One example of alternative medicine is the treatment of depression with St. John's wort, a botanical, herbal medicine, rather than with conventional antidepressant drugs.

- Complementary medicine is alternative therapy or treatment that is used along with conventional

medicine, not in place of it. An example of complementary medicine is the addition of relaxation techniques or movement awareness therapies (such as the Alexander technique, Pilates, and the Feldenkrais method) to the traditional approaches of physical and occupational therapy that are used to rehabilitate people who have had a stroke. Complementary medicine appears to offer health benefits, but there is generally no scientific evidence to support its utility.

- Integrative medicine is the combination of conventional medical treatment and CAM therapies that have been scientifically researched and have demonstrated that they are both safe and effective. An example of integrative medicine is teaching stress management and relaxation techniques to people with high blood pressure and heart disease along with the use of traditional approaches such as weight management, exercise, and prescription drugs to reduce the risks and complications of heart disease.

Despite the classification system that is outlined by the NCCAM, CAM continues to be known by a variety of names—nontraditional medicine, unorthodox medical practices, and holistic health care—and reflects a wide range of philosophies, including the need for or reliance on scientific evidence of effectiveness. Generally, alternative therapies tend to be untested and unproven, whereas complementary and integrative practices that are used in conjunction with mainstream medicine are often those with a substantial scientific basis of demonstrated safety and efficacy.

THE GROWING POPULARITY OF CAM

Many people have turned to CAM approaches out of frustration that mainstream medicine cannot meet all their expectations and needs. Some CAM users are interested in natural, as opposed to pharmaceutical, solutions to health problems, whereas others want to take charge of

FIGURE 9.1

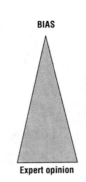

Hierarchy of evidence

Study design

BIAS

- Randomized controlled trials

- Cohort studies and case control studies

- Case reports and case series,
  non-systematic observations

Expert opinion

SOURCE: Yngve Falck-Ytter and Holger Schüenemann, "Slide 15. Hierarchy of Evidence," in *Rating the Evidence: Using GRADE to Develop Clinical Practice Guidelines*, Slide Presentation from the AHRQ 2009 Annual Conference (Text Version), December 2009. Agency for Healthcare Research and Quality, Rockville, MD. http://www.ahrq.gov/about/annualconf09/falck-ytter_schunemann.htm (accessed January 23, 2012)

their health and are seeking self-care approaches to maintaining health and wellness. Helping this movement along is information technology, which is enabling easy access to sources of CAM information on the Internet and in print and electronic media, and advertising and marketing of new CAM products and methods. Citing data from the 2002 and 2007 National Health Interview Survey (NHIS), the NCCAM reports in "The Use of Complementary and Alternative Medicine in the United States" (December 2008, http://nccam.nih.gov/sites/nccam.nih.gov/files/camuse.pdf) that 36% of American adults used CAM approaches in 2002, and 38.3% of adults and 11.8% of children used some form of CAM in 2007.

The CAM supplement to the 2007 NHIS, *Complementary and Alternative Medicine Use among Adults and Children: United States, 2007* (December 10, 2008, http://nccam.nih.gov/news/2008/nhsr12.pdf) by Patricia M. Barnes, Barbara Bloom, and Richard L. Nahin, contains questions about 36 types of CAM therapies, including those that are offered by providers—such as acupuncture, osteopathic manipulation, and chiropractic—as well as therapies that do not require a provider—such as the use of natural products (nutritional supplements and herbal remedies), special diets, and movement therapies. The survey does not ask about the use of folk remedies, such as eating chicken soup to relieve cold symptoms, or faith healing, such as praying for one's own or others' health.

CAM is used by people of all ages, although its use varies between age groups. According to the NCCAM, in 2007 about 40% of adults aged 30 to 39 years, 40 to 49 years, and 60 to 69 years said they used CAM, and more than 44% of adults aged 50 to 59 years reported using CAM during the 12 months prior to the survey. CAM use

also varies by race and ethnicity. In 2007, 50.3% of Native American adults reported using CAM, compared with 43.1% of white, 39.9% of Asian-American, 25.5% of African-American, and 23.7% of Hispanic adults.

The NCCAM indicates that in 2007 the most commonly used CAM therapies used by adults were natural products (17.7%) and mind-body therapies—deep breathing (12.7%) and meditation (9.4%). Between 2002 and 2007 there were significant increases in the use of deep breathing, meditation, massage, and yoga. Among adults who reported using natural products in 2002, the most commonly used natural products were echinacea, traditionally used to treat or prevent colds, flu, and other infections; ginseng, traditionally used to support overall health and boost the immune system; and ginkgo biloba, traditionally used to treat a variety of conditions, including asthma, bronchitis, fatigue, and tinnitus (ringing or roaring sounds in the ears), and more recently used to enhance memory. In 2007 the most frequently used natural product was fish oil/omega 3. Found in certain plants and nuts as well as in fatty fish, omega-3 fatty acids lower triglycerides and may reduce the risk of death, heart attack, dangerous abnormal heart rhythms, and strokes. The second most used natural product in 2007 was glucosamine (an amino sugar that the body produces and distributes in cartilage and other connective tissue that has been used to help prevent and treat arthritis and joint pain), followed by echinacea.

The NCCAM notes that in 2007 half of the top 10 diseases or conditions for which CAM was used were musculoskeletal problems such as back, neck, and joint pain, arthritis, and other musculoskeletal complaints. In 2002, 9.5% of people reported using CAM to treat head or chest colds; in 2007 just 2% used CAM to treat cold symptoms. According to the NCCAM, in "Herbs at a Glance: Echinacea" (July 2010, http://nccam.nih.gov/health/echinacea/ataglance.htm), this decline may be attributable to the fact that study results have been mixed in terms of echinacea's efficacy for the treatment of head or chest colds.

Children's Use of CAM

According to the NCCAM, in "Use of Complementary and Alternative Medicine in the United States," in 2007 CAM use among children was higher among adolescents aged 12 to 17 years (16.4%) than among younger children, and higher among white (12.8%) than African-American (5.9%) or Hispanic (7.9%) children. CAM use was significantly greater among children whose parents or other relatives used CAM (23.9%). It was also higher in families where the parents had more than a high school education (14.7%), in families that delayed seeking conventional medical care because of cost considerations (16.9%), and among children with six or more health conditions (23.8%). The NCCAM notes that like adults, CAM use among children most often relied on natural products, followed by chiropractic and osteopathic care, deep breathing, and yoga.

The NCCAM explains that the natural products children used most frequently in 2007 were echinacea and fish oil/omega 3. The diseases or conditions for which children most frequently used CAM therapies were back/neck pain, head or chest colds, anxiety/stress, and other musculoskeletal complaints.

Older Adults' Use of CAM

In October 2010 the AARP and the NCCAM conducted a survey of Americans aged 50 years and older to better understand their use of CAM. The results were published in *Complementary and Alternative Medicine: What People Aged 50 and Older Discuss with Their Health Care Providers* (April 2011, http://nccam.nih.gov/sites/nccam.nih.gov/files/news/camstats/2010/NCCAM_aarp%20survey.pdf). The survey finds that more than half (53%) of older adults said they had used CAM at some point during their lives and nearly half (47%) had used it during the 12 months preceding the survey. The most frequently used therapies in 2010 were herbal products or dietary supplements (37%), followed by massage therapy, chiropractic manipulation, and other bodywork (22%). (See Figure 9.2.)

FIGURE 9.2

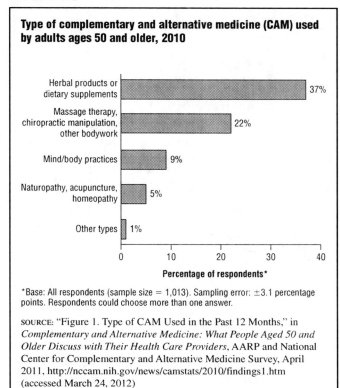

Type of complementary and alternative medicine (CAM) used by adults ages 50 and older, 2010

*Base: All respondents (sample size = 1,013). Sampling error: ±3.1 percentage points. Respondents could choose more than one answer.

SOURCE: "Figure 1. Type of CAM Used in the Past 12 Months," in *Complementary and Alternative Medicine: What People Aged 50 and Older Discuss with Their Health Care Providers*, AARP and National Center for Complementary and Alternative Medicine Survey, April 2011, http://nccam.nih.gov/news/camstats/2010/findings1.htm (accessed March 24, 2012)

Why Do People Seek CAM?

People turn to CAM for many different reasons. One of the most attractive features of CAM is an emphasis on the "whole person," rather than on simply the diseased organ or body part. CAM therapies and practitioners tend to consider patients as human beings rather than as simply physical bodies, and nearly all emphasize the mind-body connection and pay attention to emotional wellness and spirituality.

Some patients seek alternative therapies when conventional medicine fails to relieve their symptoms or when traditional treatment produces unpleasant side effects. In "Rethinking the Evidence Imperative: Why Patients Choose Complementary and Alternative Medicine" (*Leukemia and Lymphoma*, vol. 49, no. 2, February 2008), Isla Carboon of the University of Melbourne details many of the reasons that patients seek CAM. She observes that even though CAM use has been linked to distrust of conventional medicine, there are many other motivations. Carboon suggests that some cancer patients using CAM not only believe that it may benefit the course of treatment for their disease but also choose CAM as a way to regain control of their treatment. In some instances, they may see CAM as a last resort or as a way to sustain hope when conventional treatment fails to reverse the course of their disease or relieve their symptoms.

Other CAM users cite bad experiences with conventional medical treatment, historically poor communication and interactions with physicians, the impersonality of traditional medical care, and the desire for practitioner-patient partnerships that are characterized by shared decision making (rather than traditional physician-patient relationships in which physicians assume sole responsibility for decisions about patient care) for their interest in CAM.

According to the AARP/NCCAM survey, in 2010 more than three-quarters (77%) of Americans aged 50 years and older said they use CAM to prevent illness or enhance overall wellness and nearly as many (73%) said they use it to "help reduce pain/treat painful condition." (See Figure 9.3.) More than half (59%) used CAM to treat a specific health condition and 53% used it to supplement conventional medical treatment. In general, the use of CAM increased with educational attainment. (See Figure 9.4.)

The AARP/NCCAM survey finds that in 2010 family and friends were the most commonly cited source of information about CAM therapies, followed by the Internet and physicians. The percentages of survey respondents citing these sources increased from 2006, whereas the percentages citing publications and radio/television decreased between 2006 and 2010. (See Figure 9.5.)

FIGURE 9.3

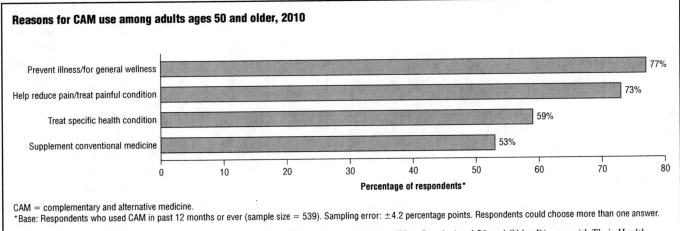

Reasons for CAM use among adults ages 50 and older, 2010

CAM = complementary and alternative medicine.
*Base: Respondents who used CAM in past 12 months or ever (sample size = 539). Sampling error: ±4.2 percentage points. Respondents could choose more than one answer.

SOURCE: "Figure 4. Reasons for CAM Use," in *Complementary and Alternative Medicine: What People Aged 50 and Older Discuss with Their Health Care Providers*, AARP and National Center for Complementary and Alternative Medicine Survey, April 2011, http://nccam.nih.gov/news/camstats/2010/findings2.htm (accessed March 23, 2012)

FIGURE 9.4

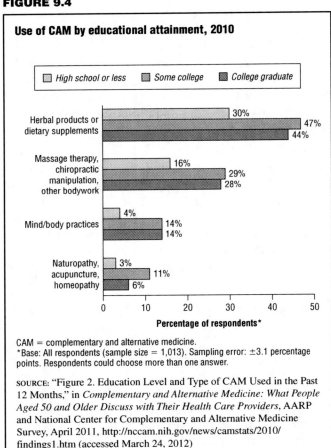

Use of CAM by educational attainment, 2010

CAM = complementary and alternative medicine.
*Base: All respondents (sample size = 1,013). Sampling error: ±3.1 percentage points. Respondents could choose more than one answer.

SOURCE: "Figure 2. Education Level and Type of CAM Used in the Past 12 Months," in *Complementary and Alternative Medicine: What People Aged 50 and Older Discuss with Their Health Care Providers*, AARP and National Center for Complementary and Alternative Medicine Survey, April 2011, http://nccam.nih.gov/news/camstats/2010/findings1.htm (accessed March 24, 2012)

FIGURE 9.5

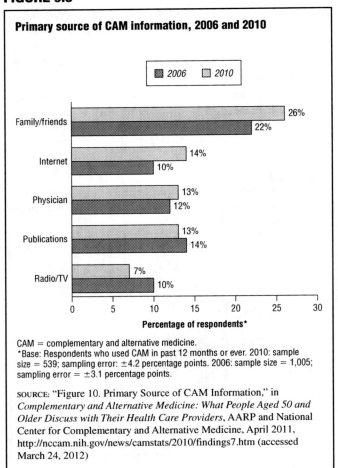

Primary source of CAM information, 2006 and 2010

CAM = complementary and alternative medicine.
*Base: Respondents who used CAM in past 12 months or ever. 2010: sample size = 539; sampling error: ±4.2 percentage points. 2006: sample size = 1,005; sampling error = ±3.1 percentage points.

SOURCE: "Figure 10. Primary Source of CAM Information," in *Complementary and Alternative Medicine: What People Aged 50 and Older Discuss with Their Health Care Providers*, AARP and National Center for Complementary and Alternative Medicine, April 2011, http://nccam.nih.gov/news/camstats/2010/findings7.htm (accessed March 24, 2012)

People from All Walks of Life Use CAM

Besides people who distrust or question conventional medical treatment, there are other groups that make frequent use of CAM. Gwen Wyatt et al. observe in "Complementary and Alternative Medicine Use, Spending, and Quality of Life in Early Stage Breast Cancer" (*Nursing Research*, vol. 59, no. 1, January–February 2010) that as much as 80% of women with breast cancer use CAM therapies to improve their quality of life during cancer treatment. Wyatt et al. find that biologically based therapies (primarily nutritional supplements) and mind-body therapies were used most often by a majority of the sample. By contrast, fewer women used therapies in the other three major CAM categories: manipulative and body based, energy, and alternative medicine systems.

Cancer patients are not, however, the only ones to seek CAM treatment. In "Any Difference? Use of a CAM Provider among Cancer Patients, Coronary Heart Disease (CHD) Patients and Individuals with No Cancer/CHD" (*BMC Complementary and Alternative Medicine*, vol. 12, no. 1, January 12, 2012), Agnete E. Kristoffersen, Arne J. Norheim, and Vinjar M. Fonnebo report that a survey of people in Norway found that the proportion of cancer patients seeing a CAM practitioner was not statistically different from patients with coronary heart disease (CHD) or individuals without cancer or CHD. The researchers do not find widespread use of CAM among cancer patients—only 8% reported visiting a CAM practitioner during the 12 months prior to the survey—and they observe that their findings are only slightly lower than the rates that are reported by other surveys, such as a United Kingdom study that reported just 9.2%.

Lauren M. Denneson, Kathryn Corson, and Steven K. Dobscha examined CAM use among U.S. military veterans with chronic pain and published their findings in "Complementary and Alternative Medicine Use among Veterans with Chronic Noncancer Pain" (*Journal of Rehabilitation Research and Development*, vol. 48, no. 9, 2011). The researchers find that 82% of subjects reported using at least one CAM therapy during the past year and nearly all (99%) expressed a willingness to try CAM treatment for pain. The most preferred CAM treatment was massage therapy and the least preferred was chiropractic care.

In "Complementary and Alternative Medicine Use for Treatment and Prevention of Late-Life Mood and Cognitive Disorders" (*Aging Health*, vol. 5, no. 1, February 2009), Helen Lavretsky of the University of California, Los Angeles, notes that mood disorders (such as depression) and cognitive problems (such as mild memory impairment) associated with aging are among the most common reasons people turn to CAM therapies. These therapies are generally nutritional supplements such as St. John's wort, omega-3 fatty acids, and ginkgo biloba.

CAM Use in Traditional Medical Settings

In the 21st century many CAM practices have joined the ranks of mainstream medicine. The Institute of Medicine finds in *Complementary and Alternative Medicine in the United States* (2005) that the integration of CAM and conventional medicine is occurring in many settings including hospitals, physicians' offices, and health maintenance organizations.

In the press release "More Hospitals Offering Complementary and Alternative Medicine Services" (September 7, 2011, http://www.aha.org/presscenter/pressrel/2011/110907-pr-camsurvey.pdf), the American Hospital Association reports that in response to consumer demand, an increasing number of hospitals offer CAM. In 2007, 37% of hospitals offered one or more CAM therapies; by 2011, 42% offered CAM therapies. Almost three-quarters (72%) of the hospitals offering CAM services were located in urban areas. Of the hospitals surveyed, the overwhelming majority (85%) said the primary motivation to provide CAM services was consumer demand; however, more than two-thirds (70%) indicated that the decision to offer CAM was also based on its "clinical effectiveness."

Another example of the acceptance of CAM use in traditional medical settings concerns the collaborative clinics that combine acupuncture and primary care at Oregon Health and Science University, which is described by Joanne Wu in "Integration of Acupuncture into Family Medicine Teaching Clinics" (*Journal of Alternative and Complementary Medicine*, vol. 15, no. 9, September 2009). More than three-quarters of the primary care physicians had referred patients to acupuncture; the majority of these patients were referred for pain relief.

TYPES OF CAM

The NCCAM categorizes CAM practices into four domains. There is some overlap between these CAM domains:

- Mind-body interventions—mind-body medicine is a range of practices that aims to use the power of the mind to influence the symptoms of disease and healing. Increasingly, this type of alternative medicine has gained acceptance among medical professionals. Mind-body therapies—such as support groups for people suffering from a variety of medical problems; relaxation techniques; and art, dance, and music therapies—are now widely used by practitioners of conventional medicine. Less widely accepted mind-body techniques include meditation, breathing, hypnosis, and prayer.

- Biologically based therapies—this type of treatment uses organic (naturally occurring) substances such as herbs, food, and vitamins to treat symptoms of disease and improve health and wellness. Examples of biologically based therapies include dietary supplements, herbal remedies, and the hotly debated use of hormones such as human growth hormone and dehydroepiandrosterone (the most plentiful steroid hormone in the body) to combat disease and to slow aging.

- Manipulative and body-based practices—movement therapies, manipulative methods, and bodywork are another type of CAM. Examples of these methods are massage therapy, chiropractic, and osteopathic manipulation (also referred to as craniosacral manipulative therapy).

- Energy medicine—these techniques aim to influence energy fields that practitioners of this form of CAM believe exist in and around the body. Also called biofield therapies, some are "touch" therapies and others do not involve direct contact with any part of the body. Reiki and qigong are examples of biofield therapies. Other forms of energy therapies known as bioelectromagnetic-based therapies use magnetic energy, electromagnetic fields, pulsed fields, alternating current, or direct current fields to influence "energy flow."

The NCCAM also considers whole medical systems. Many of these alternative medicine systems developed before conventional Western medicine or independent of it. Alternative medicine systems are based on different beliefs and philosophies and, as a result, approach both diagnosis and treatment of disease quite differently from traditional Western medicine. Examples of alternative medicine systems that began in Western cultures are homeopathy and naturopathic medicine. Alternative medicine systems that developed in other cultures include acupuncture, Ayurvedic medicine, and traditional Chinese medicine.

ALTERNATIVE MEDICINE SYSTEMS

Practically every culture has a medicine system; some developed more than one system, tradition, or philosophy to explain the causes of disease and suggest therapies to relieve symptoms. This section considers two alternative medicine systems that had their origins in Western culture (homeopathy and naturopathic medicine) and three that developed in non-Western cultures (acupuncture, Ayurvedic medicine, and traditional Chinese medicine).

Homeopathic Medicine

Homeopathic medicine (also called homeopathy) is based on the belief that "like cures like" and uses very diluted amounts of natural substances to encourage the body's own self-healing mechanisms. If taken in higher doses or in stronger concentrations, the natural substances that are used by homeopathy to stimulate self-healing would likely produce the symptoms the diluted substances aim to relieve.

Homeopathy was developed by the German physician Samuel Hahnemann (1755–1843) during the 1790s. First experimenting on healthy subjects and himself, Hahnemann discovered that he could produce symptoms of particular diseases by injecting small doses of various herbal substances. This discovery inspired him to try another experiment: giving sick people extremely diluted formulations of substances that would produce the same symptoms they suffered from in an effort to evoke natural recovery and regeneration.

Hahnemann believed that homeopathic remedies—substances that caused symptoms similar to those caused by the disease but not diluted forms of the disease-causing agents—worked by activating the "vital force," the organizing energy system that governs health in a human being. There is no comparable belief in Western medicine, but the idea of vital force bears some resemblance to the Ayurvedic concept of prana and to qi in Chinese medicine.

Homeopathy gained a foothold in the United States during the 1830s, when it appeared able to stem some epidemics, such as cholera (a devastating infectious disease that produces severe diarrhea), but by the 1900s it fell out of favor as traditional medical practice experienced greater success treating the diseases of the day. During the 1970s there was renewed interest in homeopathy in the United States, and by 2010 believers credited homeopathy with gentle, effective, and nontoxic treatment of many infections, emotional problems, and learning disorders. Even though proponents assert that homeopathic medicine speeds healing, it cannot treat traumatic injuries, such as broken bones, or genetic diseases.

Claudia M. Witt et al. looked at how patients receiving homeopathic treatment fared over the course of eight years of follow-up and published their findings in "How Healthy Are Chronically Ill Patients after Eight Years of Homeopathic Treatment?—Results from a Long Term Observational Study" (BMC Public Health, vol. 8, December 17, 2008). Having followed 3,709 patients, the researchers find that, in general, the patients had improved based on self-reports of their complaints and quality of life measures. The greatest improvements were seen in younger patients, females, and those with greater disease severity at the onset of treatment.

Naturopathic Medicine

As its name suggests, naturopathic medicine, or naturopathy, uses naturally occurring substances to prevent, diagnose, and treat disease. This alternative medicine system, one of the oldest, has its origins in Native American culture and draws from Greek, Chinese, and Indian philosophies of health and illness.

Naturopathy was introduced in the United States by the German physician Benedict Lust (1872–1945), and its popularity rose, declined, and was rekindled during the same period as homeopathy. Lust opened a school of naturopathic medicine in New York City. He and James Foster, a physician in Idaho who used natural healing techniques, christened their blend of herbal medicine, manipulative therapies, homeopathy, nutrition, and psychology naturopathy.

The overarching principles of modern naturopathic medicine are "first, do no harm" and "nature has the power to heal." Naturopathy seeks to treat the whole person because disease is seen as arising from many causes rather than from a single cause. Naturopathic physicians are taught that "prevention is as important as cure" and to view creating and maintaining health as equally important as curing disease. They are instructed to identify and treat the causes of diseases rather than acting only to relieve symptoms. Naturopathy also requires practitioners to serve as teachers to encourage patients to assume personal responsibility for their health and actively participate in self-care.

Naturopathic physicians' treatment methods include nutritional counseling and the addition of dietary supplements, herbs, or vitamins to a patient's diet; hydrotherapy (water-based therapies, usually involving whirlpool or other baths); exercise; manipulation; massage; heat therapy; and electrical stimulation. They are trained to prescribe herbal medicines and homeopathic remedies, perform minor surgical procedures such as setting broken bones, and offer counseling services to help patients resolve emotional problems and modify their lifestyles to improve their health and wellness. Because naturopathy draws on Chinese and Indian medical techniques, naturopathic physicians often use Chinese herbs, acupuncture, and Ayurvedic medicine to treat disease.

The NCCAM reports that even though there is scant published research examining the efficacy of naturopathy as a system of treatment, some studies have been conducted to evaluate the individual therapies that are frequently recommended by naturopathic physicians. For example, diet and lifestyle changes have proved extremely valuable in treating heart disease and diabetes, and the use of acupuncture to treat pain has gained widespread acceptance. Ryan Bradley and Erica B. Odberg note in "Naturopathic Medicine and Type 2 Diabetes: A Retrospective Analysis from an Academic Clinic" (*Alternative Medicine Review*, vol. 11, no. 1, March 2006) that control of blood sugar and other vital statistics in patients receiving naturopathic care is comparable to published national averages. Bradley and Odberg assert that naturopathic physicians prescribe lifestyle changes that are supported by a high level of evidence of efficacy. In this study, 100% of patients received dietary counseling, 69% were taught stress reduction techniques, and 94% were prescribed exercise. Patients additionally received prescriptions for botanical and nutritional supplementation, often in combination with conventional medication, and there is mounting evidence of their value in treatment.

Similarly, in "Naturopathic Care for Anxiety: A Randomized Controlled Trial ISRCTN78958974" (*PLOS One*, vol. 4, no. 8, August 31, 2009), Kieran Cooley et al. find that naturopathic care (NC) consisting of dietary counseling, deep breathing relaxation techniques, a standard multivitamin, and the herbal medicine ashwagandha (*Withania somnifera*), when compared with psychotherapy (PT), was effective in reducing moderate to severe anxiety. Cooley et al. conclude, "Both NC and PT led to significant improvements in patients' anxiety. Group comparison demonstrated a significant decrease in anxiety levels in the NC group over the PT group. Significant improvements in secondary quality of life measures were also observed in the NC group as compared to PT."

Acupuncture

Acupuncture is a Chinese practice that dates back more than 5,000 years. Even though Sir William Osler (1849–1919) called acupuncture the best available treatment for low back pain during the late 1800s, it was not widely used to treat pain in the United States until the 1970s. Chinese medicine describes acupuncture—the insertion of extremely thin, sterile needles into any of 360 specific points on the body—as a way to balance *qi* (also called *chi*), the body's vital life force that flows over the surface of the body and through internal organs. Traditional Western medicine explains the acknowledged effectiveness of acupuncture as the result of triggering the release of pain-relieving substances called endorphins, which occur naturally in the body, and neurotransmitters and neuropeptides, which influence brain chemistry.

There have been many studies on acupuncture's potential usefulness, but historically the results have been mixed due to complexities with study design and size. For example, a 2009 systematic review, "Evidence from the Cochrane Collaboration for Traditional Chinese Medicine Therapies" (*Journal of Alternative and Complementary Medicine*, vol. 15, no. 9, September 2009) by Eric Manheimer et al., considered 26 studies of acupuncture and concluded that, even though they suggested benefit, most of the studies were of poor quality. Nonetheless, there are many reports of acupuncture's effectiveness in reducing postoperative and chemotherapy nausea and vomiting as well as in the treatment of addiction, stroke rehabilitation, headache, menstrual cramps, tennis elbow, fibromyalgia, osteoarthritis, low back pain, carpal tunnel syndrome, and asthma.

Richard W. Rosenquist et al. explain in "Practice Guidelines for Chronic Pain Management: An Updated Report by the American Society of Anesthesiologists Task Force on Chronic Pain Management and the American Society of Regional Anesthesia and Pain Medicine" (*Anesthesiology*, vol. 112, no. 4, April 2010) that in 2010 the American Society of Anesthesiologists Task Force on Chronic Pain Management and the American Society of Regional Anesthesia and Pain Medicine issued updated guidelines on pain management. The guidelines, which are intended to assist patients and practitioners make informed health care decisions, observe that rigorous research—clinically comparing acupuncture techniques with sham acupuncture—found no difference in pain relief for patients with low back pain. Despite these findings, the expert task force suggests that acupuncture should be considered along with conventional therapy such as drugs, physical therapy, and exercise to treat low back pain.

Ayurvedic Medicine

Ayurvedic medicine (also called Ayurveda, which means "science of life") is believed to be the oldest medical tradition and has been practiced in India and Asia for more than 5,000 years. With an emphasis on preventing disease and promoting wellness, its practitioners view emotional health and spiritual balance as vital for physical health and disease prevention. Ayurveda also considers diet, hygiene, sleep, lifestyle, and healthy relationships as powerful influences on health.

Practitioners aim to balance the three *doshas*—fundamental human qualities that they believe reside in varying concentrations in different parts of the human body. The *doshas* are thought to be disturbed by improper diet, sleep deprivation, travel, coffee, alcohol, or excessive exposure to the sun and are balanced with diet, exercise, detoxification (ritual cleansing of toxins), yoga, spiritual counseling, herbal medicine, breathing exercises, and chanting.

In "Theories and Management of Aging: Modern and Ayurveda Perspectives" (*Evidence-Based Complementary and Alternative Medicine*, February 20, 2009), Hema Sharma Datta et al. explain that from the Ayurvedic perspective, proper diet, exercise, and lifestyle can create a balance of the essences—*prana* (the life energy that governs respiration and circulation), *ojas* (the essence that is responsible for immune function and intelligence), *tejas* (the essence of a subtle fire or energy, which governs metabolism through the enzyme system), and *agni* (the central fire or energy source in the body that promotes digestion and assimilation of nutrients)—and ensure health and long life.

Traditional Chinese Medicine

Traditional Chinese medicine (TCM) combines nutrition, acupuncture, massage, herbal medicine, and qigong (exercises to improve the flow of vital energy through the body) to help people achieve balance and unity of their mind, body, and spirit. TCM has been used for more than 3,000 years by about one-fourth of the world's population, and in the United States it has been embraced by naturopathic physicians, chiropractors, and other CAM practitioners.

One diagnostic technique that is noticeably different from Western medicine is the TCM approach to taking pulses. TCM practitioners take pulses at six different locations, including three points on each wrist, and pulses are described using 28 distinct qualities. Reading the pulses enables practitioners to evaluate *qi*.

TCM views balancing *qi* as central to health, wellness, and disease prevention and treatment. TCM also seeks to balance the feminine and masculine qualities of yin and yang using other techniques such as moxibustion (stimulating acupuncture points with heat) and cupping (increasing circulation by putting a heated jar on the skin of a body part).

Herbal medicine is the most commonly prescribed treatment; herbal preparations may be consumed as teas made from boiled fresh herbs or dried powders or in combined formulations known as patent medicines. More than 200 herbal preparations are used in TCM, and several, such as ginseng, ma huang, and ginger, have become popular in the United States. Ginseng is supposed to improve immunity and prevent illness; ma huang is a stimulant used to promote weight loss and relieve lung congestion; and ginger is prescribed to aid digestion, relieve nausea, reduce osteoarthritic knee pain, and improve circulation.

Many modern pharmaceutical drugs are derived from TCM herbal medicines. For example, ma huang components are used to make ephedrine and pseudoephedrine. GBE, which is made from ginkgo biloba, is used to treat cerebral insufficiency (lack of blood flow to the brain).

Research to determine the effectiveness of TCM has focused on the efficacy of specific herbs and combinations of herbs. For example, *Tripterygium wilfordii* (thunder god vine) has been used to treat autoimmune and inflammatory disorders such as arthritis. In "Evidence of Effectiveness of Herbal Medicinal Products in the Treatment of Arthritis—Part 2: Rheumatoid Arthritis" (*Phytotherapy Research*, vol. 23, no. 12, December 2009), Melainie Cameron et al. report that three studies compared preparations of *Tripterygium wilfordii* to placebos and returned favorable results in terms of their ability to relieve symptoms of arthritis.

MIND-BODY INTERVENTIONS

Mind-body interventions—such as meditation, progressive relaxation, hypnosis, deep breathing exercises, and yoga—are practices based on the belief that the mind, body, and spirit are connected to one another and to environmental influences. The NCCAM observes in "What Is Complementary and Alternative Medicine?" that mind-body medicine recognizes the relationship between stress, altered mental states, and illness and aims to improve physical, mental, and emotional well-being. According to Kenneth R. Pelletier (1946–), a clinical professor at the University of Arizona School of Medicine and author of *The Best Alternative Medicine: What Works? What Does Not?* (2000), the guiding principles of mind-body medicine are:

- Stress and depression contribute to the development of, and hinder recovery from, chronic diseases because they create measurable hormonal imbalances.

- Psychoneuroimmunology explains how mental functioning provokes physical and biochemical changes that weaken immunity, lowering resistance to disease.

- Overall health improves when people are optimistic and have a positive outlook on life. Health and wellness are harmed by anger, depression, and chronic stress.

- The placebo effect (improved health and favorable physical changes in response to inactive medication such as a sugar pill) confirms the importance of mind-body medicine and is a valuable intervention.

- Social support from family, friends, coworkers, classmates, or organized self-help groups boosts the effectiveness of traditional and CAM therapies.

This section looks at two types of mind-body interventions: meditation and biofeedback. Other commonly used mind-body interventions include music and dance therapies, cognitive behavioral therapy, hypnosis, guided imagery and visualization, and a Chinese exercise discipline called tai chi chuan.

Meditation

Historically, meditation has been used in religious training and practices and to enhance spiritual growth, but it is also a powerful self-care measure that may be used to relieve stress and promote healing. Transcendental meditation, an Indian practice that involves sitting and silently chanting a mantra (a word repeated to quiet the mind), aims to produce a healthy state of relaxation.

During the 1960s the cardiologist Herbert Benson (1935–) studied meditation, and he and his colleagues at Harvard University Medical School showed that people who meditate can reduce heart and respiration rates, lower blood levels of the hormone cortisol, and increase alpha waves (smooth, regular electrical oscillations in the human brain that occur when a person is awake and relaxed). Benson developed a relaxation technique loosely based on transcendental meditation that he dubbed the "relaxation response," and this technique quickly gained recognition in the United States and Europe.

There have been many studies performed to evaluate physical and psychological responses to meditation, and its benefits are universally accepted in the CAM and conventional medical communities. Research has focused on understanding how meditation works and the conditions it may help relieve.

In *Meditation Practices for Health: State of the Research* (June 2007, http://www.ahrq.gov/downloads/pub/evidence/pdf/meditation/medit.pdf), Maria B. Ospina et al. review research on a variety of meditation practices. An analysis of 813 research studies finds favorable therapeutic effects of meditation, such as:

- The ability to lower heart rate and blood pressure readings

- Reduction in stress, anxiety, and pain

- Reduction in intraocular pressure (pressure inside the eye)

- Reduction in cholesterol levels

- Increase in breath holding time

Table 9.1 lists the characteristics, including postures, breathing, and attention, of various types of meditation. It also describes the training that is involved in each kind of meditation practice and the recommended frequency of practice.

In "Meditation: An Introduction" (June 2010, http://nccam.nih.gov/health/meditation/overview.htm), the NCCAM states that meditation may exert its beneficial effects by reducing activity in the sympathetic nervous system (the system that mobilizes the body to respond in a "fight or flight" response when under stress) and increasing activity in the parasympathetic nervous system, which slows heart rate and breathing and dilates blood vessels to improve circulation.

Biofeedback

Biofeedback training is designed to help people learn to regulate body functions such as heart rate and blood pressure. Generally, sensitive monitoring devices are attached to the individual to measure and record a variety of physical responses such as skin temperature and electrical resistance, brain-wave activity, and respiration rate. There are also devices to monitor other functions such as bladder activity and acid in the stomach. By observing their own responses and following instructions given by highly trained technicians, most people are able to exert some degree of conscious control over these body functions. Biofeedback is especially effective for helping people learn to manage stress, and it has become a mainstream medical treatment for conditions such as high blood pressure, asthma, migraine headaches, and some types of urinary and fecal incontinence (inability to control bladder or bowel functions).

Dana L. Frank et al. observe in "Biofeedback in Medicine: Who, When, Why and How?" (*Mental Health in Family Medicine*, vol. 7, no. 2, June 2010) that "biofeedback therapy is a process of training as opposed to a

TABLE 9.1

Characteristics of various meditation practices

Meditation practice	Main components	Breathing	Attention	Spirituality/belief	Training	Criteria for success
Mantra meditation						
TM®	Sitting (no prescribed posture) Personalized Sanskrit mantra Eyes closed	Passive, unconnected to repetition of mantra No description of breathing	Attention directed to prescribed mantra Mantra repeated silently	No specific spiritual or religious beliefs required	Taught in 4 consecutive days (preceded by two 1-hour lectures and a 5–10 minute interview) in a 1-hour training session and three 1.5 hour group sessions. Individual instruction Practiced twice daily, 15–20 min/session Instruction by qualified TM® teacher	Proper technique as judged by experienced TM® teacher; no specific criteria
Relaxation response	Comfortable posture (sitting, kneeling, squatting) Eyes open or closed Can also include body scan and information sessions	Passive, but mantra is "linked" to exhalation Nasal	Attention focused on the breath Mantra repeated silently Thoughts are ignored	No specific spiritual or religious beliefs required	Taught in 5-min training session Individual instruction Practiced twice daily, 15–20 min/session and not before 2 hrs after a meal	Proper technique according to subjective evaluation and measured against reported effects of RR
Clinically standardized meditation	Comfortable seated posture Sanskrit mantra or individually chosen mantra Eyes open initially and focused on pleasant object, then closed for repetition of mantra	Passive, unconnected to repetition of mantra	Attention directed to individually chosen mantra (1 of 16) Mantra repeated aloud and then at decreasing volume until it is repeated silently Thoughts recognized, but not focused on	No specific spiritual or religious beliefs required	Taught in 2 1-hr lessons Individual instruction or training manual and audio tapes Practiced twice daily for 20 min/session	Proper technique according to subjective evaluation and measured against reports of effects of CSM
Mindfulness meditation						
Vipassana	Cultivation of a "mindful" attitude Seated posture	Passive Nasal	Attention is focused on the breath (first on the inhalation and exhalation, then shifted to rims of the nostrils) or on bodily sensations	No specific spiritual or religious beliefs required	No specific training period given Session should last no longer than one can comfortably sit Novice meditators no longer than 20 min	Proper technique determined by experienced meditator or by self-evaluation
Zen	Specific seated postures (lotus or half-lotus), positioning of hands, mouth and tongue Eyes half closed and focused on point on floor	Active Inhale through nose, exhale through mouth and nasal only Many breathing patterns	Attention focused on counting of breath, on a koan or "just sitting." Breath counted by 1 of 3 methods No attempt to focus on single idea or experience	No specific spiritual or religious beliefs required; however, attitude of nonpurposefulness is essential	No specific training period given Sessions may last from several minutes to several hours	Successful practice determined by experienced teacher; specific personal experience of the true nature of reality
MBSR	Cultivation of a "mindful" attitude Prescribed postures Seated meditation Body scan (supine posture) Hatha yoga postures	Active (diaphragmatic breathing) and passive	Seated meditation: attention focused on breath as it passes edge of nostrils or on rising and falling of abdomen Body scan: attention focused on somatic sensations in the part of the body being "scanned." Hatha yoga: attention focused on breath and the sensations that arise as different postures are assumed	No specific spiritual or religious beliefs required; however, strong commitment and self-discipline are essential	Taught in an 8-week course involving weekly 2–3 hr classes and 45-min sessions at home 6 days a week with homework exercises After course, practiced daily for 45 min Group instruction by an experienced MBSR practitioner	Successful meditation requires the technique be taught by an teacher experienced in mindfulness meditation; achievement of successful health outcomes

TABLE 9.1

Characteristics of various meditation practices [CONTINUED]

Meditation practice	Main components	Breathing	Attention	Spirituality/belief	Training	Criteria for success
MBCT	Based on MBSR program Cultivation of "decentered" or "mindful" perspective Seated meditation Body scan	Passive	Seated meditation: attention focused on breath as it passes edge of nostrils or on rising and falling of abdomen Body scan: attention focused on somatic sensations in the part of the body being "scanned."	No specific spiritual or religious beliefs required	Taught in an 8-week course involving weekly 2-hr classes and 45-min sessions at home 6 days a week with homework exercises Program taught in 2 main components: (1) teaching of mindfulness, (2) learning to handle mood shifts Group instruction by an experienced practitioner of mindfulness meditation	Successful meditation requires the technique be taught by an teacher experienced in mindfulness meditation; successful prevention of depressive relapse as determined by clinical evaluation
Yoga						
Kundalini yoga, Sahaja yoga, and Hatha yoga (many styles)	Emphasis of components vary among "schools" but can include ethical observances, physical postures, breathing techniques, concentrative and mindfulness meditation	Active and passive Techniques vary	Awareness for all techniques is centered on the breath Some techniques also focus on posture	No specific spiritual or religious beliefs required unless the ethical component is included	Regular daily practice from 15 min to several hours; instruction by an experienced Yogi or Guru; may take several years or longer to properly execute asanas and pranayama	Successful technique is judged by the individual or Guru against the standards for posture and breathing and against reported benefits of successful practice
Tai Chi						
Yang, Chen, Sun, Wu (Jian Qian), and Wu (He Qin) styles	A routine of slow, deliberate movements (movements and postures vary among schools) Body relaxed, upper body erect, not bending Mouth closed, teeth not clenched	Active Nasal	Attention is focused on movement and on one's internal energy (qi)	No specific spiritual or religious beliefs required	Routines vary in number of postures and duration Classical Yang-style Tai Chi includes 108 postures and takes approximately 20–25 min to complete; practice also includes a 20-min warm-up and 10-min cooldown Should practice everyday	Proper movement and posture as judged by experienced Tai Chi teacher
Qi Gong						
Many techniques	Meditation Prescribed posture for seated meditation Movements practiced in a relaxed stationary position Breathing exercises	Active Techniques vary	Attention is focused on the "elixir field" and on the inhalation and exhalation of the breath	No specific spiritual or religious beliefs required	Practiced twice daily for 20–30 min with no single session exceeding 3 hr	Proper movement and posture as judged by experienced Qi Gong teacher Safe practice requires instruction by experienced Qi Gong teacher

TM® = The Transcendental Meditation Program
MBSR = Mindfulness-Based Stress Reduction
MBCT = Mindfulness-Based Cognitive Therapy

SOURCE: Maria B. Ospina et al., "Table 4. Characteristics of Included Meditation Practices," in *Meditation Practices for Health: State of the Research*, AHRQ Publication No. 07-E010, June 2007. Agency for Healthcare Research and Quality, Rockville, MD. http://www.ahrq.gov/downloads/pub/evidence/pdf/meditation/medit.pdf (accessed January 24, 2012)

treatment" and that consumer acceptance of clinical bio-feedback training continues to grow. The researchers report that biofeedback has demonstrated efficacy for a host of medical conditions, including anxiety, attention deficit/hyperactivity disorder, chronic pain, constipation, headache, and motion sickness.

BIOLOGICALLY BASED THERAPIES

The principal treatments in biologically based therapies are herbal medicines and remedies, dietary supplements, and the use of hormones to combat disease and improve health. Because herbal medicines are used in a variety of other CAM practices, such as homeopathy, naturopathy, Ayurveda, and TCM, this section describes a hotly contested biologically based therapy: the use of dietary supplements.

Dietary Supplements

Most CAM practitioners and many conventional medical practitioners agree that food sources are the best way to obtain nutrients. They also agree that it is difficult for many people to get sufficient quantities of specific vitamins or minerals from their daily diet. For example, many researchers and nutritionists feel that the diets of most Americans do not contain enough chromium and that most women do not consume adequate amounts of iron. Furthermore, the CAM principle of treating each patient as an individual with unique physiologic and biochemical needs suggests that some individuals may need more of specific nutrients than others.

Advocates of dietary supplements believe the recommended dietary allowances (RDAs) are too low for some vitamins and minerals, and they observe that it is difficult to obtain higher than the RDA of certain vitamins without also consuming an excess of fat and calories. An example of this dilemma is vitamin E, an antioxidant that is found in high-fat vegetable and seed oils. For men to get the RDA (15 international units [IU]) of vitamin E, they would have to, according to Pelletier in *Best Alternative Medicine*, eat "248 slices of whole wheat bread, 16 dozen eggs, or 20 pounds of bacon." Several studies suggest that far higher doses—20 to 30 times greater than the RDA—may protect against heart disease or some cancers, but to obtain such doses from diet alone is impossible.

Another current controversy is whether to prescribe diets supplemented with specific vitamins for people without established vitamin deficiencies. Critics of dietary supplements believe that people should attempt to obtain as many needed nutrients from food sources as possible, without relying on dietary supplements. Furthermore, there is no consensus about dosages higher than the RDAs, although it is known that some vitamins and minerals, such as vitamins A and E and chromium,

are toxic in high doses. For example, more than 400 IU of vitamin E taken daily may increase the risk of stroke, and high doses of vitamin E are generally not advised for people taking medications to reduce blood clotting.

Eric A. Klein et al. confirm in "Vitamin E and the Risk of Prostate Cancer" (*Journal of the American Medical Association*, vol. 306, no. 14, October 2011) the risks that are associated with vitamin E. Based on the results of a population study, the researchers find that rather than reducing the risk of developing prostate cancer, vitamin E consumption increased the risk. A study of 35,000 healthy men aged 50 years and older found that those who took 400 IU of vitamin E per day had a 17% increase in prostate cancer.

Table 9.2 lists the characteristics and conditions that a dietary supplement must meet to conform with the legal and regulatory requirements of the U.S. Food and Drug Administration (FDA). Unlike drugs, dietary supplements are considered to be foods; as a result, they go to market with far less testing and scrutiny and without FDA approval.

The legislation governing supplements, the Dietary Supplement Health and Education Act of 1994, also established the Office of Dietary Supplements (ODS) at the NIH. The mission of the ODS (2010, http://ods.od.nih.gov/About/MissionOriginMandate.aspx) is "to strengthen knowledge and understanding of dietary supplements by evaluating scientific information, stimulating and supporting research, disseminating research results, and educating the public to foster an enhanced quality of life and health."

ARE DIETARY SUPPLEMENTS EFFECTIVE? Many dietary supplements have undergone rigorous testing to determine whether they are effective for the conditions they claim to address. However, some research questions the efficacy of several popular dietary supplements, and research continued in 2012 in an effort to resolve these questions. For example, the combination of glucosamine

TABLE 9.2

About dietary supplements

Dietary supplements were defined in a law passed by Congress in 1994 called the Dietary Supplement Health and Education Act (DSHEA). According to DSHEA, a dietary supplement is a product that:

• Is intended to supplement the diet
• Contains one or more dietary ingredients (including vitamins, minerals, herbs or other botanicals, amino acids, and certain other substances) or their constituents
• Is intended to be taken by mouth, in forms such as tablet, capsule, powder, softgel, gelcap, or liquid
• Is labeled as being a dietary supplement

SOURCE: "About Dietary Supplements," in *Using Dietary Supplements Wisely*, National Institutes of Health, National Center for Complementary and Alternative Medicine, March 2010, http://nccam.nih.gov/health/supplements/wiseuse.htm#about (accessed January 25, 2012)

(thought to play a role in cartilage formation) and chondroitin (which helps give cartilage elasticity, taken as a supplement to relieve arthritis pain) was found to be no more effective than a placebo. In "The Effect of Glucosamine and/or Chondroitin Sulfate on the Progression of Knee Osteoarthritis: A Report from the Glucosamine/Chondroitin Arthritis Intervention Trial" (*Arthritis and Rheumatism*, vol. 58, no. 10, October 2008), Allen D. Sawitzke et al. report the results of the NIH-sponsored Glucosamine/Chondroitin Arthritis Intervention Trial, which found that the combination of these supplements was no more effective than placebo in slowing the joint space loss and the loss of cartilage in the knees of people with osteoarthritis.

Another study, André Kahan et al.'s "Long-Term Effects of Chondroitins 4 and 6 Sulfate on Knee Osteoarthritis: The Study on Osteoarthritis Progression Prevention, a Two-Year, Randomized, Double-Blind, Placebo-Controlled Trial" (*Arthritis and Rheumatism*, vol. 60, no. 2, February 2009), arrives at a different conclusion. The researchers find that, among people with knee osteoarthritis, a supplement containing two forms of chondroitin sulfate (CS) did significantly reduce joint space loss and knee pain when compared with placebo. Kahan et al. conclude that "the long-term combined structure-modifying and symptom-modifying effects of CS suggest that it could be a disease-modifying agent in patients with knee [osteoarthritis]."

Roger Chou et al. report in "Analgesics for Osteoarthritis: An Update of the 2006 Comparative Effectiveness Review" (*Comparative Effectiveness Review*, no. 38, October 2011) that in 2011 the Agency for Healthcare Research and Quality (AHRQ) issued an updated report that compared the benefits and harms of oral nonsteroidal anti-inflammatory drugs (NSAIDs), acetaminophen, chondroitin, and glucosamine, and topical agents, such as cream containing capsaicin for osteoarthritis. According to Chou et al., the AHRQ reviewed the results of 273 studies and concluded that "there were no clear differences between glucosamine or chondroitin and oral NSAIDs for pain or function" and that several rigorous trials suggest that glucosamine has some "small benefits over placebo for pain."

Similarly, in "Echinacea Species (*Echinacea angustifolia* (DC.) Hell., *Echinacea pallida* (Nutt.) Nutt., *Echinacea purpurea* (L.) Moench): A Review of Their Chemistry, Pharmacology and Clinical Properties" (*Journal of Pharmacy and Pharmacology*, vol. 57, no. 8, August 2005), Joanne Barnes et al. review research that assessed the safety and effectiveness of echinacea for the prevention and treatment of upper respiratory infections. The researchers observe that several, but not all, clinical trials of echinacea preparations reported effects better than those of a placebo.

Barnes et al. caution that the evidence of echinacea's effectiveness is not conclusive because the studies are not comparable—they included different patient groups and tested various different preparations and doses of echinacea. Klaus Linde et al. conducted a comprehensive review that assessed the available evidence from clinical trials investigating the effectiveness of echinacea extracts for the prevention and treatment of the common cold and reported their findings in "Echinacea for Preventing and Treating the Common Cold" (*Cochrane Library*, vol. 1, January 25, 2006). The results from Linde et al. are consistent with those of Barnes et al., suggesting that some echinacea preparations may be better than a placebo, for both treatment and prevention of colds, and may be more effective for treatment when taken at the onset of symptoms.

SOME DIETARY SUPPLEMENTS MAY BE HARMFUL OR INEFFECTIVE. Because many dietary supplements are naturally occurring and available without a prescription, many consumers mistakenly believe that using them could not possibly be harmful. This is not the case, because dietary supplements have the potential to interact unfavorably with specific foods and medicines or even cause harm when taken on their own. The FDA has issued warnings and advised caution about the use of some dietary supplements. For example, in "Warning on Body Building Products Marketed as Containing Steroids or Steroid-Like Substances" (December 8, 2011, http://www.fda.gov/ForConsumers/ConsumerUpdates/ucm173739.htm), the FDA notes that in July 2009 it cautioned consumers to stop using any bodybuilding products marketed as dietary supplements that may contain steroids or steroid-like substances because of their potential to cause serious liver injury, stroke, kidney failure, and pulmonary embolism (blockage of an artery in the lung).

In 2011 the FDA issued "HCG Diet Products Are Illegal" (January 13, 2012, http://www.fda.gov/ForConsumers/ConsumerUpdates/ucm281333.htm), which was a warning about human chorionic gonadotropin (HCG is a hormone produced by the placenta during pregnancy) supplements that are promoted to speed weight loss. HCG is approved by the FDA as a prescription drug for the treatment of female infertility; however, it is not approved for direct-to-consumer sale for any purpose.

MANIPULATIVE AND BODY-BASED METHODS

Manipulative therapies, such as osteopathic manipulation and chiropractic, and body-based methods (also known as bodywork), such as therapeutic massage, are CAM practices that have been tremendously popular during the last two decades. Barnes, Bloom, and Nahin find that in 2007 nearly 18.1 million adults and 743,000 children received massage therapy during the year prior to the survey. The AARP/NCCAM survey indicates that in 2010 nearly one-quarter (22%) of adults aged 50 years and older had used some form of bodywork during the 12 months preceding the survey. (See Figure 9.2.) Enthusiasm for these CAM practices is at least in part attributed to their demonstrated ability to relieve aches and pains that are associated with musculoskeletal injuries and stress more effectively than treatment that is prescribed by conventional medical practitioners. As a result, these therapeutic modalities have made inroads into mainstream medicine.

In "Massage for Low Back Pain: An Updated Systematic Review within the Framework of the Cochrane Back Review Group" (*Spine*, vol. 34, no. 16, July 15, 2009), Andrea Furlan et al. review 13 trials of massage for back pain. In two of the studies, massage proved more effective than a sham therapy, and eight studies compared massage with other back pain treatment. These studies found that in terms of pain relief, massage was comparable to exercise and that it was superior to treatments involving joint mobilization, relaxation therapy, physical therapy, acupuncture, and self-care education. Furlan et al. conclude that "massage might be beneficial for patients with subacute and chronic nonspecific low back pain, especially when combined with exercises and education."

Amy T. Wang et al. recount in "Massage Therapy after Cardiac Surgery" (*Seminars in Thoracic and Cardiovascular Surgery*, vol. 22, no. 3, Autumn 2010) their experiences with massage therapy of cardiac surgery patients at the Mayo Clinic in Rochester, Minnesota. The researchers observe that following surgery, patients experience pain, anxiety, and tension that not only cause the patient to suffer but can also "impair immune function and slow wound healing." Wang et al. opine that massage therapy can effectively relieve these postoperative problems, thus enabling patients to realize the full benefits of surgery.

Chiropractic

In "About Chiropractic" (2012, http://www.acatoday .org/level1_css.cfm?T1ID=42), the American Chiropractic Association (ACA) defines chiropractic as "a health care profession that focuses on disorders of the musculoskeletal system and the nervous system, and the effects of these disorders on general health. Chiropractic care is used most often to treat neuromusculoskeletal complaints, including but not limited to back pain, neck pain, pain in the joints of the arms or legs, and headaches." Doctors of chiropractic (also known as chiropractors) do not use or prescribe pharmaceutical drugs or perform surgery. Instead, they rely on adjustment and manipulation of the musculoskeletal system, particularly the spinal column.

Many chiropractors use nutritional therapy and prescribe dietary supplements, and some use a technique known as applied kinesiology to diagnose and treat disease. Applied kinesiology is based on the belief that every organ problem is associated with the weakness of a specific muscle. Chiropractors who use this technique claim they can accurately identify organ system dysfunction without any laboratory or other diagnostic tests.

Besides manipulation, chiropractors also use a variety of other therapies to support healing and relax muscles before they make manual adjustments. These treatments include the following:

- Heat and cold therapy to relieve pain, speed healing, and reduce swelling
- Hydrotherapy to relax muscles and stimulate blood circulation
- Immobilization such as casts, wraps, traction, and splints to protect injured areas
- Electrotherapy to deliver deep-tissue massage and boost circulation
- Ultrasound to relieve muscle spasms and reduce swelling

According to the ACA, in "General Information about Chiropractic Care" (November 4, 2008, http://www.acatoday .org/pdf/Gen_Chiro_Info.pdf), chiropractic is the third-largest specialty group of health care professionals after medicine and dentistry. Visits to chiropractors are most often for the treatment of low back pain, neck pain, and headaches. Critics of chiropractic are concerned about injuries that result from powerful "high velocity" manual adjustments, and some physicians question chiropractors' abilities to establish medical diagnoses. Others worry that people seeking chiropractic care instead of traditional allopathic (conventional) medical care may be foregoing lifesaving diagnoses and treatment.

EFFECTIVENESS OF CHIROPRACTIC. In "Chiropractic: An Introduction" (October 2010, http://nccam.nih.gov/ health/chiropractic/introduction.htm), a review of the relevant literature, the NCCAM notes that most patients seek chiropractic treatment for shoulder, neck, or back pain. The NCCAM's assessment of the available research is that spinal manipulation, which may also be performed by physical therapists, osteopaths, and some conventional medical doctors, may provide relief from low back pain. Spinal manipulation appears to be safe and as effective as conventional treatments. The NCCAM reports that a 2010 review of the evidence for manual therapy treatment for a range of conditions concluded that "spinal manipulation/mobilization may be helpful for several conditions in addition to back pain, including migraine and cervicogenic (neck-related) headaches, neck pain, upper- and lower-extremity joint conditions, and whiplash-associated disorders." The review also named conditions for which spinal manipulation/mobilization appears not to be helpful, such as asthma, hypertension, and menstrual cramps, and identified disorders for which the evidence is still inconclusive, such as fibromyalgia, mid-back pain, sciatica, and premenstrual syndrome.

ENERGY THERAPIES

Energy therapies that purport to influence energy fields in and around the body are among the CAM practices that arouse the most suspicion from the conventional medical community. Some skeptics attribute the health benefits reported by patients who have received energy therapies to the placebo effect (a perceived beneficial result that occurs from the therapy because of the patient's expectation that the therapy will help). Despite a widespread lack of understanding and acceptance from traditional health care practitioners, some hospitals and pioneering practitioners are incorporating energy therapies into their treatment programs.

Reiki

An ancient Japanese technique, Reiki is bioenergetic healing that is intended to restore physical, emotional, mental, and spiritual balance. The unique therapy takes its name from two Japanese words. *Rei* means higher power, wisdom, and all that exists, and *ki* is the life force, or the energy that runs through all living things.

Based on the teachings of Mikao Usui (1865–1926), Reiki is a universal healing vibration that flows through the practitioner to the client. Practitioners act as a channel for Reiki energy, and as it passes through practitioners, it acts to strengthen and harmonize them simultaneously as it heals their clients.

There are more than a dozen styles of Reiki, each with its own subtle variations. Students studying with Usui Reiki masters receive a series of "attunements" and may progress through three levels or degrees of training. Level I connects the practitioner to the Reiki channel and initiates the flow of healing energy. Level II teaches distance or remote healing. Level III initiates the practitioner to the role of master and teacher.

Some practitioners use a variety of other therapies, including meditation, prayer, chanting, breathing, and movement education. Most often performed as hands-on bodywork, Reiki is believed by its therapists to convey energy to calm nerves, relax muscles, and ease pain. During the second level of training, practitioners learn to deliver Reiki energy remotely, over long distances.

There are many case studies describing the effectiveness of Reiki to reduce anxiety and relieve discomfort, but as of 2012 there were few published reports of rigorous research designed to determine its efficacy. In "A Systematic Review of the Therapeutic Effects of Reiki" (*Journal of Complementary Medicine*, vol. 15, no. 11, November 2009), Sondra vanderVaart et al. find all of the studies on Reiki lacking in rigor. Even though nine of 12 trials reported a significant therapeutic effect, the reviewers conclude that "the serious methodological and reporting limitations of limited existing Reiki studies preclude a definitive conclusion on its effectiveness. High-quality randomized controlled trials are needed to address the effectiveness of Reiki over placebo." In another study, Sondra vanderVaart et al. report in "The Effect of Distant Reiki on Pain in Women after Elective Caesarean Section: A Double-Blinded Randomised Controlled Trial" (*BMJ Open*, vol. 1, no. 1, February 2011) the results of a 2010 randomized control trial of distant Reiki to relieve pain following Caesarean delivery. The researchers find that it had no significant effect on pain; however, they note that women who received Reiki had lower heart rates than women in the untreated control group.

In "Effects of Reiki on Autonomic Activity Early after Acute Coronary Syndrome" (*Journal of the American College of Cardiology*, vol. 56, no. 12, September 2010), Rachel S. C. Friedman et al. find that Reiki improved heart rate variability and the emotional state in patients who were hospitalized for acute coronary syndrome. Friedman et al. hypothesize that the beneficial effects of Reiki may be due to "the presence of another person, the presence of a person with healing intention, the light touch technique, or a combination of factors" and call for additional research to gain an understanding of its mechanism of action.

NCCAM-funded research considers some of the as yet unanswered questions about Reiki, including:

- How does it work?

- Is Reiki a safe and effective treatment for chronic pain?

- Can Reiki relieve anxiety and improve the well-being of patients with diseases such as cancer and the acquired immunodeficiency syndrome?

- Can Reiki help control blood sugar levels, improve heart function, or relieve nerve pain in people with type 2 diabetes?

COMPLEMENTING TRADITIONAL MEDICINE. Clinics and hospitals across the United States offer Reiki to women in labor, surgical patients, and those suffering from pain, anxiety, sleep disorders, headaches, asthma, and eating disorders. According to the Center for Reiki Research (2012, http://www.centerforreikiresearch.org/), 68 hospitals and clinics in the United States offered patients Reiki treatments in 2012.

In conventional medical settings, Reiki is usually presented as a method to reduce stress and promote relaxation, thereby enhancing the body's natural ability to heal itself. To gain credibility with traditional physicians and other mainstream professionals, Reiki therapists often downplay the spiritual benefits of the practice and avoid mentioning other CAM practices.

Even though its effectiveness has not been documented in scientific studies, Reiki has gained acceptance because it is viewed as a complement, rather than as an alternative, to traditional Western medicine. Considered to be safe by many health care practitioners, it is well received by patients who seem to respond favorably to the time and attention, as well as to the healing energy, offered by Reiki therapists.

IMPORTANT NAMES AND ADDRESSES

Alzheimer's Association
225 N. Michigan Ave., 17th Floor
Chicago, IL 60601-7633
(312) 335-8700
1-800-272-3900
URL: http://www.alz.org/

American Academy of Child and Adolescent Psychiatry
3615 Wisconsin Ave. NW
Washington, DC 20016-3007
(202) 966-7300
FAX: (202) 966-2891
URL: http://www.aacap.org/

American Academy of Pediatrics
141 Northwest Point Blvd.
Elk Grove Village, IL 60007-1098
(847) 434-4000
FAX: (847) 434-8000
URL: http://www.aap.org/

American Association of Suicidology
5221 Wisconsin Ave. NW
Washington, DC 20015
(202) 237-2280
FAX: (202) 237-2282
URL: http://www.suicidology.org/

American Cancer Society
250 Williams St. NW
Atlanta, GA 30303
(404) 320-3333
1-800-227-2345
URL: http://www.cancer.org/

American Chiropractic Association
1701 Clarendon Blvd.
Arlington, VA 22209
(703) 276-8800
FAX: (703) 243-2593
E-mail: memberinfo@acatoday.org
URL: http://www.acatoday.org/

American College of Obstetricians and Gynecologists
PO Box 70620
Washington, DC 20024-9998
(202) 638-5577
1-800-673-8444
URL: http://www.acog.org/

American Diabetes Association
1701 N. Beauregard St.
Alexandria, VA 22311
1-800-342-2383
E-mail: askada@diabetes.org
URL: http://www.diabetes.org/

American Heart Association National Center
7272 Greenville Ave.
Dallas, TX 75231
1-800-242-8721
URL: http://www.americanheart.org/

American Lung Association
1301 Pennsylvania Ave. NW, Ste. 800
Washington, DC 20004
(202) 785-3355
1-800-548-8252
FAX: (202) 452-1805
E-mail: info@lung.org
URL: http://www.lungusa.org/

American Parkinson Disease Association
135 Parkinson Ave.
Staten Island, NY 10305
(718) 981-8001
1-800-223-2732
FAX: (718) 981-4399
E-mail: apda@apdaparkinson.org
URL: http://www.apdaparkinson.org/

American Psychiatric Association
1000 Wilson Blvd., Ste. 1825
Arlington, VA 22209
(703) 907-7300
1-888-357-7924
E-mail: apa@psych.org
URL: http://www.psych.org/

American Psychological Association
750 First St. NE
Washington, DC 20002-4242
(202) 336-5500
1-800-374-2721
URL: http://www.apa.org/

Arthritis Foundation
PO Box 7669
Atlanta, GA 30357-0669
1-800-283-7800
URL: http://www.arthritis.org/

Autism Society of America
4340 East-West Hwy., Ste. 350
Bethesda, MD 20814
(301) 657-0881
1-800-328-8476
URL: http://www.autism-society.org/

Centers for Disease Control and Prevention
1600 Clifton Rd.
Atlanta, GA 30333
1-800-232-4636
E-mail: cdcinfo@cdc.gov
URL: http://www.cdc.gov/

Cystic Fibrosis Foundation
6931 Arlington Rd., Second Floor
Bethesda, MD 20814
(301) 951-4422
1-800-344-4823
FAX: (301) 951-6378
E-mail: info@cff.org
URL: http://www.cff.org/

Epilepsy Foundation
8301 Professional Pl.
Landover, MD 20785
1-800-332-1000
FAX: (301) 577-2684
E-mail: ContactUs@efa.org
URL: http://www.epilepsyfoundation.org/

Huntington's Disease Society of America
505 Eighth Ave., Ste. 902
New York, NY 10018
(212) 242-1968
1-800-345-4372
FAX: (212) 239-3430
URL: http://www.hdsa.org/

March of Dimes Birth Defects Foundation
1275 Mamaroneck Ave.
White Plains, NY 10605
(914) 997-4488
URL: http://www.modimes.org/

Muscular Dystrophy Association
National Headquarters
3300 E. Sunrise Dr.
Tucson, AZ 85718
1-800-572-1717
E-mail: mda@mdausa.org
URL: http://www.mdausa.org/

National Center for Complementary and
Alternative Medicine
National Institutes of Health
9000 Rockville Pike
Bethesda, MD 20892
(301) 519-3153
1-888-644-6226
FAX: 1-866-464-3616

E-mail: info@nccam.nih.gov
URL: http://www.nccam.nih.gov/

National Center for Health Statistics
3311 Toledo Rd.
Hyattsville, MD 20782
1-800-232-4636
E-mail: cdcinfo@cdc.gov
URL: http://www.cdc.gov/nchs/

National Fibromyalgia Association
2121 S. Towne Centre Pl., Ste. 300
Anaheim, CA 92806
(714) 921-0150
FAX: (714) 921-6920
URL: http://www.fmaware.org/

National Mental Health Association
2000 N. Beauregard St., Sixth Floor
Alexandria, VA 22311
(703) 684-7722
1-800-969-6642
FAX: (703) 684-5968
URL: http://www.nmha.org/

National Multiple Sclerosis Society
733 Third Ave., Third Floor
New York, NY 10017
1-800-344-4867
URL: http://www.nmss.org/

National Osteoporosis Foundation
1150 17th St. NW, Ste. 850
Washington, DC 20036
(202) 223-2226
1-800-231-4222
URL: http://www.nof.org/
FAX: (202) 223-2237

National Tay-Sachs and Allied Diseases
Association
2001 Beacon St., Ste. 204
Boston, MA 02135
1-800-906-8723
FAX: (617) 277-0134
E-mail: info@ntsad.org
URL: http://www.ntsad.org/

Sickle Cell Disease Association of America
231 E. Baltimore St., Ste. 800
Baltimore, MD 21202
(410) 528-1555
1-800-421-8453
FAX: (410) 528-1495
E-mail: scdaa@sicklecelldisease.org
URL: http://www.sicklecelldisease.org/

United Network for Organ Sharing
700 N. Fourth St.
Richmond, VA 23219
(804) 782-4800
FAX: (804) 782-4817
URL: http://www.unos.org/

RESOURCES

The Centers for Disease Control and Prevention (CDC) tracks nationwide health trends and reports its findings in several periodicals, especially in the *Advance Data* series, the annual *HIV Surveillance Reports*, and the *Morbidity and Mortality Weekly Reports*. The CDC's National Center for Injury Prevention and Control provides data about deaths and disability that are caused by accidents and violence. The National Center for Health Statistics (NCHS) provides a complete statistical overview of the nation's health in its annual *Health, United States*. The NCHS periodicals *National Vital Statistics Reports* and *Vital and Health Statistics* detail U.S. birth and death data and trends.

The National Health Interview Surveys offer information about the lifestyles, health behaviors, and health risks of Americans. The CDC publishes *Health Risks in the United States: Behavioral Risk Factor Surveillance System*—the results of surveys in each state asking adults questions about a wide range of behaviors affecting their health. The National Health and Nutrition Examination Survey (NHANES), which is conducted by the National Institute of Mental Health (NIMH) and the NCHS, also helps to characterize the health and well-being of Americans. Working with other agencies and professional organizations, the CDC helped create Healthy People 2020 (http://www.healthypeople.gov/2020/default.aspx), which serves as a blueprint for improving the health of Americans during the second decade of the 21st century.

Mental health and illness in the United States were detailed in the landmark report *Mental Health: A Report of the Surgeon General* (1999) and in follow-up reports, including *Mental Health: Culture, Race and Ethnicity* (2001) and *Achieving the Promise: Transforming Mental Health Care in America* (July 2003). In addition, the Center for Mental Health Services reports data describing the nation's mental health status and services in its periodic *Mental Health, United States*. The NIMH provides detailed information about mental health research and treatment of mental illness. The Harvard School of Medicine's *National Comorbidity Surveys* and the NIMH publication *The Numbers Count: Mental Disorders in America* (August 2009) provide estimates of the incidence and prevalence of mental disorders.

The National Institutes of Health provides definitions, epidemiological data, and research findings about a comprehensive range of medical and public health subjects. The National Center for Complementary and Alternative Medicine defines and describes a range of alternative, complementary, and integrative medical practices. The National Institute of Environmental Health Sciences provides information about environmental hazards and behaviors that jeopardize health.

Medical, public health, and nursing journals offer a wealth of disease-specific information and research findings. The studies cited in this edition are drawn from a wide range of professional publications, including the *Annals of Internal Medicine*, *Archives of General Psychiatry*, *Circulation*, *Journal of the American Medical Association*, *Journal of Physical Activity and Health*, *Lancet*, and *New England Journal of Medicine*.

The American Cancer Society's *Cancer Facts and Figures, 2011* (2011) provided valuable data, as did the Alzheimer's Association, the American Diabetes Association, the American Heart Association, the American Lung Association, and the National Osteoporosis Foundation, all of which are excellent resources for information about the epidemiology of diseases, treatments, and clinical trials. Many other professional associations, voluntary medical organizations, and foundations dedicated to research, education, and advocacy related to other specific medical conditions and disabling diseases proved to be useful sources for up-to-date information in this edition.

INDEX

Page references in italics refer to photographs. References with the letter t following them indicate the presence of a table. The letter f indicates a figure. If more than one table or figure appears on a particular page, the exact item number for the table or figure being referenced is provided.

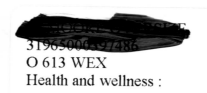